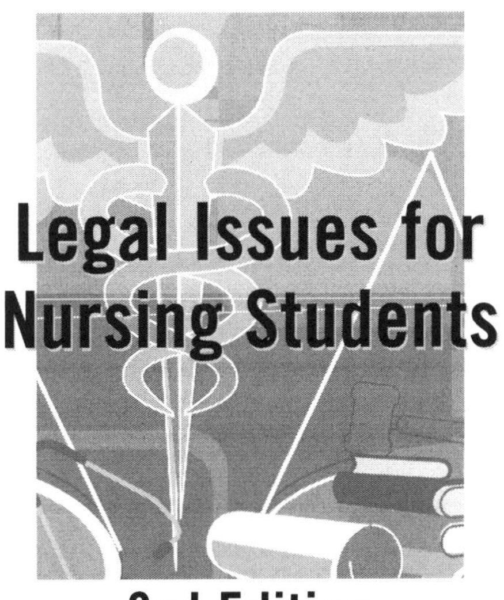

Legal Issues for Nursing Students

3rd Edition

Thanks go to students and colleagues for their feedback, recommendations and contribution to the recognition of difficulties and anxieties they identified in understanding and using legal concepts in nursing practice.

Legal Issues for Nursing Students

Applied principles

3rd Edition

Pam Savage
RN., RM., DipN (Lon)., BA., MHPEd., Dip Law
Barrister at Bar, New South Wales

Pearson Originals is an imprint of Pearson Australia, a division of Pearson Australia Group Pty Ltd. It has been established to provide academics throughout Australia and New Zealand with fast and efficient access to the printing, warehousing and distribution services of Australia's leading educational publisher, ensuring a smooth supply channel to your campus bookseller.

For more information about the **Pearson Originals** service, contact the Editorial Department, Pearson Australia, Suite 1001, Level 10, 151 Castlereagh Street, Sydney, New South Wales 2000. Telephone: 02 9454 2200.

Custom Project Management Team Leader: Jill Gillies
Custom Specialist: Nicki Barlow
Project Manager: Lisa D'Cruz
Production Controller: Brad Smith

ISBN 978 1 4886 1118 6

Printed and bound in Australia by The SOS + Print Media Group

Pearson Australia
Suite 1001, Level 10
151 Castlereagh Street
Sydney NSW 2000
www.pearson.com.au

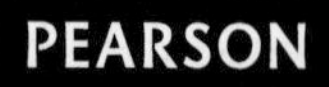

Contents

Preface

The aim of this book is to provide to undergraduate nursing students an introduction to the law as it applies to their practice and an opportunity to explore not only legal issues but also the governance issues that must be understood to practise in a safe and competent manner.

The book is the result of a number of years of experience in teaching undergraduates, graduates and overseas trained nurses about legal concepts and health care in Australia. As a practising nurse working with health staff in urban and remote environments, the constant refrain among practitioners is anxiety about the nurses' vulnerability to legal consequences that could arise from any, or all, actions they take in the course of practice.

This work does not explore to any extent the legal reasoning that underpins legal doctrine. Rather, the focus is upon areas of law and the rules that give direction to practice with the aim to give practitioners awareness and confidence that their actions and decisions would satisfy legal scrutiny.

There is no doubt that health practice carries great responsibility and the learner has the obligation to acquire a huge amount of knowledge and skills while functioning under great pressure to achieve standards of practice to be a professional. It is hoped that this introductory text will contribute to that essential knowledge in a practical and efficient manner.

As all professionals accept the obligation to continue to develop their knowledge and commit to lifelong learning, further studies in law relevant to future practice will build upon this introductory text.

Pam Savage
September 2011

New to this edition

The aim of this book is to provide to undergraduate nursing students an introduction to the law as it applies to their practice and an opportunity to explore not only legal issues but also the governance issues that must be understood to practise in a safe and competent manner. As it is the intersection of professional standards with legal expectations that are the most likely used sources for investigation and hearings, these standards for professional practice, codes and guidelines enforced by the professional regulating authority and used by courts are a major focus.

This third edition has included a number of nurse tribunal findings to highlight the legal and professional expectations that exist and demonstrate the consequences of failing to satisfy professional standards. The professional governance arrangements and codes and guidelines that dictate standards are explained in the context of legal powers and related to legal doctrine.

Legislation relevant to current nursing practice and professional ideology are reported and the intent and purpose of these laws is explained. Changes to legislation are explained in the context of nursing work.

A number of "practice assignment questions" are new additions to this text, these can be used by both lecturers and students. The aim is to give students an opportunity to apply learning as they progress by considering posed questions. These assignments directly relate to chapter content and can be used to promote class discussion or give opportunity to rehearse and practice examination techniques.

Table of abbreviations

AHPRA	Australian Health Practitioner Regulation Agency
AAT	Administrative Appeals Tribunal
AC	Appeal cases
ALJ	Australian Law Journal
All ER	All England Law Reports
ALR	Australian Law Reports
ANMAC	Australian Nursing and Midwifery Accreditation Council Limited
ARTG	Australian Register of Therapeutic Goods
AVCC	Australian Vice Chancellor's Committee
CLR	Commonwealth Law Reports
Cwlth	Commonwealth
EN	Enrolled Nurse
J	Judge
JD	Justice Department
LQR	Law Quarterly Review
NHMRC	National Health and Medical Research Council
NSWR	New South Wales Reports
QB	Queens Bench
RN	Registered Nurse
SASR	South Australian State Reports
TGA	Therapeutic Goods Administration
UN	United Nations
WHO	World Health Organization
WLR	Weekly Law Reports

Introduction: why study philosophy, ethics and legal issues?

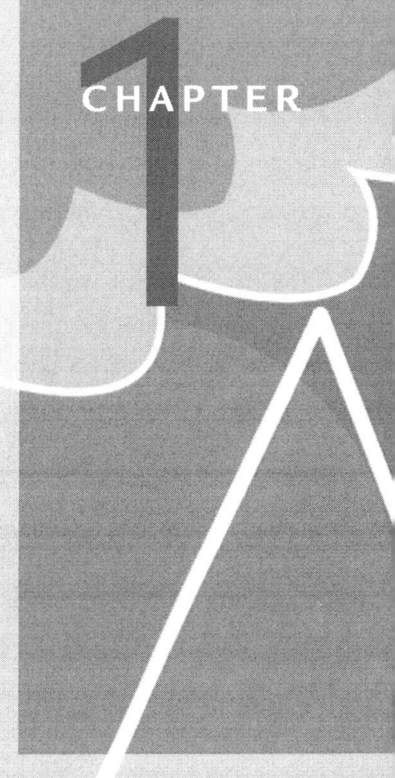

Learning outcomes

After studying this chapter you should be able to:

- Articulate the differences between legal and ethical concepts.
- Discuss the relevance of legal and ethical concepts to professional practice.
- Identify the links between legal concepts and policies governing practice.
- Describe the role of the law in providing direction for health care practice.
- Relate Codes governing nursing practice to legal and ethical concepts.

Overview

This book aims to provide direction for practice in health care environments recognising that in fact the law does not specifically focus upon all aspects of that practice to give health professionals rules to work by in all situations.

For example, the rules aimed to overcome institutional risks to clients are not necessary in private homes, therefore we have to consider the context of our work and recognise that anything from level of education, comprehension, environment, prior experience and resources can change the way a situation is evaluated by the law. This creates uncertainty. Health staff want clear and simple rules to avoid legal risks. However, a professional has the responsibility for assessing, applying knowledge and taking responsibility for their own decisions and interventions.

- A health professional is not a lawyer but by practising to the highest standards of their profession with some insight into their legal obligations and legal expectations the professional will as an individual be less likely to find themselves in professional or legal difficulties.

Law is a discipline in its own right; it has its own traditions and jargon, and the skills acquired rest strongly on taught legal reasoning. This is why lawyers give complex answers to what to us seem simple questions. The inclination of most people is to judge a situation on the basis of 'fair or not fair'. In legal proceedings the subtle or historical arguments founded on a legal principle can be very confusing when findings involve complex arguments and results that go against 'perceived wisdom'. What is suitable and considered legally sound in one circumstance may not be in another.

For a lawyer there are many variables that must be considered – this is the lawyers' professional responsibility. Nurses and other health professionals, in their real-world situations, do not have time to contemplate complex legal aspects, but rather are responsible for satisfying a professional responsibility in relation to care, treatment and interventions, often in difficult situations. In relation to the many complex situations to which our practice can expose us, there is no way we can routinely refuse to do something until we have checked our legal risks for every little thing. We need to be alert to the areas of particular risk, know when a situation does have legal ramifications and why that situation has obligations, then we can make an informed decision based on sound reasoning, rather than 'jumping in at the deep end'.

As a citizen and a professional you do have legal obligations and you probably take it for granted that there are penalties should you fail to adhere to these. This is the focus of this text. While some understanding of legal concepts and the legal system is essential, here the aim is to highlight the general and specific law and professional governance aspects that can provide guidance to the health professional.

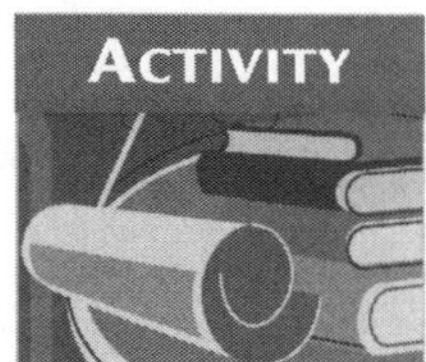

Activity

- List some activities you are anxious about in your professional practice because you fear legal consequences.

Keep this list handy. As you progress through each chapter occasionally refer to your list; this will help you focus on content in order to answer your own questions and hopefully lessen your anxiety about the legal consequences of health professionals' activities.

Why study philosophy, ethics and legal issues?

Health professionals often feel vulnerable about legal and ethical issues. They recognise that their work carries moral obligations, there are conflicting demands, rules and regulations and often real anxiety about 'just where they stand' in relation to these pressures. It is not rare for the student or qualified professional to hear or say, 'Can I do that, and is it legal?' In fact the law, nebulous and complex as it is, is often used by managers and teachers to set boundaries on behaviour, to restrict and restrain people from doing something until they are proven competent or the activity is approved.

This threat of legal consequences can inhibit and dismay people. It can be used as a blunt weapon by management to control and limit risks, and fear of or confusion about the law can be used to coerce and manipulate. The law by its very existence is meant to control and provide order and certainty in society. However, when health professionals are faced with questions about 'is this fair', or 'can I do this' the moral, ethical and legal aspects of their work are being addressed. Recognising and adhering to one's own conscience may not be sufficient to meet the standards expected of a professional as there are often many competing interests and expectations that must be met.

Understanding the foundations of governing rules and policies can assist health professionals in judging situations and give them confidence that they are making decisions and behaving within acceptable limits – not because they are 'scared of being found out and facing the consequences' but because they have taken the time to consider objectively their own skills, abilities and beliefs, others' needs and expectations and the rationale for policies, rules and regulations before taking steps into murky waters.

Every person is under pressure to conform to their family, tribe, cultural and social environment. Rules exist that define responsibilities, expectations and obligations. These rules are imposed explicitly with codes of practice or rulebooks or implicitly through modelled behaviour within groups. Deviation from these expectations or 'norms' has consequences. Depending upon the way a society interprets the degree of deviation there may be severe penalties. Over time codes of behaviour or rules can become 'law', with clear penalties. Structures are put in place to enforce these rules and particular groups or individuals in the society are empowered to take action and sanction any failure to adhere to the rules.

Formal education may take on the responsibility to teach these rules of behaviour so that there is less chance that an individual will remain ignorant of these laws or become, through their actions, deviant in the eyes of their society.

This conformity to rules may be fluid or rigid. Social behaviours may be condoned or condemned at different times in history. Religious and cultural aspects underpin many of the rules and social constructs that aim to promote harmony between and within groups.

When two different cultures or two individuals have different sets of rules there is a tendency for each to assume the other is 'wrong', 'deviant' or 'uninformed'. When individuals hold opinions about 'right and wrong' these may be a source of conflict and misunderstanding.

- Societies are complex and the rules for behaviour and the reasons for these and why they exist is worthy of investigation. That is the work of a philosopher.
- The standard of behaviour and how people should relate to the needs of society and others is the interest of the ethicist.
- Formal rules may be very complex and need interpretation and clarity and hence specialists are required; these are the lawyers and judges.

To highlight the difference between what is fair and what is legal consider the case study below (developed from *Norton v. Argonaut Insurance Company (1962)*).

Case study

J, an RN with many years' experience, worked normally in administration at a medium-sized hospital in a regional area. During a flu epidemic the facility was so short staffed that J was asked to work in the paediatric ward on a busy am shift.

J had to do a medication round for her allocated patients. One of these, seven-year-old Paul, was scheduled for heart surgery at 10 am. The surgeon's orders were for pre-operative 0800 hours, Digoxin 0.75 mg oral to be administered.

J looked up the drug and noted that this was far in excess of the normal dose. J checked with the senior RN, who was surprised and suggested J must check with the medical officer. Paging the resident J discovered he was already in theatre, scrubbed with the prescribing surgeon. J called theatre and asked the charge nurse to go and speak to the resident and J gave all the details of the problem.

The charge nurse reported back to J that the surgeon, not the resident, had in fact answered the query and was furious at the delay of medication and yes the order was correct and it must be given immediately or surgery would be postponed.

J remained unhappy; she gathered notes and orders and went to theatre, gowned and masked, and interrupted the surgeon to bring his attention to the medication order and asked him to check that the dose was correct. The surgeon was furious. He not only insisted the order was correct but demanded it be given and blamed J for now delaying the child's surgery for an hour pending drug action.

J gave the drug. The child died. The case went to court as a wrongful death. The surgeon, resident and J were charged.

Outcome

J was found guilty. The surgeon was chastised by the judge for his actions but no guilt was attributed to either doctor.

This case study is based upon quite an old legal case. For the purposes of this book the case has been summarised and updated but the findings continue to affect practice.

Every nurse who has read this scenario is amazed and affronted. 'That's not fair' is their comment. However, stand back from the issue and analyse it from a very objective perspective. What is the bottom line?

J was guilty on the basis *that in spite of her professional knowledge and belief that the drug dosage was unsafe and probably incorrect, she still went ahead and gave the drug.* The fact that J was subjected to inappropriate intimidation and language from the surgeon, despite the accepted pressures of the situation, despite the fact that J tried everything to check and confirm, J was guilty because her professional responsibility was to refuse to give something she knew was dangerous and was outside of her professional expertise.

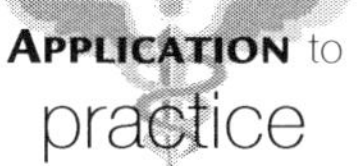

Application to practice

Policies about drug checking, medication orders and the right to refuse to implement an order that lies outside of professional competence, knowledge or conviction have evolved. In fact professional codes of practice explicitly or implicitly direct health professionals to adhere to such standards. Institutions have since been found liable for situations where circumstances have driven staff to work outside of their competence.

Ethics and law are similar but different

In Western history both concepts have grown from a root source of intellectual inquiry to become formal structures of learning and work, and each now has many branches that relate to and give direction to our society in all aspects of life.

There have always been laws, written and unwritten. There have always been penalties and sanctions visited upon wrongdoers. There are many branches of the law, some of which have died over time, and new areas of law continue to develop.

As groups developed and societies became stable, cultural and religious doctrines developed and the reasons for human behaviour and the expectations of what could be human potential, rather than what were the rules governing people, became an area of inquiry. This is the source of ethics.

- Ethics is about human potential, behaviour and expectations of what is good and socially worthy.
- Law is about rules and the consequences or penalties imposed should someone fail to adhere to what society expects.

It is obvious, then, if a society has expectations for good behaviour that promotes harmony and stability that society may well have laws to enforce that behaviour.

- This is the blurred line between ethics and law.

Philosophy is the study of why people, society and groups behave or believe in certain standards and manage their relationships in particular ways. By studying the religious, economic and historical development of a society the philosopher tries to explain how the fabric of that society has been woven. This investigation can then help understand and even predict how individuals will react to pressures and circumstances that occur. This questioning about how and why people think and act in order to promote and maximise individual potential or improve societies is the focus of the philosopher. There have been many famous and many forgotten philosophers. The need to find a language to explain their thinking and interpretations has led to a specialised field of study and ethics is one branch of this evolving, dynamic tree.

The study of law has also developed from a background of ancient rules and their interpretation. Specialised language drawn from various cultures has been incorporated into this field. Some laws are universal. Killing another person is an example of this. Yet there are exceptions: war, self-defence or to save the life of another may enlist sympathy and avoid the otherwise automatic sanction of gaol or a death sentence in some societies but not in others.

Some laws reflect the cultural expectations of a group. If everyone agrees that defacing a gravestone is a terrible thing, or spitting on the sidewalk is a dangerous thing, then making the action illegal and applying a penalty such as a fine is an example of a law that may be imposed on every individual in that group.

Here again, the interest of philosophers in why some rules exist, why others persist and yet others disappear over time means that their questions about the society and the way it manages its affairs blend the language of philosophy with the language of law. Neither language is very clear to the uninitiated.

What is clear to the health worker, whether a novice or experienced, is that their society imposes expectations about their behaviour and their interactions with the dependent and vulnerable people for which they are responsible. These expectations may be formal, clear and specific to professional practices and health institutions. However, laws may also be general; society has rules that everyone must obey. Some laws relate to a particular area of work only and these dictate how and when certain activities must be carried out; for example, there are standards that must be met and failure to satisfy these standards means that penalties will be imposed.

Because professional groups want to ensure that the behaviour of their members is above reproach and reflects the best of human potential in all professional endeavours, ethical expectations may be imposed. Codes of ethical practice promoting behaviours that society deems 'best' are taken up by a professional group to provide clear and usually very high standards. Meeting these standards allows the individual to be part of this select and (usually) respected group. These standards may be higher than those of the general society. The codes are often directive in that they specify what behaviours are and are not acceptable to the group.

The particular laws and ethical codes that relate to health professionals must be understood. Failure to meet standards may result in loss of professional status or legal penalties. Because the standards of behaviour expected are often higher than those of the general society it is a challenge to meet these. Unless you understand them and the rationale for them, it would be impossible to meet that challenge.

Laws ancient and modern become guidelines to behaviour. If we know there will be consequences for actions we may take time to consider our actions and avoid reacting to provocations. If the penalties are to be avoided then dictating just how things must be done can give day-to-day direction for activities.

- This is where policies and procedures fit into the health system.

No one wants to suffer the legal consequences for failing to satisfy legal requirements. Therefore, ensuring that everyone adheres to a strict policy, adopts behaviours that limit risks and takes steps to record and report relevant information giving proof of attempts to avoid doing a wrong can lessen the risk of unwanted outcomes and the attendant sanctions.

Ethics in a nutshell

Health professionals are recognised and usually registered by a professional body which often has a statutory responsibility to govern those professionals and to protect the public. Many of the rules governing the right to practice and standards of practice reflect the blurred lines between ethics and law. Most undergraduate courses either combine law and ethics or present law and ethics as two separate subjects. This short overview of ethics is included to provide an insight into some of the concepts and the jargon upon which ethics is founded. Your ability to interpret the rationale and the intention of professional codes of ethics and other professional governance documents relies on understanding these concepts.

The first thing to accept is that in ethics there is never one absolutely right answer. This can drive students mad. We all seek certainty and reassurance that our choices, problem solving and interactions are based on sound reasoning and proven principles. However, ethics is about people. How we think and the social, religious, cultural and family influences that lead us to a way of reasoning what is right or wrong, good or bad, fair or unfair affect our ethical viewpoint. Our opinions about justice, truth and honesty change as we grow up and adapt, through experience and exposure, to other ideas and learning. Therefore ethics is not a static and limited field of inquiry.

Ethical decisions may differ in their quality and validity over time. What was 'the only way to act' in the 1800s depended on social class, gender and where you lived but this has little relevance today. Belief in outside influences being the driving force for established rules of behaviour may conflict with the belief that we are all independent of each other and we make our own rules. People may have quite different rules within their family or group about whom they will respect and how they will act compared to those rules and behaviours they choose to adopt at school, work or university.

Western thinking and the history of how Western society approaches ethics and the resolution of ethical problems have its origins in ancient Greece. Pythagoras, who lived around 530 BC, believed that we were merely living to carry out the wishes of the Divine Being. This belief premised that all actions and the relevance of our lives, of being good or worthy, were beyond an individual's ability without that individual becoming a 'vessel' of God. (Mitchell, Kerridge & Lovat 1996)

Plato, another Greek philosopher, later held the same views. Both Plato and Pythagoras were Mystics. Plato's philosophy contemplated the social and political structures in light of this essential divine concept. The closer you were to God the better you would be at interpreting and implementing God's rules, and the better person you would be. This would lead to a just and ethical society. As it happens, Plato believed that the ruling classes were best placed to interpret and impose the rules. Lower classes, as a natural consequence of the way God planned it, were meant to be ruled and needed the governing classes to set the rules and intervene with God on their behalf. This belief system, in the language of philosophy, laid the ground for an ethical knowledge base called *absolutist*, *ontological* or *deontological*. These terms are key concepts within philosophy.

This view of reality about how the good and bad in the world resulted from man accepting or failing to accept divine rules was not a universal belief. There were philosophers such as Protagoras who took what we now might call a 'scientific approach' to explaining why people act as they do. Protagoras proposed that people behave in good and worthy ways because it suits them to do so. The choice of how to behave is based upon a realistic assessment of here and now, what the benefits or consequences to oneself are in a particular situation. No one individual or group had all the answers; there was no absolute rule or right to dictate to others the way to do things or behave. To come to the best conclusion involved discussing and debating and questioning. An inclusion of others through education and debate in order to gain insight and answers meant there would be a cohesive and harmonious society. Shared values and agreement grew out of being willing to examine reality and work out for one's self what was a good or right solution. This belief system, in the language of philosophy, laid the ground for an ethical knowledge base called *utilitarian*, *situationist*, *consequentialist* or *teleological* ethics. These terms are also key concepts within philosophy.

Protagoras' denial of divine rule occurred after Pythagoras died and before Plato was born. Plato's philosophy was opposed to Protagoras; he worked to discount the notion of self-rule. For Plato a ruling class and divine law were essential to avoid social breakdown and anarchy. It is easy to see how this philosophy was attractive to the ruling elite. It was taken up by the Romans and from there incorporated into Christianity. The obligation to accept a hierarchical structure of the Church and a society based upon the divine right to rule held by those in power was upheld by writers like Saint Augustine (AD 400) and was the prevailing philosophy, directing what was ethical behaviour and the rules of law, right up until the Renaissance.

Aristotle was a student of Plato. He had adhered to Plato's philosophy although he was interested in exploring the natural world and, as a result of balancing what Plato said and what he actually saw, he proposed that human will did not always depend on divine law for its expression; people could make good decisions and act in good ways without recourse to God. By the thirteenth century Aristotle's theory became a key philosophical ideal in a world now experiencing new ideas through contact with Islamic scholars and writers. More educated people had doubts about the way the Church explained the world in light of their own scientific inquiry and explanations for their findings. Aristotle's premise that we can express our will and learn from our own endeavours gave the new 'scientific' believers of the time a way to balance the conflicts created by what the Church ordained and what they perceived as real.

St Thomas Aquinas merged the concepts of Aristotle with Church doctrine. Although the Church was the final arbiter of God's will that did not mean people lacked a conscience and a person's own perceptions did enable them to act independently and take a stance based on their own conscience. This belief system, in the language of philosophy, laid the ground for an ethical knowledge base called *relativist*, *proportionist* or *deonto-teleological.*

- Can you see how the blending of the philosophies created a blended type of philosophical label? Rather than being confused by the new words, can you see how these labels explain the philosophical beliefs to which they relate?

Since the Renaissance the gradual growth of science, that is, seeking answers in nature instead of accepting that all was divine law, opened the way for large and small changes to society. The rejection of Plato's belief 'that lower orders lacked the ability for self-rule' brought about revolutions to depose the 'divinely created ruling classes'. The demand by Martin Luther for the right of the individual to answer directly to God split the established Church when he raised questions about papal authority. Plato's and Protagoras' philosophies continued to give direction to opposing viewpoints. Their threads were incorporated into later philosophical works. Arguments about whether the individual was the source of ethics and reason, whether the human condition was intrinsically good or bad, why and how circumstances can mould a person to create a 'good', 'moral' or 'bad', 'depraved' person were explored by many famous writers.

In the final analysis, the question remains. Is ethical behaviour (our notion of good and worthy action) a standard which comes from God so that the rules are not negotiable but *absolute*, or are there in nature certain 'laws of nature' and we can choose, depending on the situation and circumstances, the best way to act (*relativist*), or is ethics simply a case of personal choice, a matter of doing and acting in particular ways because things work better if that is the way we go (*utilitarian*)?

As individuals you can believe and argue and choose the philosophy that makes sense to you. As health professionals, however, you will deal with people who may be just as convinced their view is the only one that makes sense. One person might believe that something is always right or always wrong and nothing, ever, can change that. Another might believe that while there are things that are always going to be right or wrong, certain situations or circumstances may mean, for that particular case, an action is not so clearly right or wrong. Or you may be working with someone who holds the view that no one has the answers and any rule about right or wrong is only opinion, so if it feels good, do it.

Further, as a professional you are identifying with a group. You are accepting that within reasonable limits the philosophy of that group will reflect your own philosophy; that the perceptions of what is right and wrong, acceptable and unacceptable the group holds are valid and, while these may alter over time, they should be a good fit with your own belief system.

As health professionals we do not need to explore the complexities of philosophical thought and language but we do need to understand the belief system that creates our ideals, ethical boundaries and individual conscience. By recognising that we can all perceive the world differently and through exploring the philosophical position of a person, group or society we can better understand why they have certain views, rules and beliefs. The philosophical terms are simply a shorthand way to describe these ways of making sense of the world.

Activity

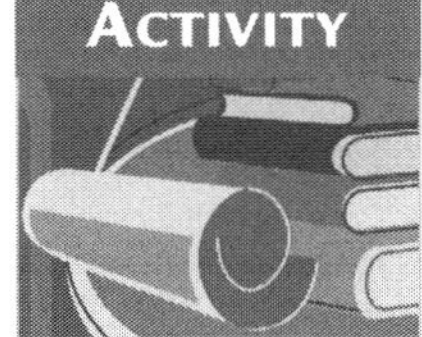

Consider these current ethical issues that particularly affect professionals.

Abortion

This ethical issue raises a dilemma for many people. Does a woman have the right to terminate a pregnancy for reasons she deems are important to her or is the action so against nature or divine law that it can never be acceptable? There are three clear philosophical belief systems that underpin the dilemma posed.

What about the professional who recommends the procedure in light of the pregnant woman's circumstances. Does a scientific, objective analysis of a situation really provide a sound ethical reason to make such a suggestion? What about the staff involved in the procedure? Do their own beliefs have a place; can they ethically refuse or ethically provide the intervention?

Euthanasia
Ask yourself how euthanasia poses an ethical dilemma and to whom?

Organ transplants
What about organ transplantation – what ethical questions are raised in your own mind concerning issues of availability, resources, age of donor and age of recipient?

Research
Are the risks associated with testing of drugs on animals or people worth the benefits? Who gains and who loses in experimental situations?

- How would an absolutist approach these questions?
- How would a utilitarian see the issues?

As we progress the aim is to explore how we can recognise what is an ethical dilemma and identify what actually creates an ethical dilemma. Once a dilemma has been identified, what approaches can we take to analyse and balance competing interests or determine the best course of action that has the least ethical risk?

- What strategies are involved in ethical decision making and when should they be used?

Respect for the individual and protection of the individual, group and society against forces that may take advantage of, damage or demean the rights and potential of others lies at the root of behaving in an ethical way. Sometimes our own beliefs, culture or good intentions blind us to another point of view. Some terrible actions and persecution have been taken against individuals or groups based on what, at a given time, was seen as sound and ethical reasoning.

- Can you think of an example in history where actions were taken that are today viewed with great regret or disgust?

What no one wants during their professional life is to find themselves carrying out an action that results in disapprobation, loss of standing or sanctions. This has happened to many professionals. Think about methods of controlling unruly clients that were once employed, about how babies were taken for adoption from unmarried mothers, about experiments on poor, confused or incarcerated people.

Professionals have power and this power must be used ethically. Not every situation is governed by a law, policy or rule. Caring for individuals carries the burden of being an advocate and defender of rights. If different belief systems and philosophies do exist then the professional must have skills to balance and respect these.

Ethics, health ethics, bioethics

What's in a name? For our purposes here, not a lot. However, we need to understand terminology to be able to contribute as equals in an ethical debate. Health professionals often find themselves arguing with each other about a moral issue. Each may be acting as an advocate for a different member of a family or patient. The conflict arising out of resource limitations affecting staff numbers, quality of care provision, access to services and every other aspect of health work are common sources of ethical debate.

> The theories people hold about their everyday work – the subjective theoretical framework in which they operate – can affect their interpretation of what they do. Health workers' understanding of their practice affects both their performance and their attitudes towards those for whom they are caring (Seedhouse, 2001).

To be able to articulate an argument, be understood and enter into a dialogue rather than have a confrontation relies on there being a mutual recognition of the issues and the way we describe needs, problems or solutions. Unless we can identify the underpinning philosophy and the driving forces giving individuals and groups their perspective we risk being unable to find a point of agreement. When one party uses jargon to perplex and confuse another party, relying on creating a sense of insecurity to gain the high ground, the moral issue has been lost in a situation of competition.

Ethics is about words, and often very emotive and value-laden considerations have to be articulated. Professionals usually try to adopt a rational, scientific approach to problem solving; they may feel a need to distance themselves from emotional issues and can do so by using jargon and their position of 'power' to promote their point of view.

Basically health workers are committed to achieving health goals. Doctors work towards achieving a diagnosis and cure, nurses participate in these activities and promote positive outcomes by focusing upon care. Health promotion and community health services often focus on prevention of illness or loss of health through education and lifestyle strategies. Paramedic interventions aim to maintain life and reduce further injury pending treatment and hopefully a cure. Paramedical specialists such as physiotherapists and occupational therapists participate to a larger or smaller degree in all these activities while focusing on a particular patient need.

However, unless there is a moral dimension in the provision of health care the way is open for conflict between groups and depersonalising the service and the client. This can lead to a denial of basic human rights in the name of treatment. Depending on the underpinning theory of health care work and the ethical dimension included in the education and practice of each group the language used to discuss issues may differ.

Bioethics is the study of ethics as the field relates to health care. Bioethicists specialise in translating and relating the theories of health to the theories guiding moral behaviour in health care. Bioethicists address health and health research controversies and raise awareness of these controversies. Some authors have devised strategies to examine problems or have developed codes of ethical practice to ensure professionals know the behaviour expected in real life when competing interests arise.

Bioethics is 'applied' ethics. The focus tends to be on determining the most suitable ethical solution to a specific health issue. Bioethics is less concerned with the theories and social or religious moral systems that underpin values, or with emotions, opinions or personal belief; rather it identifies agreed ways of investigating issues, establishing ways to analyse problems that have a moral dimension and achieving an objective assessment in order to make an ethical decision.

- Codes of professional ethics and codes for ethical research give direction to and policies for health professionals to adhere to in order to satisfy expected standards. Some are very precise as to what is expected while others are less specific.

Nuremberg Code

Until the Nuremberg trial of doctors for actions involving extreme research and violation of all basic ethical principles against prisoners in German concentration camps, there were no 'codes' guiding physicians or researchers other than the Hippocratic Oath. Until then it was assumed that ethical behaviour was intrinsic to a physician and there would never be morally repugnant medical practitioners. World War II changed that.

The focus of the judges in drawing up the Nuremberg Code, which was part of the judgment, was to ensure the rights of people involved in research. The judges felt that the traditional oaths of physicians, such as the Hippocratic Oath, were insufficient to achieve this. The Nuremberg Code was the first document of its kind and the 10 points set out by the judges form the basis for all ethical codes for research practice; however, the value system (philosophical ideals) that underpin it are strongly deontological, that is, there is a foundation belief that the rights of the individual are 'God given', that there is an absolute moral imperative to respect these rights.

While the Nuremberg Code was an important historical document and set the trend for research and eventually all health ethics, there were instances where later researchers failed to adhere to these standards. For example, some researchers argued that participant knowledge about their study, in order to gain informed consent, would in fact foil the purposes of the study.

Over time professional organisations have developed codes that take a more utilitarian view of matters. While the primary aims of the Nuremberg Code were respected, the balance between scientific gains and participant harm or lack of full understanding about the purpose and uses of the research was basically a matter left to up to the researcher.

The discussion below describes a controversial research that raised many ethical questions and did breach the Nuremberg Code.

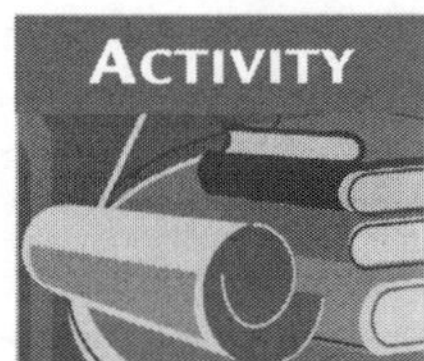

Activity

- Read this and take some time to reflect on both the ethical issues and the very interesting research findings.

Milgram's Obedience Research

American social psychologist Stanley Milgram (1933–84) carried out research on people to explore human behavior when obeying authority figures. The experiment was undertaken in 1961. After publication there were questions about ethical issues and these have since led to the development of research guidelines and professional governance for all research.

At the time of his experiment, the trials of WWII German war criminals were underway and many of the defendants had insisted they had only been following orders. This was the defense of even very senior Nazi leaders.

Milgram wanted to see if people really could be ordered to undertake actions that were considered 'evil' and if they would obey someone in authority who demanded that they 'kill' an innocent person.

Milgram devised an experimental test that sought to answer the question of whether inherently decent people could be made to do evil acts by someone in authority. His logic was that if ordinary people can be induced to follow orders to commit atrocious acts, atrocities are produced by social situations rather than by evil individuals.

Milgram's Experiment

Subjects were volunteers (over 1,000 people) who responded to a newspaper article offering money in return for their participation in a laboratory experiment at Yale University. The subjects were assured they could leave at any time during the experiment and they would still be paid. When the experiment was happening, some participants wanted to withdraw, but they told they had no choice; they had to continue.

The experiment required subjects to play the role of teachers. They were supervised and directed to teach a 'victim', the learner, who was really an actor, connections between words.

The supervisor was the authority figure. The subjects were required to provide a word and the learner had to give a correct answer. If the learner gave an incorrect answer, the subject/teacher was required to administer an electric shock. For the first error, the subject/teacher was instructed to deliver a 15-volt shock as punishment. The subject/teacher had to follow a protocol of increasing the intensity of subsequent shocks for every error. Increases in voltage of 15 volts were to be given until the maximum of 450 volts was reached. A shock of 330 volts is fatal.

The set up included monitors and electronics, noises and lights that gave the illusion that a shock was actually being delivered. In fact there was no shock. The victim/learner pretended that they were being administered shocks and would scream and beg for the subject/teacher to stop. The supervisor would prompt the subject/teacher to continue. These prompts progressed from a mild 'Please continue' through to 'the experiment requires that you continue' to insisting 'It is absolutely essential you continue' to a demand 'You have no other choice, you must go on!'.

The researchers wanted to see what level of shock would be reached before the subject/teacher refused to continue to 'teach'.

The subjects were very distressed, many begging the supervisor to let them stop administering the shocks. However contrary to the expectations of the researchers, most subjects continued to obey. They were distressed and some were crying but they continued to follow the protocol and keep increasing the voltage and administering the shocks.

Ethical Issues Arising from Milgrams' Experiment

At the time there were few ethical guidelines and, as with all original research, the outcomes were unpredictable. However Milgram was investigated and questions about the morality of the study were raised.

- *There was deception of the subjects. They were told they were teachers and that the shocks were real.*
- *Their consent was not informed.*

Milgram and more contemporary researchers have argued that if people knew the purpose of the research their behavior would be different. This is always an ethical research dilemma and the value of the findings must be balanced against the purpose of deception.

There were other deceptions.

- *Subjects were told that the experiment was concerned with the effects of shock on learning and its true purpose was not disclosed.*
- *They were misled into believing that the 'victim' was another subject rather than a confederate of the researcher.*
- *Most important, they were deceived into thinking that they were administering dangerous levels of shock to another human being.*
- *The subjects were paid. This can create an obligation to fulfill a contract.*

The primary ethical objection is that Milgram exposed participants to an extremely stressful experience without alerting them to this possibility in advance.

Subjects were told they could withdraw at any time but in reality they were strongly pressured to continue. There were reports of participants being so stressed their symptoms were similar to a nervous breakdown.

Milgram had undertaken immediate and intensive debriefing of all subjects when they had completed the experiment. It has been suggested that this debriefing had a positive effect when subjects were asked to evaluate their experience. Subjects were on the whole positive about their experiences after the debriefing. The majority (84%) were glad that they had the opportunity of participating in the experiment, 15% were neutral and 1% regretted participation. Three-quarters of the subjects said that they had learned something of personal importance from the experience (Barber, 2002).

- Does it surprise you that ordinary people would do this? It surprised the researchers and the experiment was repeated many times to confirm findings. Conditions were altered with various situations; allowing the subject to see the victim, at other times only hear the victim. Teachers and victims might be in the same room or separated by a wall or glass. However overwhelmingly subjects obeyed the authority figure.
- Have you ever wondered how normal people fall into behaving in unethical ways? The risk of being 'socialised' by a group or coerced by rules into adopting dangerous or negative attitudes towards others is important to everyone. We learn from our teachers and superiors. We model behaviour and perform in the same way we are taught. Dismissing the needs of the client because they are 'complainers' or giving more attention to one client over another who has been classed as being 'less worthy' for whatever reason are examples of how innocently and sometimes reluctantly we might adopt practices that an outsider would see as unethical.

APPLICATION to practice

Application to practice

An experiment was carried out on nurses. It found that 95% of nurses (twenty-one out of twenty-two) were prepared to give excessive doses of an unlisted drug to their patients when ordered to do so. The order was given over the phone by a doctor who claimed to be 'Dr Smith in Psychiatry'. There was a doctor of the same name on the hospital staff list, but none of the nurses had ever met him. Findings from this and later research warrants serious consideration. These nurses' obedience to an authority figure overrode policies and protocols for drug administration, for telephone orders and safe practice. While the drug administered was only glucose so there were no risks to patients, the experiment did support Milgram's findings.

Activity

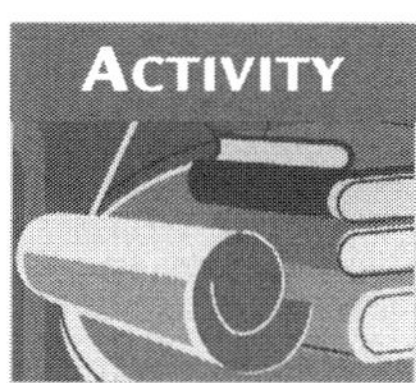

- In your own words can you articulate why there is sometimes confusion about what is law and what is ethics?

Declaration of Helsinki

With the continued, rapid development of research in psychology, sociology and medicine there were other studies and clinical trials that failed to adhere to the Nuremberg Code. It was argued by many researchers, however, that the code did not actually address 'the increasing contentious issue of Clinical Research in Patients with Illness'. (*British Medical Journal*, 1996: 1448) The Declaration of Helsinki 1964 took on this problem. Below is an extract from the declaration: (*BMJ*, 1996: 1448)

> It is the mission of the physician to safeguard the health of the people. His or her knowledge and conscience are dedicated to the fulfilment of this mission.
>
> The Declaration of Geneva of the World Medical Association binds the physician with the words, 'The Health of my patient will be my first consideration,' and the International Code of Medical Ethics declares that, 'A physician shall act only in the patient's interest when providing medical care which might have the effect of weakening the physical and mental condition of the patient.'

The purpose of biomedical research involving human subjects must be to improve diagnostic, therapeutic and prophylactic procedures and the understanding of the aetiology and pathogenesis of disease.

National Health and Medical Research Council publications

The National Health and Medical Research Council (NHMRC) in Australia has adopted the Declaration of Helsinki and developed codes and guidelines to ensure research activities meet ethical standards. These are much more prescriptive than the Declaration of Helsinki.

Requirements for informed consent, the right to withdraw from research by a participant, monitoring of research, ethics approval before research begins are all spelt out and the professional must provide extensive and accurate information about proposed research.

The publications below can be found at <https://www.nhmrc.gov.au/guidelines/publications/e72>.

- *National Statement on Ethical Conduct in Research Involving Humans*
  This statement consists of a series of guidelines made in accordance with the *National Health and Medical Research Council Act 1992*.
- *Human Research Ethics Handbook* – commentary on the *National Statement on Ethical Conduct in Research Involving Humans*
  The handbook complements the NHMRC *National Statement on Ethical Conduct in Research Involving Humans*, which is the primary guideline for ethics committees and researchers alike.

- *Australian Code for the Responsible Conduct of Research (2007)* Developed jointly by the National Health and Medical Research Council, the Australian Research Council and Universities Australia, the Code has broad relevance across all research disciplines. It replaces the *Joint NHMRC/AVCC Statement and Guidelines on Research Practice (1997)*. The statement and guidelines exist to guide institutions in developing their own procedures and guidelines by providing a comprehensive framework of minimum acceptable standards.
- *Values and Ethics: Guidelines for Ethical Conduct in Aboriginal and Torres Strait Islander Health Research* (PDF format 310kb)

Professional organisations, such as nurse registration bodies, may develop their own codes to ensure their members know and adhere to the standards expected of them. Many are general statements while others specify actions to take in particular instances and give direction for the work and client relations that the profession undertakes. Some identify the sanctions or discipline that may be taken should a member fail to satisfy professional ethical standards. The Nursing and Midwifery Board of Australia adopted and rebranded the governing codes for nurses and midwives when professional health regulation became a national responsibility.

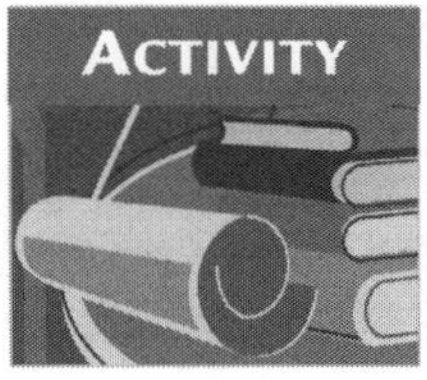

Activity

- Find the Code of Ethics for Nurses in Australia if you do not already have a downloaded copy. It is recommended you find and keep the NMBA publications handy

Note the preamble: *this code has been developed from the United Nations' Universal Declaration of Human Rights, International Covenant on Economic, Social and Cultural Rights and International Covenant on Civil and Political Rights; the World Health Organization's Constitution and publication series entitled Health and Human Rights; and the United Nations Development Programme Human Development Report 2004: Cultural liberty in today's diverse world.*

The underpinning philosophy for this document is clearly related to those developments since the Nuremberg Declarations discussed above.

This is evident in the stated purpose of the document.

The purpose of the *Code of Ethics for Nurses in Australia* is to:

- identify the fundamental ethical standards and values to which the nursing profession is committed, and that are incorporated in other endorsed professional nursing guidelines and standards of conduct
- provide nurses with a reference point from which to reflect on the conduct of themselves and others
- guide ethical decision-making and practice, and
- indicate to the community the human rights standards and ethical values it can expect nurses to uphold.

Here then is the nurse's guideline to ethical practice reflecting the philosophy and attitudes that the profession embraces and in fact will demand. Failure to satisfy these standards opens the way for professional sanctions and the documents may be used by the public or a legal hearing to establish what the professional benchmark for ethical behaviour is. Individual beliefs are not denied in such a code but the individual is given clear direction about how to act within their professional capacity.

Application to practice

APPLICATION to practice

It is all very well accepting that the nursing profession is guided by and adheres to a Code of Ethics. Reading the ethical value statements is unlikely to raise controversy or dismay. However in practice situations these guidelines are assumed knowledge and when you find yourself in a difficult situation and ethical questions arise, how do you react?

The concept of accountability is important. These codes are just words unless the individual accepts personal, professional responsibility to adhere to these standards. It is all very well suggesting breaches of the code will lead to sanctions but that assumes someone is monitoring ethical situations and reports the breach and that the failure is proven or admitted to.

In our work we deal with vulnerable and stressed clients and families. They need to rely on our skills and determination to provide support and communication that best meet their needs. Sometimes that might not be possible. There are occasions when providing full and complete information to a person may precipitate a collapse, so do we lie? Do we avoid the truth? Do we ignore the request for information?

Ethical issues/problems/dilemmas are situations in which there are conflicting moral claims. In some of these situations people:

- Do not know what the ethically right thing to do is.
- Do not agree about the ethically right thing to do.
- Can find no satisfactory solution or there are two equally unsatisfactory solutions.
- Know what the ethically right thing to do is, but do not want to act on this.

This brings us back to the concept of accountability. What ethical steps should be followed when we are faced with a dilemma? Realistically the baseline for judging and monitoring individual health workers relies on the fact the health worker has integrity. It is:

- Always assumed individual and profession will act to benefit clients and avoid harm.
- Always expected that a professional fulfils their duty of care and enhances their own practice.

However:

- Failure to comply with standards are difficult to police and discipline.
- There are limits to the powers of professional regulatory bodies.

Accountability relies on these concepts, there is an expectation the individual and organisations monitor themselves and their colleagues in order to protect the vulnerable. This is the concept of self-regulation. It is:

- Expected that the professional is capable of monitoring their own and colleagues behaviour to reflect ethical and professional standards.
- Expected that professional is active and committed to remaining up to date and competent.
- Expected that organisations meet accreditation and are committed to contemporary expectations of knowledge.

Recall the information about bioethics above. The work of a number of bioethicists has focused on developing practical approaches to problem solving ethical dilemmas and most health workers adopt these principle based approaches to issues.

Bioethical principles give us a way to categorise and isolate issues. Beauchamp and Childress (2009) developed what have become the most commonly accepted bioethical principles.

These are:

- the principle of respect for autonomy,
- the principle of non maleficence,
- the principle of beneficence
- the principle of justice.

Your question is always: "What is the ethically right action to take in a given situation"? Then you consider these principles.

- Autonomy- competent adult patient's right to decide
- Non Maleficence = Do No Harm- very old medical/nursing ethical principle. However we need to understand in various contexts just what is the meaning of harm? An operation to save life actually requires harm through surgery.
- Beneficence = Do Good- Again, what is the meaning of good? If we satisfy a request that has health risks, the good is might be a happier patient but at what cost?
- Justice – fair distribution of burdens/benefits in society.

Later ethicists have added to these.

- Veracity = Rule of Truth Telling. Should we always tell the truth? What is Truth?
- Rule of Promise Keeping- Is there anything that might justify not keeping a promise we have made?

How you decide what is the ethically right thing to do, will depend on how you ethically define the situation and which values and bioethical principles you use. Reference to your ethical code establishes there is a clear standard expected.

In health situations we tend to accept an act is ethical if it brings about the Greatest Good.

This does **NOT** say the act must bring about good for **EVERYONE**

Think about this for a moment. Can you think of situations where the benefit and satisfaction of one person's needs will fail to satisfy another?

Scenario

The elderly person begs to be allowed to return to their own home rather than transfer to an aged care environment is a situation we often encounter. The family and health staff know this would lead to disaster and risks. Yet the patient expects us to be their advocate, they are convinced they will manage.

What do we do ethically if one of these principles/rules conflicts with another principle?

Here the question of client autonomy needs to be considered. Is the client competent and able to make choices?

Yes they are, that this choice puts them at risk is to their mind of no consequence. Life is all about risk.

Going home will be good; it is to the benefit of this client right to choose and preference.

The obvious risk of harm and family fears for their loved one are an issue.

What if the worst happens and questions about the decision to let them return to a risk situation put the health staff in the spotlight and they are found to have failed in their responsibility to protect a vulnerable person?

- Which ethical principle would you allow to determine the ethically right choice?

Aim: make decisions and live with them.

There are tools we can use to help us in our decision making processes. An ethical framework gives direction for undertaking logical and careful steps in solving problems.

Ethical frameworks

Many authors have presented ethical decision making frameworks. These all have the same focus. There are clear steps to logically identify and clarify the issue and the final decision is one that is reached rationally. Good documentation will show later that the decision was, in light of the circumstances and investigations at the time, fair and unbiased.

1. Collect, analyze, and interpret the data or information
2. State the dilemma clearly
3. Consider the choices of action based on ethical principles.
4. Analyse the advantages and disadvantages of each action.
5. Make a decision that resolves the dilemma (Aiken, 1994, cited in Clark, 2002).

Activity

- Consider this second ethical decision making framework.

Examine the ethical dilemma.
Thoroughly comprehend the possible alternatives available.
Hypothesize ethical arguments.
Investigate, compare, and evaluate the arguments for each alternative.
Choose the alternative you would recommend.
Act on your chosen alternative.
Look at the ethical dilemma and examine outcomes while reflecting on the ethical decision (Mastrian, McGonigle, Mahan, & Bixler, 2011, p. 313)

Can you see the similarity to the first framework? Do a search to find the decision making framework that fits your personal approach to problem solving and keep it for future reference.

Summary

This chapter has tried to separate concepts that are bound up in the historical and philosophical traditions of law and ethics. Nursing practice draws on many science and humanities subjects and the demand for nurses to be able to identify their legal and moral obligations is high. Nursing occurs in many environments and care is provided to people with varying needs, abilities and expectations. Holistic approaches require us to consider the needs of the client across many dimensions so it will be inevitable that dilemmas will arise and a desire to have a 'one size fits all rule' is understandable but not possible.

As professionals there is an expectation that we have the knowledge and skills to assess not only the needs of the client but the context within which those needs arise. As you progress through this book, always keep in mind that the legal reasoning that underpins cases, legislation and policies is subject to this issue of context. We need to be alert to the fact the boundaries of our practice, the decisions we take and the actions we implement are always context bound. What is reasonable in one time and place will not necessarily be reasonable in another circumstance. Professional reasoning, professional assessment and professional documentation that considers the context, and which gives a rationale for our work, is a communication skill we need to develop. Clear and unambiguous facts, lucid and accurate reports and evaluation of our actions will give anyone who questions or reviews our work and behaviour valuable and reliable information. Gaps will only raise doubts about the accuracy or integrity of the author of notes and poor explanations or limited engagement with our clients can lead to loss of trust and it is the clients' perceptions of us as professionals we need to meet. By satisfying these obligations the risk of legal and professional investigations are minimised.

Practice assignment question

The aim is to get you to apply learning as you progress by considering posed questions.

This question is a series of scenarios and the whole assignment of 4 responses relates to the first 4 chapters to be answered in its entirety. Scenarios 3 and 4 are to be found in Chapter 4.

Scenario 1 Length 400-500 words
Apply the bioethical principle of beneficence to the dilemma below.

RN Kate is currently a post graduate Masters student who is required to design and undertake a research project as part of her studies. You are a new RN, recently employed at the same aged care facility, often working with Kate. Kate tells you she has an idea for her research project but is going to try it out before putting up a proposal. Her intention is to identify among residents two groups; the first will have a history of smoking and alcohol use, the second will have no reports of this in their medical history. Kate will design memory and physical stamina tests and compare the two groups.

Scenario 2 Length 400-500 words
Apply the bioethical principle of non maleficence to the scenario.

Kate has identified 10 residents who were or are, currently smokers or regular users of alcohol and a group of 10 who have no history of use. They are all between 80-84 years of age. Her tests will be 3 quizzes testing recall, arithmetic and language use plus a series of physical activities: walking 300 metres, muscle strength with lifting bar bells and flexibility tests with bending and stretching. Pre and post physical tests she will take BP and pulse. Kate will record and compare the capacity of each group.

Sources

Barber, N., (2000) 'Milgram's obedience research', *Encyclopedia of Ethics in Science and Technology*, Infobase Publishing, New York.

Beauchamp, T., & Childress, J., (2009) *Principles of biomedical ethics* (6th edition). New York: Oxford.Johnstone, M. (2009). *Bioethics: a nursing perspective*. Sydney, NSW: Elsevier.

British Medical Journal, Nuremberg doctors' trial, Declaration of Helsinki (1964) Recommendations guiding physicians in biomedical research involving human subjects. *British Medical Journal* 1996; 313: 1448–1449.

Clark, D.A., (2002) "Development ethics: a research agenda", *International Journal of Social Economics*, Vol. 29 Iss: 11, pp.830–848.

Kerridge, I., Lowe, M., & Stewart, C. (2013). *Ethics and law for the health professions.* Sydney, NSW: Federation Press.

Kings College London, (2013) MPhil/PhD Nursing Research/Midwifery Research/Health Studies Research Programme Handbook 2013-14 Florence Nightingale School of Nursing & Midwifery.

Mastrian, K. G., McGonigle, D., Mahan, W. L., & Bixler, B. (2011). *Integrating technology in nursing education.* Boston, Mass: Jones and Bartlett.

NMBA codes and guidelines available from http://www.nursingmidwiferyboard.gov.au/Codes-Guidelines-Statements/Codes-Guidelines.aspx

Seedhouse, D., (2001) *Health: The Foundations for Achievement*, 2nd edn, John Wiley & Sons, New Jersey.

Seedhouse, D., & Lovett, L., (1992) *Practical Medical Ethics*, John Wiley & Sons, Chichester.

Storch, J.I., Rodney, P. & Starzomski, R. (2004) *Toward a Moral Horizon: Nursing Ethics for Leadership and Practice*, Pearson Education Canada, Toronto.
Tschudin, V., (2003) *Ethics in Nursing: The Caring Relationship*, 3rd edn, Butterworth Heinemann Elsevier Science Limited, Edinburgh.
White, B. C. & Zimbelman, J. A. (2005) *Moral Dilemmas in Community Health Care*, Pearson Longman, New York.

Case

Glynace H. Norton et al. v. Argonaut Insurance Company et al. No. 5601, Court of Appeal of Louisiana, First Circuit 29 June 1962

Law and the health professional

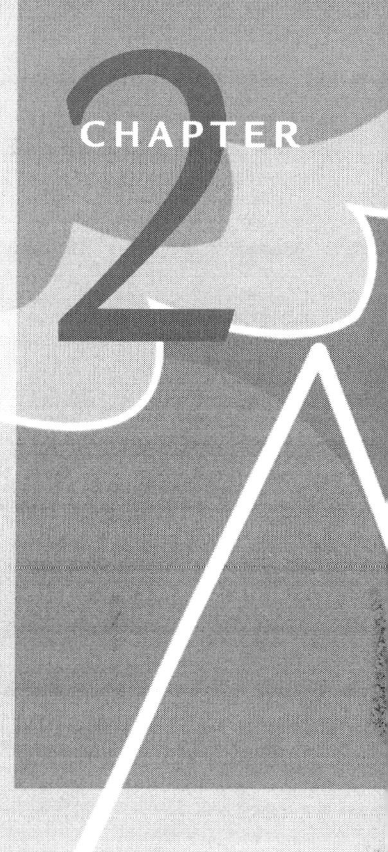

Learning outcomes

After studying this chapter you should be able to:

- Demonstrate an understanding of the Australian legal system and relevant statutory bodies that create or interpret law and policies for health professionals and health agencies.
- Discuss the relationship between legal institutions, professional governance and professional standards.
- Display an understanding of key legislation affecting health policies and procedures.
- Describe the role of the law in providing direction for health care practice.

Overview

Students are often confused about whether there is such a thing as health law. There are textbooks on health law yet a lawyer will tell you there is no such thing as health law.

The law in Australia does not have an identifiable area like taxation law or constitutional law for health-related matters. There are, however, many Acts of Parliament and legal cases that provide rules and findings in relation to health issues. These come from various sources and when grouped together for convenience give the health industry a complex wealth of legal information. This is where the term 'health law' has come from. For the health professional, understanding the general areas of law that impinge upon professional practice and the specific law that directly affects practice provides both guidelines and certainty where it might otherwise be a matter of opinion whether to act or not to act.

Lawyers need to understand the sources of law and devote much time and effort in establishing the validity, relevance and breadth of law in relation to issues at hand. This focus, using specialised and sometimes arcane language, means that the outsider often has great difficulty in following arguments or understanding the results of hearings where protagonists argue their point. It means the public is often stunned at the result of a case where the outcome 'was a foregone conclusion – everyone knows he did it'. The rules of law and procedure may affect the outcome or the judgment may be so insightful that future decisions or accepted ways of doing things are never going to be the same again.

For the health professional it is important to know where the laws that affect practice as well as daily life come from and just when and how these laws are upheld. Unless the professional can identify the difference between what is legal and what is not legal and can adhere to practices that limit the risk of harm, as defined by the law, the professional will be liable for the penalties of being found wanting.

Health professionals are likely to be mobile throughout their careers. They work in every state and territory and often overseas. The Australian system of laws, the structure of the court system and those courts' ambit of responsibility varies between states due to legislation. The professional has an obligation to work within the law and professional guidelines. Knowing where to find specific information and relating this to their current or planned future environment is an essential skill.

The Australian legal system in a nutshell

- The actual sources of the laws are the *legislature*, that is, federal (Commonwealth) and state Parliaments, and the courts, that is, *common law*.

Legislation

Elected representatives make up the Parliament (federal or state) and they can pass 'primary' legislation on matters that fall within Parliaments' particular powers (these powers come from the Australian Constitution). Legislation may also provide for 'delegated' or 'subordinate' legislation. Specific institutions responsible for governing specific areas can be created and given limited powers. The Nurses Registration Board is an example. Also, powers can be given to allow for future alterations or adaptations to regulations to ensure currency in the rules the agency is responsible to oversee. This avoids every little change having to go back to Parliament for approval.

There are many commissions and professional and quasi legal bodies that have been given responsibilities to carry out investigations, give approval or set standards and take action to protect the public from activities recognised as having risks. An example is the Therapeutic Goods Tribunal, which has powers to approve and regulate medicines.

Common law

The second main source of law in Australia is the common law, or 'judge-made' law. It is a body of law, made up of a number of specialised branches which have been built up, evolving from and incorporating ancient rules, laws brought by conquerors who imported their system into Britain, English Kings and Parliaments. These are expressed in the decisions of various courts. Judges are required to follow precedent, which means that 'like cases should be decided alike'. This gives certainty and limits the chances of an individual or personal interpretation of law. However, as society changes judges need to consider many variables and this requires flexibility as well as consistency. The system has checks and balances; the right of appeal exists to raise issues or questions of law that may not have been anticipated in the first instance.

The legal system in Australia follows the Westminster system and has developed upon the imported law of England. For much of our history the final arbiter for legal conflicts was the Privy Council, the highest British court. Australia now has its own High Court. However, the procedural rules, traditions, language and processes are very similar in all countries which have taken up the common law.

It is an adversarial system. Protagonists are represented by lawyers, arguments are presented and the judge and jury are the mediators and final decision makers. In criminal cases the prosecutor is the legal representation for the state and the defendant is the accused person. In civil cases the person claiming injury is called the plaintiff and the opposition is the defendant.

While the right to go to court is not automatic and there are numerous procedural rules, the basic premise of the Westminster system is that everyone is presumed innocent until proven otherwise and everyone is entitled to a fair, impartial and unprejudiced hearing. This concept is called *Natural Justice* and extends to all legal, administrative and disciplinary institutions.

Activity

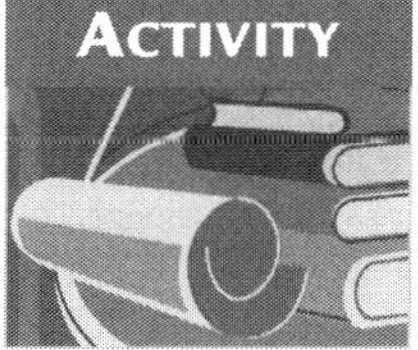

- What in your own words does common law mean?
- What is the difference between an adversarial system and an inquisitorial system?
- If you were accused of a wrongdoing and yet were not told exactly what the charges were before being asked to present your defence, this would be a denial of what?
- Can you think of how, in relation to direct health care activities, communication and labelling might lead to someone being accused of being a 'bad nurse' or 'difficult patient' but without that individual being aware they have been labelled?

Jurisdiction

Every state has a court hierarchy, each level being strictly limited as to the matters it can take on. Different courts have different jurisdictions.

At the lowest level of the court hierarchy are Local or Magistrate's Courts (in some states, years ago these were called Courts of Petty Sessions). These are presided over by a magistrate who is a qualified and experienced lawyer. There are no juries; the jurisdiction is (generally) limited to minor matters but every state and territory has legislation that specifies these limits. Magistrates are involved in presiding over Licensing Tribunals, they can be appointed as the coroner in investigations of suspicious or unanticipated deaths and preside over Children's Courts and Mental Health Tribunals. It is the Magistrate's or Local Courts that handle the bulk of cases in each state.

Next there are District Courts (in some states called County Courts), which are presided over by a judge. The judge may be assisted by a jury or not, depending on the case at hand. These courts exist in the larger states; smaller states and territories do not have this level due to population size. District Courts are also governed by state legislation limiting the range of matters they can deal with, but they usually have jurisdiction over most civil and criminal cases except the most serious crimes, such as murder.

The District Court, Federal Court (which specialises in trade practices, constitutional and administrative issues) and the Family Court sit at the same level in the hierarchy, the last two being more recent and specialised creations. All can hear appeals arising from a case.

In every state and territory there is a Supreme Court. This court has, like the Magistrate's and District Courts, *original jurisdiction*, that is, it can hear a case for the first time, and also has *appellate jurisdiction*. Appeals from the Supreme, District or Magistrate's Courts can be made to have a Full Court hearing composed of three judges. The right to appeal a court decision is not automatic, as the grounds for the appeal are governed by law and procedures differ at the hearing.

The High Court, as the name suggests, is the most senior court in Australia. There is a Chief Justice and six other judges who hear original disputes and appeals from all states and territories. However, in this court the focus is on matters of constitutional, national or public importance. Recall that the common law is bound by precedent – future cases are based upon the law as it was stated in previous cases. High Court judgments carry the most 'weight'. Matters of legislation, disputes between the Commonwealth and states, civil and criminal issues are heard and this court's judgments and arguments explaining these set the rules for the future.

Figure 2.1 Summary of the Australian court system

- Federal laws are administered by federal courts. These are:
  The High Court
  The Federal Court
  The Family Court

  The federal system also include commissions and tribunals such as the Human Rights and Equal Opportunity Commission, the Australian Industrial Relations Commission, the Social Securities Appeals Tribunal and the Administrative Appeals Tribunal.

- State laws are administered by state courts. These may be called slightly different names in different states but their jurisdiction is similar throughout Australia. These are:
  The Magistrate's Court
  The County/District Court
  The Supreme Court

  The state system also includes tribunals and commissions such as Civil and Administrative Tribunals, the Equal Opportunity Commission and the Victims of Crime Assistance Tribunal.

- The High Court is the final court of appeal from both the state and federal court systems.

Source: Attorney-General's Department (2004).

Optional reading

For an extensive but easy to understand coverage of the legal system in Australia go to <http://www.dfat.gov.au/facts/legal_system.html> or <http://australia.gov.au/topics/law-and-justice/courts-and-tribunals> (accessed 6 August 2014).

Case law

As discussed earlier, when a case is heard the judge is obliged to follow earlier judgments. This relates to criminal and civil cases, and also to specialised courts and tribunals. What is important to realise is that there is often no precise legal answer to questions raised in law. Cases are heard by judges or magistrates, with or without juries. In recent years the costs, time and variables jury hearings introduce into cases has led to a reduction in the number of jury hearings.

Decisions made by judges bind the parties of that case unless the judgment is overturned by a higher court on appeal. However, even if there has been no appeal, later courts may overrule prior judgments. There are some cases that result in judgments that carry far more weight than others. The principles of law that come out of these, especially from the High Court of Australia, carry great weight and give direction to later judgments.

These principles and the interpretation of actions or circumstances, findings of fault or inappropriate behaviour give direction to individuals and institutions. If there are others functioning in the same way as the defendant and if the judge declares that the defendant's actions were faulty or dangerous, then of course this will give direction to people who, while not party to the case, are doing the same or similar things.

- Policies grow out of case law.

In coronial inquests all the facts known about the deceased person's cause of death are examined. This examination is inquisitorial in nature. The rules of evidence and court procedures do not have any bearing here. Anyone and any circumstance can be called upon to provide information. The cause of death may have been the result of unsafe work practices, mechanical failures or predictable (if someone had just given it some thought) reasons. The findings will be taken up by industries and prevention strategies will be put in place. Policies will be implemented to ensure this type of tragedy does not occur again.

There is an area of common law that grew out of a need to overcome the rigidity created by rules of precedent. Known as *Equity*, it has become a distinct area of case law and disputes are resolved by applying reason and conscience to the specific problem at hand. This area of common law has its own particular rules and remedies but, from a health professional perspective, actions in Equity might relate to contractual agreements, where one party has taken advantage of another, unconscionable dealings, fraud, mistake, undue influence, breach of confidence or trust funds.

There are a number of branches of the common law. However, at this stage for our purposes the common law can be classified as either criminal law or civil law.

Criminal law is a body of law that has a moral, community value and social protective element. The need to protect society, uphold agreed values and standards of behaviour and protect individuals and property is incorporated into the criminal law. Not all behaviour that falls outside of the agreed 'moral majority' will be sanctioned by the law; equally there are some acts that have no 'moral imperative' which are sanctioned.

Driving without a seatbelt, retail shopping hours, parking and speeding offences are punishable by the state, through fines or gaol sentences. None of these actions have a real moral aspect but all have been deemed illegal by Acts of Parliament (legislation). Other offences may have a moral or value aspect. Pornographic material, obscene telephone calls, crimes against a person are examples. The organ of the state responsible for maintaining the law and bringing wrongdoers before the courts to answer for their actions is the police.

Civil law provides the *individual* with a course of action to achieve compensation or recognition for a wrong done to them. The wrong may not be against the law as we understand it as a crime, but the wrong has caused a type of loss or hurt that the courts will recognise. In a civil suit, the wronged individual (the plaintiff) is looking for redress or monetary compensation for the suffering inflicted by a specific individual or group. There needs to be an identified wrongdoer (defendant) for a civil action to be brought.

Legislation

While there are many rules, procedures and cases to refer to, there will never be a rule for every circumstance. Meanings of words change with time, their interpretation and social changes affect the law. Parliament may decide to reduce the 'uncertainty' of having judges make decisions with all these variables and instead create *legislation* to deal with the matter.

There are quite a number of Commonwealth and state Acts of Parliament (statutes) that directly relate to health care. However, finding and understanding legislation can be difficult. If there have been amendments over time, working out just what has changed and whether it will affect policies or procedures currently in place, whether it affects only one state or all of Australia, is often an issue.

Legislation can be created whether or not there is a dispute in the courts, and often the aim is to prevent problems. Recall the fact that parliaments can delegate responsibilities; they can create statutory bodies such as a professional board or councils. When these bodies make rules and impose these, this is *delegated legislation*. Professional licensing bodies set standards, register those who meet standards and take action against the members who fall short. Registering bodies have an obligation to protect the public and do so through education, monitoring performance, hearing complaints and taking action within the limit of their delegated powers.

The language of court actions

In a civil action or claim the person or party bringing the case is called the *plaintiff*. Civil law cases are usually initiated by a document called a *plaint* (or sometimes a writ) and the person who must answer or defend the claim is called the *defendant*. When a case is cited it is the name of the plaintiff that is shown first – plaintiff v. defendant.

In some circumstances the person bringing the case may be called the *applicant*, and the person answering or responding is called the *respondent*. This is true of cases heard in the Family Court. In situations such as those often heard in the Family Court where government, community or welfare representatives are interested parties (as the matter is one of great public interest), these third parties may be listed in the court record as an *intervener*.

Once a judgment is handed down on the initial hearing it can be appealed. The person bringing the appeal action is called the *appellant*. The other party is called the *respondent*. When appeals are cited in the higher court the appellant's name is first. For example, the initial case will be cited *Jones v. Smith*. As Smith was unhappy about the judgment, which went against him, he decided to appeal, and the citation for this case will be *Smith v. Jones*.

Note the 'v.'. This is an abbreviation of versus. Recall that common law is adversarial – the parties to a case are against each other and every court case is recorded as *X versus Y*. Many cases do not name the party but use initials only to preserve the anonymity of people in the court record.

Activity

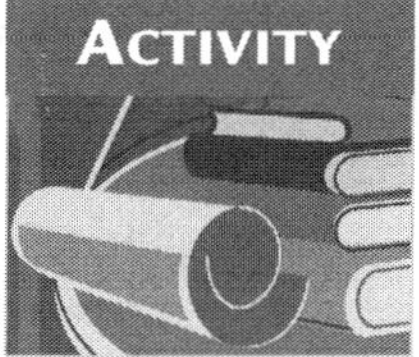

The High Court of Australia is now the final court of appeal for all Australian states and territories.

- What exactly does this mean?
- What is the meaning of these terms:
  Defendant
  Plaintiff
  Appellant
  Respondent

Check your answers against those given below to make sure you understand these important concepts.

Until the creation of the High Court of Australia the final court of appeal for decisions of Australian courts was the Privy Council. When a case is decided it is usual to appeal to the next level in the hierarchy. In particular circumstances direct appeal to the High Court can be granted. These are matters of public concern, often related to government activities or questions about constitutional powers.

Plaintiff: The person who or entity that initiates a civil lawsuit.
Defendant: The person who or entity that is sued.
Appellant: The party initiating an appeal of the decision of a lower court.
Respondent: The party against whom the petition is filed.

Government, judiciary and health

While the focus of your studies is not legal history or legal procedure, there are key concepts in the historical structure of the Australian legal system and the manner in which issues are dealt with that relate to health issues.

A number of references have already been made to the Australian Constitution. Constitutional law is in fact a specialised branch of law. It is the Constitution that frames the form of government and the courts and the Constitution sets limits on the powers, roles and functions of these institutions.

Most citizens understand that we have both state and federal parliaments in Australia. State and the federal parliaments comprise elected representatives and in our parliamentary system the relationship between federal and state governments and the limits on their powers to provide and manage health care systems is controlled to a large extent by the Constitution.

Another important issue is that the Constitution dictates that there is a separation of powers between the legislature (parliamentary members who propose and formulate laws), the executive (elected representatives who implement those laws) and the judiciary (courts which apply the common law and interpret legislation created by Parliament). This separation of powers is aimed at ensuring the courts have independence from political interference.

The Commonwealth government can only enact legislation under the powers granted by the Constitution. Commonwealth legislation takes precedence over state legislation to the extent that there is inconsistency between federal and state laws. It is not unknown for the federal parliament to enact legislation to limit or prohibit state legislation using its constitutional powers.

Regulation of health matters is not directly granted by the Constitution to the Commonwealth government. The authors of the Constitution had identified that health was a state issue and gave responsibility to the federal parliament only for health in the territories and for those issues that had relevance nationally, such as quarantine matters. In reality, the fact that taxation is now primarily a federal responsibility gives the Commonwealth control over the allocation of funding. This and the existence of a national health insurance scheme has given the Commonwealth greater powers in the area of health. It is through funding grants to the states that the Commonwealth controls what would otherwise be a state responsibility.

The Commonwealth *does* have the right to regulate health professionals and thus health care and so it has directly, or in cooperation with state Acts, great influence over the provision of care and regulation of health matters. There is cooperation between state and Commonwealth government legislation especially in relation to health. The need for uniform standards, uniform funding and qualifications and skills of staff for health services and the desire for equality and equity in access to health services means that the states share powers with the Commonwealth on many matters.

- State legislation and federal legislation takes precedence over case law.

Parliament may enact legislation that ensures public concerns are met, while the courts are bound by rules that insist on certain limits. Courts may deal with each sentence differently, for example gaol versus community service sentences for theft. Public concern about length of sentences for certain crimes has led to mandatory sentencing legislation. This means that there is a specific sentence that must be awarded for specific crimes.

Most legislation affects future actions, that is, it applies only to events occurring after it has been enacted. However, occasionally legislation is retrospective. This type of legislation may aim to catch people who have taken advantage of a legal loophole or results from a finding in a court case where the judge constrained by the rules of the law has not been able to impose a sentence that reflected the attitude and desire for justice the court and public felt were valid.

Legislation can be changed or repealed. Parliament can insert new clauses to include new technical advances or remove a provision that has no relevance. Repeal can involve a whole Act or part of an Act. Sometimes legislation is created to be in force for a specific period only; National emergencies often give impetus to the creation of specific statutes but they are needed only for the duration of the emergency.

Most of us rarely have reason to refer to a statute; however, there are many Acts specific to health so there may be an occasion for health professionals to do so. Statutes can be purchased from the Government Printer; most institutions have relevant legislation kept in each department or the institution's library or you can use the Internet to search either Commonwealth or state legislation resources. A site with links to every state and territory where you can search for your own state's legislation is <www.aph.gov.au/library/intguide/law/auslaw. htm>.

Below are some examples of Commonwealth and State Acts that relate to health work.

Protecting laws

For example:

Australia has enacted federal (Commonwealth) laws to prevent discrimination on the basis of race, sex, age and disability. The objective of the legislation is positive rather than negative: to engender respect for individuals and to promote human rights rather than merely to impose a prohibition.

Laws that protect individual rights and interests must, to be effective, incorporate a proscriptive element that imposes certain penalties for non-compliance, but they are not essentially proscriptive in their thrust.

Equal opportunity legislation, for example, may prohibit certain conduct on the part of employers, landlords and others that is held to amount to unlawful discrimination, but the philosophy underpinning the legislation is that of protecting individuals against discrimination.

Another example:

Legislative Response to Failures of mental health services.

Victoria's amended *Mental Health Act* provides an example of national responses to failures.

> "...people with mental illness should: ... be provided with high quality and timely care according to professionally accepted standards ... be provided with care designed for them to live, work and participate in the community wherever possible ... be provided with appropriate and comprehensive information about their illness and treatment ... be involved in the development of their ongoing treatment plan wherever possible have their treatment plan regularly reviewed and revised" [*Mental Health Act 1986 (Vic)] Every state in Australia has since 2000 enacted new Mental Health legislation that embraces such principles.*

Disability Legislation:
In December 2008, the Federal Government tabled draft Disability Standards to improve access to premises for persons with disabilities, and introduced legislation to implement recommendations of the Productivity Commission from 2004 to improve the operation of the Disability Discrimination Act.

The states and territories also have existing programs to address issues of discrimination.

Protecting patient rights

An example:

Freedom of Information Act 1982 (Qld), Freedom of Information Regulation 1992 (Qld)

These Acts establishes a statutory avenue through which an individual can access their personal medical/health records held by a public authority. The object of this Act is to extend as far as possible the right of the community to have access to information held by Queensland government.

Protecting people's health

Such Acts are current in each state and territory, examples- *Environmental Protection Act 1994 (Qld)*

Environmental Protection (Waste Management) Policy 2000 (Qld)

Environmental Protection (Waste Management) Regulation 2000 (Qld)

All health facilities in Queensland have an obligation to comply with this Act by taking appropriate measures to minimise or eliminate environmental hazards.

There are specific provisions dealing with clinical and related waste.

Protecting the public

An example:

Health Rights Commission Act 1991(Qld)

The Health Rights Commission was established by this statute and its role is to oversee, review and improve the quality of health care in Queensland.

It receives complaints about all health services, including private health services.

The Commission also has an educative role, to make health consumers more aware of their rights and to encourage informed participation in the management of their health problems.

The Act places an emphasis on resolving complaints through conciliation and negotiation rather than through litigation.

Regulating health services

Again, every State Parliament has enacted equivalent statutes for these examples:

Health Act 1937 (Qld)

Health Regulations 1996 (Qld)

Health (Drugs and Poisons) Regulations 1996 (Qld)

This is the primary piece of legislation regarding the regulation of public health within Queensland.

The Act is divided into 7 parts and deals with issues including powers of government officers, responsibilities of local and state government in relation to public health, prevention/notification/treatment of disease/disability, and a number of miscellaneous provisions.

Protecting Australia

An example: *Quarantine Act (Cwth)*

Section 51(ix) of the Commonwealth Constitutions has been used to support the *Quarantine Act 1908. Section 4 of that Act states:*

'Quarantine has relation to measures for the inspection, exclusion, detention, observation, segregation, isolation, treatment, sanitary regulation and disinfection of vessels, persons, goods, things, animals or plants, and having their object the prevention of the introduction or spread of diseases or pests affecting man, animals or plants.'

Control of Drugs and Devices

Therapeutic Goods Act 1989 (C'wth)

The objects of this Act are to do the following, so far as the Constitution permits: a) provide for the establishment and maintenance of a national system of controls relating to the quality, safety, efficacy and timely availability of therapeutic goods that are:

- used in Australia, whether produced in Australia or elsewhere; or
- exported from Australia;
- to provide a framework for the States and Territories to adopt a uniform approach
- to control the availability and accessibility, and ensure the safe handling, of poisons in Australia

Privacy and confidentiality

The *Privacy Act 1988* (C'wth) governs the manner in which 'personal information' is handled by Commonwealth agencies.

Confidentiality does not provide an ethical or legal obligation to keep any and all information secret in every circumstance.

Instead it centers on a duty to use particular information – typically identified through some form of notification or through the nature of the context in which it is imparted – only for the purposes for which it was provided. Justice will on occasion override that duty, for example to preserve the life of a medical patient or the patient's associates or for national defence or law enforcement.

Reading an Act of Parliament

When Parliament finally approves or enacts a statute it is published in a particular format. The statute will have a number and a title and be divided into sections. Depending on the size of the Act there may be subsections, such as schedules dealing with specific classes of things. At the beginning there will be an explanation of how the Act is arranged; this shows what is included in each section. For very long Acts there may also be a table of contents.

An important part of an Act is the section where there is an *interpretation* of the terms and meanings used. This ensures that the reader has a clear understanding of key terms. For example, the *Queensland Dental Technicians and Dental Prosthetists Registration Act 2001* is clear about what constitutes a dental technician just as the *Medical Practitioners Act 2001* specifies what is meant by medical practitioner for the purpose of that statute.

If you need to read legislation, first determine if it is still in force. Referring to the *Lunacy Act 1898, Lunacy (Amendment) Act 1952* or even the *Lunacy (Amendment) Act 1955* is not just a case of seeing 'old' dates and assuming it has been superseded; some legislation remains on the books for decades and the issue is whether it has been repealed and if there is new legislation in force. Often the copy of an Act lying around an office is no longer valid. This is why going to the government website is worthwhile.

State and federal governments have websites giving speedy and easy access to legislation. You need only provide a key word or cite the legislation to gain full text or summaries of current, repealed or proposed legislation.

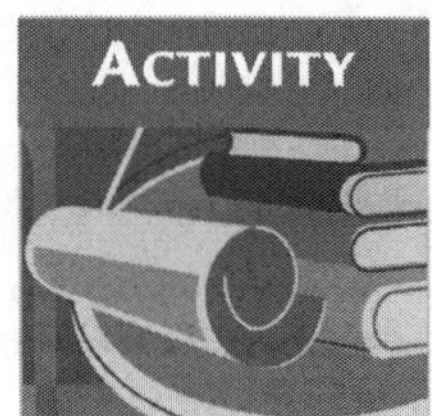

Activity

This exercise is aimed at introducing you to legal research.
While reading and interpreting an Act requires time and effort it is worth looking at one just to see how complex it is so you can see why a summary version is often valuable.

- The homepage of the website below lists various ways to find legislation. Go to the website and click on 'How to read legislation'. <http://www.comlaw.gov.au/> (accessed 6 August 2014)

Scan the document just to gain an idea of how legislation is managed and you will see reference to a number of Acts that we will be addressing in the near future. For example, at the end of the page: the *Privacy Act* 1988.
If you go back to the tabs at the top of home page and click <Acts>, a search under 'Pr' will lead you to this primary legislation but you will see that there is an Act that amends this key piece of legislation: *Privacy Amendment (Enhancing Privacy Protection) Act* 2012, No. 197, 2012.
Now go back to the tabs at the top of the document.
Click on Home.
You will see on this page 'popular titles'. Scroll down and click on Poisons Standard 2012.
It does not matter whether you have undertaken Pharmacology studies yet, you will be aware that there are rules governing medicines. The Schedule of Poisons categorises all substances including those used for therapeutic use.
This Act dictates matters of storage, labelling, prescription and uses. This information governs all aspects of medication and its distribution.

- An example of a specific Act is Health Practitioner Regulation National Law Act 2009, which can be viewed at <www.legislation.qld.gov.au/LEGISLTN/ACTS/2009/09AC045.pdf>

This state Act was duplicated in every jurisdiction in Australia. The State authorities regulating health profession registration were superseded with the creation of a National Health Regulating Authority (AHPRA).
You can go to your own State government site for legislation and find this and other specific legislation that relates to that state's laws.
Using a search facility you will see how easy it is to find any state's legislation that has relevance to nurses or other statutory regulatory organisations such as for doctors.

- Now visit the Queensland Legislation site and find Workplace Health & Safety homepage. <www.deir.qld.gov.au/workplace>
- Visit <www.deir.qld.gov.au/workplace/law/legislation/index.htm>

There you will find options to click for information that governs all workplace safety requirements. For example: Work health and safety laws Information about Queensland's work health and safety laws which came into effect on 1 January 2012.
In New South Wales similar information can be found at the official State Government site at: http://www.workcover.nsw.gov.au/newlegislation2012/Pages/default.aspx
In Victoria at: http://www.vwa.vic.gov.au/laws-and-regulations
South Australia at: http://www.safework.sa.gov.au/show_page.jsp?id=112104#.U7TvzvmSzD8

You can see from this activity that legislation alters, sometimes frequently. The Medical Insurance Acts that underpin Medicare and private medical insurance are often newsworthy items. They have been adjusted many times. Professionally the issues of insurance, what interventions are covered by insurance, who can order or perform interventions and governance issues are important to practitioners. Being able to go to the source document and understand how to find information is a valuable skill.

Health governance

Federal governance for many areas of health is through the Minister for Health and the relevant government departments. At federal level there is the Commonwealth Department of Health and Ageing.

> The Commonwealth Department of Health and Ageing provides policy advice to the Government and implements Commonwealth government health and aged care programs. The Department's mission is to lead the development of Australia's health and aged care system.

Both federal and state health departments have a range of responsibilities and this is extended by creating specialised councils, boards, registering authorities and giving them powers to implement and impose sanctions in order to achieve their work. An example is the Australian Institute of Health and Welfare (AIHW).

> AIHW is a statutory authority within the Commonwealth Health and Aged Care portfolio. The Institute's mission is 'To improve the health and well-being of Australians, we inform community discussion and decision making through national leadership in developing and providing health and welfare statistics and information'. The Institute's main functions relate to the collation and dissemination of information related to health and welfare. The AIHW works closely with other agencies which collect data, produce statistics and undertake research and analysis in the health, community services and housing assistance fields <http.//www.aihw.gov.au/about> (accessed 18 March 2011).

The AIHW is established and operates under the provisions of the *Australian Institute of Health and Welfare Act 1987*. Specific data and findings of the AIHW may be familiar to you as a result of professional or research courses you have taken and include:

- Australian Institute of Health and Welfare 1987
- Australian Institute of Health and Welfare Regulations
- Australian Institute of Health Ethics Committee Regulations
- <www.aihw.gov.au/publications>

Another important statutory body is the National Health and Medical Research Council (NHMRC).

> The NHMRC is a statutory body that reports to the Parliament through the Commonwealth Minister for Health and Aged Care. The NHMRC has statutory obligations to:
>
> - raise the standard of individual and public health throughout Australia;
> - foster the development of consistent health standards between the States and Territories;
> - foster medical research and training, and public health research and training, throughout Australia; and
> - foster consideration of ethical issues relating to health. <www.nhmrc.gov.au/about/role/index> (accessed 11 September 2006)
>
> The NHMRC provides collaborative leadership to improve the health of Australians by fostering and supporting a high quality and internationally recognised research base, providing evidence based advice, applying research evidence to health issues, and promoting informed debate on health and medical research, health ethics and related policy issues. (Source: National Health and Medical Research Council)

A final example of a specific health federal body is one you may have learnt about in relation to pharmacological products: the Therapeutic Goods Administration (TGA). This statutory body was created by the *Therapeutic Goods Act 1989,* which came into effect on 15 February 1991.

> The aim of TGA is to provide a national framework for the regulation of therapeutic goods in Australia and ensure their quality, safety and efficacy.
>
> The regulatory framework is based on a risk management approach designed to ensure public health and safety, while at the same time freeing industry from any unnecessary regulatory burden.
> <www.tga.gov.au/docs/html/tga/tgaginfo.htm> (accessed 20 July 2014)

The TGA is a unit of the Australian government Department of Health and Ageing and is responsible for administering the provisions of the legislation. Essentially, any product for which therapeutic claims are made must be entered in the Australian Register of Therapeutic Goods (ARTG) before the product can be supplied in Australia. The *Therapeutic Goods Act 1989*, Regulations and Orders, set out the requirements for inclusion of therapeutic goods in the ARTG, including advertising, labelling, product appearance and appeal guidelines. Some provisions, such as the scheduling of substances and the safe storage of therapeutic goods, are covered by the relevant state or territory legislation.

The TGA carries out a range of assessment and monitoring activities to ensure therapeutic goods available in Australia are of an acceptable standard. At the same time the TGA aims to ensure that the Australian community has access, within a reasonable time, to therapeutic advances.

State legislation and statutory authorities

Each state and territory has a Health Department. Australian territories are directly responsible to the federal government but state governments can implement legislation in any area. If there is a conflict between state and federal legislation, as long as the federal legislation is within the Constitution it will take precedence.

In all Australian states there are many licensing and regulatory bodies with specific functions and limited powers. These statutory authorities are created by Parliament to govern particular areas; many are professional organisations.

Until July 2010 each State and Territory had their own legislation creating professional regulating and professional registering authorities for many health professions. The creation of Australian Health Practitioner Regulation Agency (AHPRA) meant state legislation had to alter or be repealed. AHPRA was formed by an Act of Parliament and is bound by the Health Practitioner Regulation National Law as in force in participating jurisdictions, and its Regulations. Above you were directed to this Act.

The state nurses registration boards or councils no longer exist. There is no longer a need for states to grant delegated powers to state nurse regulating bodies. Instead, each state had to enact new legislation to accept the Commonwealth legislation empowering a National Authority. Every state and territory had to pass legislation to accept the Commonwealth National Regulating Authority.

In Queensland this new legislation was the Health Practitioner Regulation National Law Act 2009. Part 1 ss3 identifies: Objectives and guiding principles.

This section explains that the object of this law is to establish national registration and accreditation to regulate health practitioners. It clearly identifies the objective is to protect the public and allow professionals to practise in any state or territory without needing to register in each state. The law also requires registration of students who are undertaking health professional education or clinical training in a health profession.

At the time of writing, the nursing and midwifery student registration procedures have not been finalised, hence this law extends regulation of the profession to learners. The national accreditation part of the regulation means all programs for health professionals that lead to registration must adhere to national standards for content, duration, quality of teaching and clinical experience. All programs for registered health professionals will award recognition to successful applicants based on the same criteria.

This section also specifies that overseas trained health professionals will be assessed in a 'rigorous and responsive' manner.

Go to <http://www.legislation.qld.gov.au/LEGISLTN/ACTS/2009/09AC045.pdf> (accessed 20 July 2014). Review the objectives and note section 3 where it refers to both fees and restrictions. In practice the fees are individual practitioner registration fees. The costs for assessment and approval for accreditation of education and training programs are met by education providers seeking program accreditation.

This section also makes reference to the fact the law empowers (delegated authority) the regulatory authority to impose restrictions on a health profession. Note this section of the Act is not referring to powers over individuals; it could be possible that limits could be imposed on the whole profession.

The National Authority is responsible for a number of recognised professions—

(a) Aboriginal and Torres Strait Islander health practice;
(b) Chinese medicine;
(c) chiropractic;
(d) dental (including the profession of a dentist, dental therapist, dental hygienist, dental prosthetist and oral health therapist);
(e) medical;
(f) medical radiation practice;
(g) nursing and midwifery;
(h) occupational therapy;
(i) optometry;
(j) osteopathy;
(k) pharmacy;
(l) physiotherapy;
(m) podiatry;
(n) psychology.

Other legislation that has a direct bearing on health and health institutions in Queensland include:

- *Health Act 1937*
  - Health Regulation 1996
  - Health (Drugs and Poisons) Regulation 1996
- *Health Services Act 1991*
  - Health Services Regulation 2002
- *Private Health Facilities Act 1999*
  - Private Health Facilities Regulation 2000
  - Private Health Facilities (Standards) Notice 2000

No matter which state's legislation you are interested in it is a simple matter to search that state's *State Law* website. Select **Online Publications**. Check the 'Notes' for the date of the publication.

So it is obvious that there is a wealth of legislation covering many aspects of health. It is also obvious that finding, understanding and interpreting legislation is a specialised skill. On a day-to-day basis we find our actions governed by policies that have been drafted to ensure the requirements of legislation are met.

- Can you think of a policy that does this?

Every health student at some point is taught safe practice for client transfer and manual handling. Often the subject is called something like 'No Lift and Manual Handling'. Much of the theory for that subject will discuss the Occupational Health and Safety Act and the employee's responsibilities as well as explaining the various obligations and policies the employer was required to put in place. The Act is the source of law in relation to everyday procedures and policies governing your daily work.

Activity

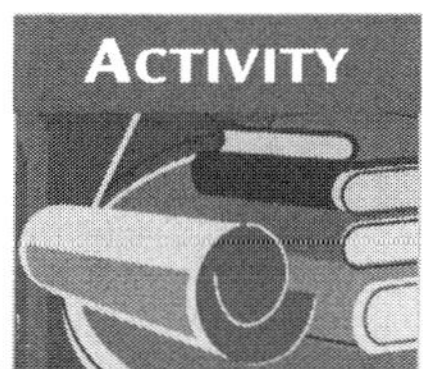

- One example of the various State Acts is Workplace Health and Safety Act 1995 (Qld). Have a look at division 3. This Act also explains the roles of staff involved in health and safety committees. The public protection aims are clearly spelt out. <https://www.legislation.qld.gov.au/LEGISLTN/CURRENT/W/WorkHSA11.pdf> (accessed 4 July 2014)

Another Act mentioned above was the *Therapeutic Goods Act 1989*, a Commonwealth Act that imposes quality controls and covers all stages of the production and retail of therapeutic substances. In relation to clinical drug trials where a new drug may be tested on humans in the clinical environment this Act has great relevance. Should a company or individual want to test a new drug not only must the research be approved by the institution's ethics committee, but the Act requires that the researcher meet the obligations of the Clinical Trial Notification Scheme.

Some states have requirements for the labelling and packaging of therapeutic substances for that state. In Queensland the Health Regulation (1996) sets these out.

Case study

A fellow nurse has returned from an overseas trip bringing with her samples of a tribal remedy she saw used in a mountain village in a remote tourist resort. This ointment made up by the villagers, she claims, will work like a miracle on the clients in the nursing home where you both work. She intends to use this remedy on the many varicose ulcers experienced by various clients.

In relation to the two Acts discussed above (*Therapeutic Goods Act 1989* and *Nursing Act 1992*), what issues would you raise with her, what position would you take in response to her request that you be part of this 'research'?

Review

The case study is about clinical drug trials where a new drug will be tested on humans in the clinical environment so this Act has great relevance. Should the

Registered Nurse (RN) want to test a new drug not only must the research be approved by the institutions ethics committee, the Act requires that the RN researcher meet the obligations of the Clinical Trial Notification Scheme.

This case study raises issues of law but also, as you will have seen from Chapter 1, issues of ethics. Health professionals are frequently involved in research which may be an informal or a clinical or theoretical study. This scenario involves not only an untested and unapproved drug, but issues of the right of the client, consent of the client and the 'power' the nurse might be abusing.

- While legislation might be in place to prevent actions it will often be the ethical dilemma that alerts a practitioner to an issue that may have both moral and legal ramifications.

The legal process

Television and movies about court cases have given us quite a bit of information about pre-court and court processes but the problem is that these are often misleading. Most court rooms are much smaller than we see in the movies, the court staff are numerous and there are rules of behaviour and dress that reflect our British legal history although some courts have abolished many of these procedures. Here we will just cover the steps in the legal process. Before any civil trial occurs there are numerous stages which are usually managed by legal representatives.

1. *Commencement* The person who wishes to initiate a legal action – the plaintiff, usually through their lawyer – files a complaint specifying the charges against the defendant. The document used to do this is called the *originating process*. For example, to start a personal injury action in the District Court the document required is a statement of claim. Another common type of originating process is a summons. To commence an action, these documents are filed in the registry of the relevant court together with the prescribed filing fee.
2. *Service* The defendant is served with a summons and the complaint. Sometimes service on another party is required to be personal which means that the document has to be delivered to the person involved and left in their presence. For many court documents, however, it will be sufficient under the rules of the court for service to occur by mail.
3. *Defence* The defendant files a response to the charges or may even file a *counterclaim*. Most courts have a procedure called judgment by default where, if the defendant does not take certain steps – judgment will be entered in favour of the plaintiff.
4. *Discovery* The lawyers embark on an information gathering and often exhaustive review of documents. This information is gathered by getting witnesses to provide depositions (written reports), interrogatories (verbal examination of key people) and researching relevant documents such as gaining access to medical files or research data.
5. *Pre-trial hearings* The court can make orders or directions for things which need to be done by the parties to prepare for the hearing. At this time the court might also consider whether the matter is appropriate

for referral to some other method of dispute resolution, such as arbitration.

6. *Trial/Hearing* If the matter has not been resolved it will proceed to a hearing before a judge. It is at the hearing that each side will have the opportunity to present its case through the testimony of witnesses and each party will have the opportunity to cross examine those witnesses.

   Courts are generally required to apply strict rules to the evidence which can be used and parties can object to certain types of evidence being given by witnesses such as opinion evidence where a witness is not qualified to give that opinion. Many tribunals are not bound by the same rules of evidence as are applied in courts.
7. *Closing statements* Legal representatives, having presented their case and examined witnesses, summarise their respective cases.
8. *Jury instruction* If there is a jury (many hearings do not involve a jury) the judge takes time to instruct the jury on points of law that are relevant.
9. *Jury deliberation* Review of the facts, evidence and case occurs and the jury votes on the verdict. The judge reports the verdict back to the parties.
10. *Verdict* If there is no jury, at the end of the hearing the judge will give a verdict and make other orders which may include orders as to the payment of costs.
11. *Appeal* Parties can elect to appeal the verdict or awards on the basis of legal issues. The case is not reheard but the appeal reviews points of law, procedure and fairness.
12. *Enforcement* There are procedures available to the court for ensuring that the court's orders are carried out. For example, if a person has been ordered to pay money it may be possible to obtain a court order for this money to be taken out of their salary.

Summary

This chapter has explained the systems of law in Australia and sources of law that govern our lives. While this information is not routinely drawn upon in our daily work it provides the foundation, the basic building blocks to further readings. Knowing that nursing has great breadth, drawing upon so many specialties to build our nursing practice, it is sometimes a source of anxiety for nurses that they do not actually understand the origins, the core of the subject. It is not very reassuring to find that no matter how many subject areas we learn about there is always someone who is a specialist who has a depth of knowledge in that particular area that we cannot match. Law is such a specialty, but our ongoing learning and ability to stay abreast of relevant and applicable law for practice requires us to be able to identify the sources of relevant laws and assess the validity of that source. Most of us will never need to go to court, examine legislation or attend a tribunal. However, as citizens and professionals we live in a world that does expect us to adhere to and know the laws governing our lives.

Practice assignment questions

Standards exist in Australia governing nursing practice. What actions can you take as a nurse to ensure that your own practice is ethical?

Relate these actions to the NMBA nursing codes and the bioethical principles of: Beneficence, non-malificience, autonomy and justice.

What is your State's legislation/Act covering workplace safety?

What Act would you search to determine the rules governing a clinical trial in your ward?

Sources

Attorney-Generals Department (2014) *Australia's Legal System*, <www. ag.gov. au/agd/ WWW/agdHome.nsf/Page/Legal_System_Australias_Legal_ System> (accessed 15 August 2014).

Cook, C., Creyke, R., Geddes, R. & Holloway, I. (2001) *Laying Down the Law*, 5th edn, Butterworths, Sydney.

Federal Magistrate's Court of Australia *Practice and Procedures*, <www.fmc.gov.au/ services/html/case_family.htm> (accessed 16 August 2014).

Forrester, K. & Griffiths, D. (2005) *Essentials of Law*, 2nd edn, Harcourt, Sydney.

Forrester, K. & Griffiths, D. (2010) *Essentials of Law for Health Professionals*, 3rd edn, Elsevier, Chatswood, NSW.

Kennedy, R. & Richards, J. (2004) *Integrating Human Service Law and Practice*, Oxford University Press, Melbourne.

MacFarlane, P. (1995) *Health Law*, 2nd edn, The Federation Press, Sydney.

MacFarlane, P. J. & Reid, S. J. (2003) *Queensland Health Law Handbook*, Queensland Department of Health, Brisbane.

McIlwraith, J. & Madden, B. (2014) *Health Care & the Law*, 6th edn, Lawbook Co., Australia.

Staunton, P. & Chiarella, M. (2003) *Nursing and the Law*, 5th edn, Elsevier, Sydney.

Staunton, P. & Whyburn, B. (1997) *Nursing and the Law*, 4th edn, Harcourt Australia Pty Ltd, Sydney.

White, B., Wilmott, L & McDonald, F. (2014) *Health Law in Australia*, 2nd edn, Thomson Reuters, Australia.

Legislation

Australian Government Department of Health and Aging.

Therapeutic Goods Administration.

Poisons Schedule 2012.

Common law: civil law torts

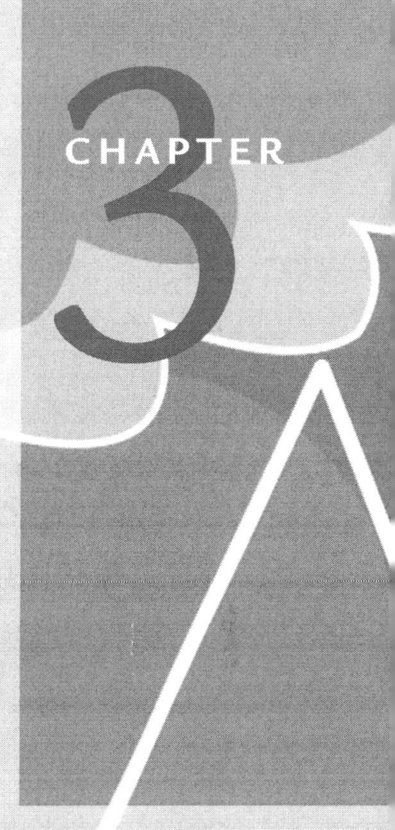

Learning outcomes

After studying this chapter you should be able to:

- Describe the role of the law in providing direction for health care practice.
- Show understanding of practices and procedures in clinical settings that reflect these policies.
- Apply legal and professional standards when assessing and responding to client needs, practice and policy situations, professional reporting and communication.

Overview

Lawyers' education involves learning about the many varied areas of the law and the relevant principles of those general and specialty areas. Health professionals' education is similar, in that we explore foundation knowledge, categorise it into various areas and build up a body of knowledge that evolves from the general to the specialist. What is more common in health is that basic principles tend to remain the same across categories. That is not always the case with law. Some areas are governed by very strict legal principles that do not have much, if any, relevance to other areas.

One of the major areas of common law is civil law. The rules of procedure, jurisdiction and the types of cases that can be heard and appealed are complex. However, it is this area of the law that has underpinned many of the rules and regulations that govern health care activities. The protection of the citizen and institutions through policies, procedures or legislation to overcome gaps has arisen as a result of findings in civil law cases.

In many states legislation has been enacted to remove any uncertainty or variables in matters that were previously civil court issues. Some states have set limits on the amount that can be paid in compensation for certain wrongs; other legislation exists that deals with business, employment and contract issues that affect individuals.

That said, the ancient rules that are embedded in the rules of civil law and the intent and purpose of this branch of common law are still valid and important in society today.

- It is important to understand the rights of an individual and the responsibilities of a citizen. For the health professional these principles extend to understanding professional responsibilities as well.

The rights of the individual citizen are often supported by the civil law. It is this system that opens the way for an individual who has been wronged to take action to enforce their rights.

Individual 'rights' is a tricky term. What are our rights in law? Are rights synonymous with 'fair'? Over time the term 'basic human rights' has gained currency. Many of these expectations have arisen as a result of court cases upholding an individual's claim that they have a 'right to clean air, safe environment, freedom from coercion, security of tenure, right to work in a safe place' and so on.

Often the issue in a case is specific to an individual, at other times the case has ramifications for the society. What is particular about civil law is that there is no 'punishment'; instead the court aims to put the wronged person back into the position they would have been in if there had been no wrong done. This is achieved by imposing costs, paying monetary compensation or ruling that the 'wrongdoer' restores property or places the wronged person (the plaintiff) back into the situation they would otherwise have been in if the other party had not done this thing.

Tort is a very old word that today only has a meaning in a legal or civil law context. It evolved from 'bent, crooked or twisted' to become, in French, the word for wrong. There are different types of tort.

Defamation

Defamation is a common law action in the ACT, South Australia, Victoria and Western Australia. In Queensland, New South Wales, the Northern Territory and Tasmania it is governed by legislation. On 1 January 2006, uniform defamation legislation was enacted in all Australian States. Now every State has legislation under the Defamation Act 2005. The 2005 Act does not define the meaning of the elements of a defamation action. Instead, they are defined by the common law, or the body of "judge-made" law that has been developed through cases decided by the courts.

The tort of defamation recognises an injury or damage to a person's reputation or character caused by the words of another person. The word defamation covers:

- Libel, the term used for words that are written.
- Slander, the term for spoken words.

High Court cases that set the precedent for defamation have tended to focus upon the emotional distress caused by statements or publications and the damage to business or personal reputation. If statements cause, or are likely to cause, injury to the reputation whether personal, professional or business, if the statements cause others to hold them up as victims of ridicule or contempt or if statements cause others to shun or avoid them then the court has found for the victim.

While our society supports the idea of freedom of expression as a basic right, this must be balanced against an individual's right to privacy, to be protected from malicious or untrue comment. There is legislation in every state designed to protect the individual from publication of material that could be argued to damage the individual unfairly or unjustly. However, like so much legislation there are subtle differences between different state Acts.

If an individual knows that a program, magazine or newspaper intends to air or publish or there has been a publication that they feel 'defames' their character they can go to court to obtain a writ to stop further publications. A writ is essential to initiate a court action, therefore to continue publishing would be seen as a 'contempt of court'. Whether or not a court action does occur, this writ will act to stop further comments.

It is important to realise that if someone tells you to your face, without witnesses, what they think of you, this is not grounds for claiming defamation. If the statement were written in a letter and never seen by someone else it cannot be defamation. However, if there was someone else present, or the item was read or heard on tape by others, the matter is public. That opens the door for an action in defamation.

It is not just the speaker or author of the comment that might be liable in an action. Failing to prevent someone else publishing a defamatory comment can get a third person into trouble. For example, one staff member puts up on the notice board a cartoon that is clearly representing another staff member. This cartoon shows that individual performing in a very negative way. Even if it is funny the cartoon is defamatory and if the notice board is in an office or work area under the responsibility of other workers or managers, leaving it there is permitting a libel. The other staff members could be found at fault if they chose to leave it in place.

Slander, speaking about another person in a manner that may affect adversely that person's reputation or standing, is not unheard of among nurses. Think about handover. Sometimes you hear statements reporting incidents that give the impression of a 'troublemaker' or that ensure a person will be considered in a poor light that could be interpreted as an effort to 'get back at' a client, family member or other staff member. This usually results in other staff members treating that person with caution or avoiding contact; such statements go to the character of a person and are defamatory.

- Consider this: We all get things off our chest and often say things about someone else who has upset us. Defamation is an issue when we move from discussing what occurred and our opinion of what happened and why, to actually stating something negative about the worth, competence, ability or credibility of another person.

It is a defence to an action in defamation if you can show that the statement or publication was true, not just that you thought it was true. There must be evidence to support your claim. The media take great care to check items and verify the accuracy of such statements.

The law does recognise particular situations where absolute freedom of speech must be protected. This is the concept of *privilege*. You often hear politicians being accused of taking advantage of 'parliamentary privilege' to state something that otherwise could be claimed to be defamatory. The law also allows people in the course of their employment to make statements that are considered to be *qualified privilege* and thus protected from an action in defamation. Discussions about clients and family between staff members that have relevance to treatment fall into this category. Giving a reference, communications between parents and teachers, lawyers and clients are all protected *if* these statements are honest and there is no underlying motive that raises doubts about the moral, social or professional validity of the comment.

Defences to defamation include:

- The statement was true. Legislation in each state differs. Some courts not only require that the statement is true but also must be satisfied it was in the public interest to make the true statement.
- The statement was merely a personal opinion, a 'fair comment' about your personal experience.
- There was a duty to provide the information. The idea of there being a duty to provide information is based on the concept of qualified privilege. If there is any hint that comments were malicious and intended to cause harm this privilege is lost. It covers things like information about a child to parent, client to family, employee to other staff member.
- Absolute privilege is a defence that exists for (a) parliamentarians when they speak under parliamentary privilege and (b) any participant in a court case, if the matter is stated in court.

In some common law countries the issue of invasion of privacy is bound up with defamation but this is not the case in Australia. Generally the courts consider the damage to reputation to be far more important than rights to privacy or even whether the statement is true.

Recall that the common law is adversarial, that is, the courts consider arguments presented by lawyers on behalf of the plaintiff (civil law) and respondent. It is up to the respondent to justify and defend their statements; the plaintiff (if they get to court) need only claim injury as a result of the respondent's action. It is a very expensive exercise. Threatening an action against someone is not the same as initiating and carrying through an action. The winner is frequently out of pocket, but it may be worth it on the basis of 'getting their reputation back' or, for example, the media will vigorously defend their right to 'free speech'.

In relation to our work this tort gives us direction for taking care about our comments and writing. We are responsible for setting boundaries on our (natural) desire to vent frustration or complain about someone or the 'system' when we are under stress. Managers and employers must document issues to satisfy their duty to report and protect the public from an employee, and they should do so with an understanding of the defences and the limitations of those defences to the tort. Here is an example of careless talk (*Schessler v. Keck* (1954)).

> An American nurse told another person that a client (a well-known caterer) was being treated for syphilis. The caterer's business was destroyed. The caterer sued and won on the basis that the statement was in fact false.

> The nurse had her facts wrong *but* in this instance it was pointed out that, even if true, any statement that would prejudice a person's professional or business standing (such as saying they were sex offenders or suffered from sexually transmitted diseases or other contagious diseases) would, in spite of their accuracy, be grounds to win a defamation case.

The Internet and email are powerful and increasingly this medium is being monitored and comments made in the electronic mode are just as likely to be called as any other documents as evidence in any form of legal action. Thinking that this medium is transitory and comments will only be known by the sender and receiver is false. Letting rip with defamatory comments about someone or failing to recognise professional boundaries in electronic correspondence can provide evidence that the author may find they need to defend should a third person access the mail. Consider this example.

> A technician working on a senior nurse manager's computer found a memo about a staff member. The manager had recorded comments about that employee's lack of professionalism, listed a number of negative behaviours and stated that she would not support this employee for promotion. The technician circulated this memo to other staff.
>
> The professional tone and language of the memo, the fact that it was the senior nurse's opinion of the employee and the issue of qualified privilege as part of the role of the senior nurse gave the court grounds to support the senior nurse, who had been taken to court by that employee when the memo was made public.
>
> The point is, whether true or not the senior nurse had to go to court to defend the statements that she believed were utterly confidential and would never become public. The nurse had an obligation to fulfil her role as manager and assess and document findings about an employee. The professional manner in which the memo was written had a powerful effect on the outcome.

Activity

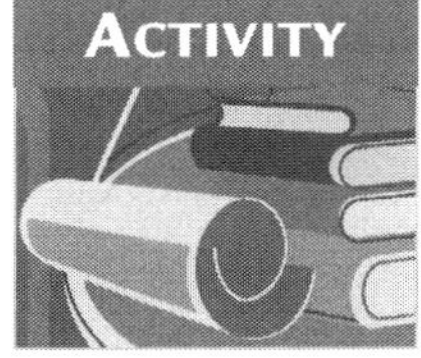

- What does the term civil law mean?
- Define defamation and give an example of defamation that might occur in a health facility.

A web resource that presents a hypothetical example of a defamation situation might be of interest. The Risks of Defamation.
<www.invivo.com.au/newsletter0811_1.html> (accessed 5 July 2014)

Mandatory reporting and defamation

Under the National Regulation legislation of health professionals in Australia, registered health practitioners, as well as employers of health practitioners and education providers, are required to report notifiable conduct to the National Agency.

Members of the public can make a notification to AHPRA about the conduct, health and performance of a practitioner or student.

Practitioners, employers and education providers are all mandated by law to report:

- notifiable conduct relating to a practitioner or
- in the case of a student, an impairment that may place the public at substantial risk of harm.

Registered practitioners and students who fail to report notifiable conduct may face disciplinary action by their National Board.

However you should be aware that you are protected from liability and defamation claims when reporting conduct of another practitioner in good faith. The National Law provides that:

- A person is not liable, civilly or criminally or under administrative process for giving information.
- The making of a notification or giving information does not constitute a breach of professional etiquette or ethics or a departure from accepted standards of professional conduct
- No liability for defamation is incurred by the person because of the making of the notification or giving information.
- The protection extends to a person who, in good faith, provided the person with any information on the basis of which the notification was made or the information was given.
- The protection also extends to cover a person who, in good faith, was otherwise concerned in the making of the notification or giving information.

AHPRA Notifications and Guidelines (2014) can be viewed at: <www.ahpra.gov.au/Notifications-and-Outcomes/Conduct-Health-and-Performance.aspx> (accessed 5 July 2014)

The tort of trespass

This is an ancient area of law. Concerned with protection of property it has evolved and changed over the centuries. Breaking into someone's home or land could be a crime but if it was for the purpose of taking a shortcut and doing no 'harm' to the property then where would the owner find protection? This area of law gave the owners of property rights that today are now limited to unlawful entry into public or private property.

An important change to this tort over the centuries has been its application to persons who are victims of force such as assault and battery, and unlawful imprisonment. This created another tort, *trespass to person*. This tort, which involves the issues of assault and battery, will be discussed in Chapter 4, on consent, as from a health professional perspective it has great relevance in relation to issues of consent. At the moment we will just deal with the concept of trespass to property.

Trespass occurs when someone enters your property or land without permission. The trespass may be deliberate or unintentional. It may include the presence of someone on the owner's property, the trespasser having left something (think dumping of rubbish) or having allowed a third person to enter. The owner has the right to remove a trespasser only after they refuse a 'reasonable request to leave'. Refusal to leave means the trespasser is now committing criminal trespass.

Owners can obtain court orders to prevent trespass; the trespasser(s) can be sued for damages and if they continue to ignore a court order they can be gaoled.

Not everyone who enters property without permission can be sued. Some public servants have the right to enter as a matter of their work. Meter readers, health inspectors, fire fighters are examples.

Sales and delivery staff are only trespassers when they refuse a request to leave.

Application to practice

APPLICATION to practice

Security and protection of a client's person and privacy is the responsibility of staff. Asking to see identification or establishing the identification of the many staff and visitors in a busy area is daunting. However, failing to check the authority of people looking at client documents or wandering around the environment leaves everyone vulnerable.

Wearing of ID is now so commonplace that no one really looks at it, but lack of ID is grounds to check. If a client asks for their visitors to be vetted to avoid or limit numbers staff must accommodate the request by explaining and asking visitors to respect those wishes and leave. Hurt feelings can be lessened by providing people opportunity to write and leave a note. Where members of the public have no clear purpose or are causing a disturbance requesting them to leave and notifying security to escort them from the premises is the usual protocol.

Emotional distress

A modern development has been the recognition of and compensation for mental distress. Traditionally the law did not recognise anything other than physical or financial damage although there have often been substantial awards as compensation for 'pain and suffering' linked to physical damage.

Other common law countries have, like Australia, gradually moved towards accepting mental distress as a cause of action in relation to proven discrimination, domestic dispute, harassment and provoked fears such as arise with misdiagnosis of disease. There is a tort of infliction of intentional emotional distress but a broader application of this has been a steady development.

An interesting case that reflects this move occurred in Queensland through the District Court: *Grace v. Purvis* (2003). This case establishes a new common law right to recover damages (similar to rights with respect to nuisance, trespass and negligence) which is additional to, and independent of, rights under existing privacy statutes.

Specifically the judge found that conduct such as:

- following, loitering near, watching or approaching a person
- contacting a person in any way, including by telephone, mail, fax, email or any other technology
- loitering near, watching, approaching or entering a place where a person lives, works or visits

- giving offensive material to a person or leaving it where it can be found by the person
- committing an intimidating, harassing or threatening act against a person, whether or not involving a threat of violence
- an act of violence, or a threat of violence, against any property

may justify an action for invasion of privacy if such conduct intruded on an individual's privacy or seclusion in a highly offensive way and caused mental, psychological or emotional harm or prevented or hindered them from doing an act they were lawfully entitled to do.

APPLICATION to practice

Application to practice

At first glance none of these behaviours would relate to nursing. The point is that there is now a right to bring an action that will be recognised by the court. Judge Skoien in this case proposed that Australian law now allows an individual to recover damages for mental, psychological or emotional harm, including embarrassment, hurt, distress and post-traumatic stress disorder caused by a deliberate act.

There have been cases where misinformation, mistakes in diagnosis, careless statements about a client's prognosis or condition have caused serious distress. While courts have been sympathetic, the lack of physical or financial damages has been a barrier at times to a successful action. In light of the changes discussed above this would not be difficult in the future.

Confidentiality

Confidentiality is *not* a tort in its own right. However, with a little thought you should see that the issues of privacy and confidentiality link to the concept of defamation and emotional distress. There is legislation that gives direction to practice for the protection of individual right to privacy.

There is a Federal *Privacy Act 1988*(C'th) and state legislation; New South Wales (NSW), Victoria and the ACT all have specific legislation that regulates the handling of personal health information in the private sector.

- Health Records and Information Privacy Act 2002 (NSW)
- Information Privacy Act 2000 (Vic)
- The Health Records (Privacy and Access) Act 1997 (ACT)

Other states have a number of statutes and guidelines encompassing privacy issues.

This means that health service providers and others in the private sector in those jurisdictions are required to comply with both federal and state or territory legislation in relation to personal health information.

As you have seen, civil law remedies exist for individuals who claim their reputation has been damaged by statements, written or verbal. Health information is personal and unauthorised access or use of it is governed by legislation and actions in tort law.

The professional obligation to respect privacy and keep information in such a manner that records are confidential is supported by many guidelines and professional standards. Researchers must explain how their findings, transcripts and participant details are kept to ensure confidentiality to satisfy the National Health and Medical Research Council guidelines, and thus their Research Ethics Committee, before any proposal is accepted. Professional ethics and codes of practice overtly recognise this is an area where high standards are imposed.

Changes in policy have occurred in relation to allowing patients to have access to their own records. In some health circumstances the client actually pays for and receives a copy of, for example, their records, x-rays, diagnostic results or medical certificates.

Often it is difficult to balance competing interests, the client's right to know and the fact that the information is a danger to the client's health (for example, a terminal diagnosis). It has been argued that unlimited access by other parties, the client included, might affect the manner in which records are maintained. Deliberate censoring of critical information about client behaviour or professional assessment might occur if the professional feared the consequences of having outsiders read them.

There has been some division among judges in Australia considering the issue of whether a client should have full access to medical records, based on the argument that they were paying for a service, creating a 'contract', and thus should have right of ownership to all information. The High Court has held that it is a matter for Parliament to legislate upon, as the common law rules can only deal with a case-by-case analysis.

Health professionals need to understand the difference between the rights to privacy and respect for a confidential information. The trust between client and staff often means that confidential, personal information is exchanged. In rare circumstances that information may be crucial to the health and wellbeing of the client and must be shared. The need to gain consent for that sharing is obvious. In practice we have obligations to constantly protect client information. Breaching confidentiality can result in complaints to the Nursing and Midwifery Board of Australia (NMBA), involvement of the Privacy Commissioner, or even legal action.

> "It is not enough anymore to assume we're maintaining confidentiality as we go about our daily work. There are too many opportunities for private information to be inadvertently read, faxed, overheard, transmitted, or otherwise unintentionally disclosed. As nurses and as leaders of the health care industry, we need to sharpen our awareness and redouble our efforts to protect our patients' rights to privacy" (American Hospital Association, 2002).

Confidentiality, social media and nurses

There have been some serious professional breaches in relation to confidentiality. These may not result in legal consequences, clients and families often remain oblivious about the fact their business and their health has been discussed by staff outside of expected professional guidelines.

These discussions may be innocent. They may be educational in their nature, sharing information and care decisions. At other times they may be pure gossip and tea room chatter. Where staff and too often students, expose themselves to professional investigation and discipline is in their use of social media. Further, the need for online communication and learning tutorials puts a burden on lecturers and students to closely monitor their discussions and online communications about clinical situations and experiences. Case studies and discussions should carefully remove identifying information.

The Privacy Act 1988 (Cth) does not regulate the handling of personal information by individuals for the purposes of, or in connection with, their personal, family or household affairs. This means that an individual acting in a personal capacity, for example, an individual who posts personal information about others on a personal 'blog' is not regulated by the Privacy Act.

The issue of personal privacy has been the subject of a number of reports focused on the use/misuse of on-line services. For example:

> "A major concern about individuals handling personal information relates to the content of information published by individuals on the internet. Individuals regularly use social networking and user-generated sites such as Facebook and YouTube to post photographs, videos and commentary that may interfere with the privacy of other individuals" (Australian Law Reform Commission, 2008).

The Nursing and Midwifery Board has published social media guidelines that reflect the codes governing nursing and midwifery practice. The Royal College of Nursing has published Social Media Guidelines for Nurses (2011) that is well worth downloading.

Privacy law

The right to privacy and the absolute expectation that personal data, medical records, financial data and credit information is kept secure and protected is the focus of extensive legislation.

There is Commonwealth legislation that covers public entities. Ongoing reforms in this area have broadened the range of obligations and responsibilities as well as including private entities. The *Privacy Act 1988* regulates the handling of personal information about individuals. This includes the collection, use, storage and disclosure of personal information, and access to and correction of that information. There have been many amendments to the Act and since 2014 the inclusion of *13 Australian Privacy Principles* replaced the former Information Privacy Principles. This has made many significant changes to the *Privacy Act 1988*. These changes commenced on 12 March 2014.

The Privacy Regulation 2013, made under the Privacy Act, also commenced on 12 March 2014.

Of less importance to health workers are other privacy laws such as:

Telecommunications Act 1997 (Cth)
National Health Act 1953 (Cth)
Data-matching Program (Assistance and Tax) Act 1990 (Cth)
Crimes Act 1914 (Cth)
Anti-Money Laundering and Counter-Terrorism Financing Act 2006 (Cth)
The Healthcare Identifiers Act 2010 (Cth)

All States have laws governing health information and protecting the privacy of all health clients. Some states consider breaches of confidentiality to be a criminal offence. The complexities of Privacy Laws, Federal and State, is a lawyer not a nursing problem however a nurse who fails to respect a client's confidentiality and who fails to treat information and documentation with care and caution is failing to satisfy legal standards and, if you refer to your professional codes, failing to satisfy professional standards.

An overview of State and Territory privacy laws (and their intersection with the Federal Privacy Act) is provided by The Office of the Privacy Commissioner at. http://www.oaic.gov.au/#1 (accessed 5 July 2014).

In New South Wales the *Privacy and Personal Information Protection Act 1998(NSW)* covers the public sector and has established an Office of the New South Wales Privacy Commissioner. Major government agencies, such as the police, are exempt from some or all of the privacy principles. All state-owned corporations, courts, tribunals and royal commissions are fully exempt. The *Health Records and Information Privacy Act 2002* deals with medical records. Other relevant legislation is:

- Privacy and Personal Information Protection Act 1998
- Health Records and Information Privacy Act 2002 (NSW)
- Freedom of Information Act 1989 (NSW)

In Victoria there is the *Information Privacy Act 2000.* It is restricted to the public sector and does not apply to health information, which is covered by the *Health Records Act 2001*. Other related legislation:

- Information Privacy Act 2000 (Vic)
- The Charter of Human Rights and Responsibilities Act 2006 (Vic)
- Freedom of Information Act 1982 (Vic)
- Public Records Act 1973 (Vic)

The ACT government agencies are notionally covered by the federal legislation, although health records were removed from the jurisdiction of the Federal Privacy Commissioner by the ACT *Health Records (Privacy and Access) Act 1997,* based on the federal privacy principles and intended to allow patients access to their own medical records in the public and private sectors. Other related legislation:

- Human Rights Act 2004 (ACT)
- Freedom of Information Act 1989 (ACT)

The Northern Territory has developed privacy legislation for the public sector only, with the *Information Act 2002.*

In Queensland the *Invasion of Privacy Act 1971* was primarily concerned with the licensing of private inquiry agents and the regulation of listening devices, as well as a number of offences relating to unlawful entry of homes. More recently there have been a number of new Acts relating to privacy law.

- Information Privacy Act 2009 (Qld)
- Right to Information Act 2009 (Qld)
- Public Records Act 2002 (Qld)

The other states (South Australia, Western Australia) have issued administrative instructions requiring broad compliance by government agencies with the federal principles but may move towards discrete privacy legislation covering public or private sector bodies. These instructions do not have the force of law and there are few supervisory or enforcement mechanisms. South Australia has a part-time Privacy Committee with some advisory and ombudsman functions.

Tasmania has enacted privacy legislation giving legal weight to former administrative instructions.

- Personal Information Protection Act 2004 (Tas)
- Right to Information Act 2009 (Tas)

Most states feature legislation that restricts reporting on aspects of the administration of justice. The proposed *National Health Privacy Code* is the result of this framework and aims to:

- safeguard the health privacy and dignity of all individuals;
- achieve national consistency in health privacy protection – across jurisdictions and between the public and private sectors; and
- take into account changes in the way personal health information is handled as a result of technological change.

In Queensland there is the *Freedom of Information Act 1992* which gives a person the right to access documents and records held by any organisation that receives government funding. There are some limitations; where medical or psychiatric information may prejudice the health of the person this may be withheld.

Generally the patient has a right to access information held directly by a medical officer or in an institution, but this right is subject to disclosure being limited to the best interests of the client. Just as important is the issue of disclosure to third parties, where information, records or verbal communications are made available to someone other than the client or to whom the client has consented to inform.

Of course there are exceptions. Infectious diseases are covered by the *Health Act 1937* (Qld), where there is a requirement to notify certain diseases and collect data for public health reasons, but this Act specifies and limits how information can be used.

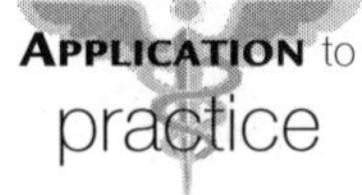

Application to practice

Policies exist in most institutions about who can release information to police, solicitors, potential employers, media representatives and family. There is often a particular staff member responsible for providing public statements or dealing with the media. This nominated person is obliged to establish why the information is being sought and determine just how much can be given, as well as verifying the identity and the requirement for information. Consent from the client is an important consideration but police investigations may override this.

Some professionals have found themselves in hot water for speaking about a matter they believed was 'public knowledge', something they had known others had discussed so assumed they too could give the information. There is a duty to maintain confidentiality whether or not others might have access.

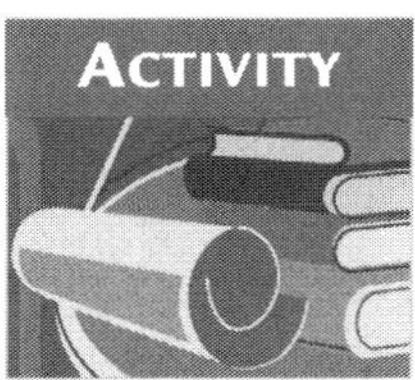

Activity

- What systems or procedures have you seen that contribute to ensuring client confidentiality is maintained?
- Can you identify where there are risks and weaknesses that may lead to loss of confidentiality?

False imprisonment

This is where someone claims to have been denied their freedom. Intentional deprivation of liberty without a just cause or excuse may even lead to criminal charges. The issues of confinement of the mentally ill client or quarantine law will be discussed later. Here the issue is when someone of sound mind has been denied their freedom.

Case law in this area explores aspects of whether there was an avenue of escape, the type of detention and form of restraint. It doesn't matter if escape was possible; if the person believed they could not leave or that there were severe penalties for leaving then this is false imprisonment.

This is an area where most facilities do have policies and procedures in place. Documentation about type and method of restraint and why, client forms agreeing they have made the decision to discharge themselves against advice, 'gate passes' or some type of document signed by the client and family for short periods of absence from care all exist.

Health staff may have to restrain a client where there is a risk to the client, to other persons or to the environment. If there is any evidence that restraint is carried out for staff convenience or staff purposes rather than for the real safety of client or others, then this will be false imprisonment.

Clients may wish to discharge themselves in spite of medical advice. The law does recognise that a person who is sick or incapable of looking after themselves may need to be detained on medical grounds. If, however, they were detained because they were a nuisance or on the grounds that restraint would 'promote a speedy recovery' rather than on sound medical evidence, this defence would not hold up. Clients may wish to leave hospital to attend to their own business or pleasure in spite of medical advice.

Some specific legislation is discussed below but generally if a person is of sound mind and has 'legal capacity' they cannot be detained against their will. Police threats, medication, withholding of treatment and staff verbal and non-verbal behaviour may cause so much anxiety and fear that the client believes they cannot leave the premises. In one case, telling a client they could not leave until the bill for health services was paid was found to be false imprisonment. Here the fear that the police would be called and the client's belief in the statements amounted to false imprisonment.

Mental health legislation exists in all states and territories giving health authorities limited powers to admit, treat and detain clients without their consent. This will be revisited in Chapter 12. There is also legislation covering suspected child abuse or neglect. A child who is at risk may be detained against the parents' wishes for protection. *The Quarantine Act 1908* is federal legislation that delegates the responsibility for detaining and treating people with particular diseases. This is a public safety issue, and people can be held onboard the ship they arrived in or at a quarantine facility.

Physical and chemical restraint

It was discussed above that a client may need to be physically restrained or medicated to lessen the risk they pose to themselves or others. Health staff may need to deal with violent and disturbed clients in many situations. Other clients may be so confused or restless, for example affected by drugs or dementia, that physical restraint is necessary.

There are policies in most facilities about the circumstances and types of physical restraint that is permitted. Satisfying documentation requirements for reassessing and checking client status is essential. The accepted grounds for restraining a patient are to protect from injury, to protect other patients from the risk of injury and to avoid unnecessary harm. It is not acceptable to restrain a patient because staff don't have the time to 'keep an eye on them'.

Restraint policies usually specify the need for consultation and a medical order. Before physical restraint is considered alternatives such as medication or consultation with relatives to identify triggers should be explored. Satisfying the client's request may resolve the situation. Needs may be stated in a confused or illogical manner, for example 'Don't leave me here, I want to sit with my mother', 'All I want is something to eat, I am going to the shop right now', yet satisfying them by recognising the key words underlying the distress is often not difficult. Fear and confusion about where and why a client is in this environment is often a precipitating cause for violence.

In emergency situations nursing staff can initiate restraint using cot sides and lamb's wool arm and leg restraints. However, satisfying policies requiring consultation, documentation, full client assessment and notification of relatives must occur in a timely manner. There have been instances of using tubular gauze coverings to encase the arms and tie the ends to the bed. The risk of client's fingers being trapped in a tear and circulation being cut off is real. Using bandages, tying down the top sheet or old-fashioned 'manacles' which are hard leather straps for hands and feet should be avoided. *Best Practice Evidence Based Practice for Physical Restraint* has been published by the Joanna Briggs Institute. This information has been included in most policies.

Recommended reading

Go to <www.joannabriggs.edu.au> (accessed 7 July 2014) and review the Physical Restraint (Part 1) and Restraint Minimisation (Part 2) documents. Another easy to read and worthwhile resource is the NSW policy document Section 4. <http://www0.health.nsw.gov.au/policies/gl/2006_014.pdf> (accessed 5 July 2014).

Finally, another informative but not specifically policy-related document that may give you a better understanding of alternatives to restraint in relation to Mental Health Services Policy statement on reducing and where possible eliminating restraint and seclusion in Queensland mental health services <www.health.qld.gov.au/mentalhealth/docs/sandrpolicy_ 081030.pdf> (accessed 5 July 2014)

Summary

This chapter has introduced and briefly explained some very substantial areas of law. The aim is to give you a general understanding of these and help you see how these legal concepts can apply to practice. Each topic has dozens of cases that explore every permutation of the law in relation to the facts of each case and the principles of the relevant law. So from a lawyer's perspective each area is worthy of considerable specialised learning and research. Our needs are much simpler, although it is important to acknowledge that we have only touched on key concepts. The variety of web sources you have been directed to have been aimed at increasing your own research abilities and broadening your clinical knowledge where this has particular legal relationships.

Sources

American Hospital Association (2002). *HIPAA Privacy Standards*. www.hospitalconnect.com/hospitalconnect/jsp/keyissues.jsp?topic=HIPAA. (accessed 7 July 2014)

Australian Government; Australian Law Reform Commission (2008) *For Your Information: Australian Privacy Law and Practice* (ALRC Report 108) Published on 12 August 2008. Last modified on 22 July 2014.

Australian Parliamentary Library; The Australian Law Reform Commission (http://www.alrc.gov.au/) (accessed 7 July 2014)

Civil and Human Rights: Privacy (http://www.aph.gov.au/library/intguide/law/civlaw.htm#privacy) (accessed 7 July 2014)

Forrester, K. & Griffiths, D. (2005) *Essentials of Law*, 2nd edn, Harcourt, Sydney.

Forrester, K. & Griffiths, D. (2010) *Essentials of Law for Health Professionals*, 3rd edn, Elsevier, Chatswood, NSW

Kelly, G. (1998) 'Editorial: Patient data, confidentiality and electronics', *British Medical Journal*, 316: 718–719.

Kennedy, R. & Richards, J. (2004) *Integrating Human Service Law and Practice*, Oxford University Press, Melbourne.

MacFarlane, P. (1995) *Health Law*, 2nd edn, The Federation Press, Sydney.

MacFarlane, P. J. & Reid, S. J. (2003) *Queensland Health Law Handbook*, Queensland Dept of Health, Brisbane.

McIlwraith, J. & Madden, B. (2014) *Health Care & the Law*, 6th ed. Lawbook Co., Australia.

Queensland Public Interest Law Clearing House Incorporated (QPILCH) http://www.qpilch.org.au/resources/factsheets/Defamation.htm (accessed 7 July 2014).

Staunton, P. & Chiarella, M. (2003) *Nursing and the Law*, 5th edn, Elsevier, Sydney.

Staunton, P. & Whyburn, B. (1997) *Nursing and the Law*, 4th edn, Harcourt Australia Pty Ltd, Sydney.
White, B., Wilmott, L & McDonald, F. (2014) *Health Law in Australia*, 2nd ed Thomson Reuters, Australia.

Cases

Groce v. Purvis (2003) QDC 151 (16 June 2003).
Schessler v. Keck (1954) 271, 588 (California).

Consent: legal principles and practice considerations

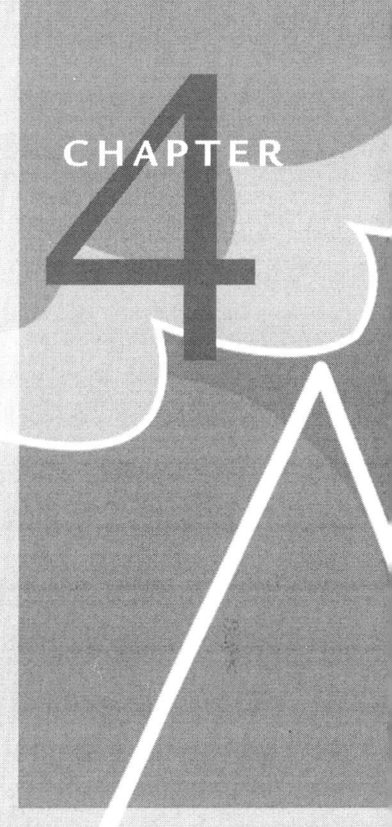

Learning outcomes

After studying this chapter you should be able to:

- Display understanding of key legislation affecting health policies and procedures.
- Describe the role of the law in providing direction for health care practice.
- Apply legal and professional standards when assessing and responding to client needs, practice and policy situations, professional reporting and communication.

Overview

By now you will have quite a lot of knowledge about the issue of consent. You have been alerted to the fact that consent is essential before you go ahead and perform care on a client. There are legal principles that regulate the relationships between the client and health professional.

In Chapter 3 in relation to the tort of trespass to property the existence of the tort trespass to person was mentioned. This is where we see the principles of assault, battery and false imprisonment come into play when an individual complains that they have suffered direct (and unlawful) interference. This interference can be either intentional or as a result of ill-considered, thoughtless or (in the general sense of the term) negligent behaviour. In trespass this negligent behaviour does not require the proof of damage, just the fact that interference occurred.

- Unlike an action in negligence where the plaintiff must prove the damage was caused by the respondent, in trespass it is up to the respondent to prove that the trespass was not intentional and that they are not at fault. Evidence of consent would go a long way to helping do this.

Not every state has a criminal code (legislation), some states deal with criminal matters through the common law (judge made law). Where crimes have been codified the issues of consent are linked to assault. The Queensland Criminal Code states:

> *Queensland Criminal Code*
> *Act No. 37, 1995*
>
> ***Division 2—Assault generally***
> **What is an 'assault'**
> **113.(1)** A person assaults anyone if, without the other person's consent—
> (a) the person applies force to the other person; or
> (b) the person—
> (i) by a bodily act or gesture, attempts or threatens to apply force to the other person; and
> (ii) is able, or appears to be able, to apply the force.
> **(2)** A person applies force to anyone if the person, directly or indirectly—
> (a) strikes, touches or moves the other person; or
> (b) applies heat, light, electrical or other energy, gas or odour to the other person to a degree that causes the other person injury or personal discomfort; or
> (c) applies force in any other way to the other person.

As you can see, reading legal text is quite an art but here in this section the authors have tried to capture every possible idea. In fact this is the standard a civil court will apply.

Before you get too anxious it is important to realise that there are exceptions and protections in both civil and criminal actions in every state and territory. The Queensland Criminal Code gives protection to doctors who proceed to give treatment to a standard expected and with the best of intentions in circumstances (such as an emergency) where it was impossible to gain the client's consent. Further, for the law to identify the interference as a criminal act, *there has to be intent to harm or a reckless indifference to the fact harm could result*. This attitude is not likely to exist among health professionals.

- Evidence of consent is a recognised defence to a civil action in negligence (the defence of 'volenti').

While lack of consent is not automatically evidence of trespass, negligence or assault, neither does every client contemplate a legal action when treatment does not achieve intended outcomes. However, if people undergo interventions or treatments they don't understand or feel they have been rushed into accepting something they would normally refuse, it can be a serious oversight if consent was not gained.

When an adverse event occurs it is often the manner in which the problem is dealt with that precipitates a legal action. The degree of damage is of course a major consideration, but when people feel that their rights have been trampled on, suspect they have been lied to or disregarded or have experienced attitudes or actions they feel amount to professional negligence, assault or failure to satisfy an agreement (contract) to provide care, there is the likelihood they will seek legal advice.

Assault and battery

- Assault is when someone deliberately creates a fear or apprehension of harmful contact.
- Battery is when the threat is actually carried out.

Often the two occur in rapid succession, a threat such as raising a weapon followed by a harmful touch (hit with the weapon), and this is then referred to as 'assault and battery'.

- The key to trespass to person is *intention*.

Not every touch without permission is assault, nor is every offensive or harming touch battery. An innocent or accidental touch or even passively obstructing another does not fall within battery. However, being obstructive, such as preventing someone passing you in a narrow doorway or passage or inhibiting their movements because it would involve an offensive, perhaps sexual or intimate, touching could fall within the tort of nuisance. To quote Chief Justice Holt: 'The least touching of another in anger is a battery' (*Cole v. Turner* (1704)).

The act must be a positive, deliberate and offensive action. Battery can even occur where no direct touch of the person is involved. An example would be practical jokes such as pulling a chair out from behind a person when they are about to sit down or pouring a bucket of water over someone.

If the person is unaware of the threat then it cannot be assault. It is awareness of the intent or threat to harm that creates assault. It does not matter that the person threatening an action has absolutely no intention of going through with it; the desire to create an apprehension of physical harm in another creates the assault.

Application to practice

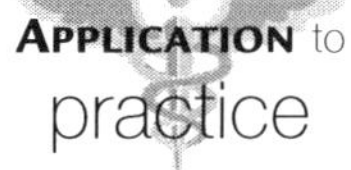

The idea of deliberately putting someone in a state of being apprehensive about an intervention because you are warning them 'this will hurt a bit' is not assault nor will the treatment be a battery unless of course there is an intention to intimidate or hurt. The professional has a duty to meet the needs of the client. It is true that sometimes things are said in jest; for example, 'I have a nice blunt needle with your name on it' could be construed as a deliberate and intentional threat. It would depend on the context, the relationship that has been established and the professional's assessment of these two essential criteria.

Sometimes an observer of these types of exchanges may judge the professional harshly, being unaware of that client–staff relationship. However, sometimes a professional used to being a 'cheerful and funny live wire' fails to assess and identify a client who is unable to see the humour in such statements due to their anxiety, discomfort, cultural background or language.

Courts have held that 'exceptional timidity' is not grounds for claiming assault but, equally, being fearless in the face of a threat does not deny the fact that assault was committed. The courts make a decision based on what a 'reasonable person' would believe was an intentional threat. A little thought will identify that 'reasonable person' in a care setting is a difficult concept to measure. Frequently patients are much more sensitive and vulnerable than normal, therefore professional assessment of the client's response to varied forms of communication would consider all the variables. Rather than going to the extremes of never making a joke or being so careful about not putting a client in fear of treatment that you muddle the facts or avoid effective treatment because it hurts, the professional assesses the situation and works to establish a clear and open communication, drawing from their repertoire of communication abilities to interact sensitively and effectively.

Questions from the real world

Q. What of the situation of a nurse with benevolent intent (that is, trying to do good)?

A. In an emergency an intervention to save, support or comfort is always allowed. Often touch is made to comfort when someone is upset. It is the context and the intent that matters. However it does not pay to be casual about it. "The law ...does not consider that an act done without a person's consent but for his benefit is deserving of reward or even of immunity from the action of trespass" (Lord Devlin 1905 Samples of Lawmaking).

Q. What about all those contacts which occur every day?

A. Innocent and inevitable contact with others is not assault. It is when proximity and deliberate invasion of a person's space or body by choice it becomes assault. The High Court referred to (and impliedly endorses) Collins v Wilcock- implied consent to 'all physical contact which is generally acceptable in the ordinary conduct of daily life.

Q. In Cole v Turner it was said that 'the least touching of another in anger is a battery'
Does this mean anger is necessary for a battery?

A. It is clear that anger/hostile intent is not necessary for a battery, which protects a person's right to determine what shall be done with their body. Medical practitioners who seek to force treatment on an unwilling patient risk civil action and perhaps prosecution for assault, unless their actions are justified under Crimes Act to prevent suicide, under some other statutory protection or unless the patient is of unsound mind and the action results from a bona fide decision by a doctor.

Consent

- Consent may be implied, spoken or written.

When the client sees you coming to administer an injection and then bares their arm and positions themselves to accept the jab, this is implied consent. Accepting their medication and swallowing it without discussion is another example of implied consent.

Experienced patients can predict what is going to be done and understand from previous information why it has to be done, and certainly for non-invasive interactions, implied consent could be assumed by the health professional. However, it is important to realise that should there be something different about this intervention or when the client expects you are about to do one thing when in fact you intend to carry out another, implied consent will not hold up.

Most of us habitually explain, even as we are initiating the steps to do something, what it is we are about to do.

- If you do not get into the habit of introducing yourself and explaining your intentions, giving the client an opportunity to ask questions and agree to it from a position of knowledge, you are failing to satisfy an expected standard.

Just because the patient has presented at hospital does not imply that they will agree to everything that is initiated or deemed to be essential.

- Communication is the key to consent.

Appropriate and clear information must be provided. The client must actually understand not only what you intend to do but why you intend to do it and, further, what the risks or benefits of this are for them, before consent is valid.

If the information given to the client is incomprehensible, if the environment is such that they cannot hear or make sense of the information, if their fear, pain or confusion interferes with understanding then, whether implied, spoken or written, the consent is not valid.

- Another key to consent is that it relates only to the specific procedure consented to.

Just because there is consent to a shower does not mean that this extends to consent to a hair trim. Even though the client has consented to surgery, should a further problem be discovered the surgeon cannot go ahead and perform a second procedure at the same time unless the possibility has been discussed and agreed to preoperatively.

Informed consent

> *Every human being of adult years and sound mind has the right to determine what shall be done with his own body* (Cardozo J in *Schleondorff v. Society of New York Hospitals* (1914)).

While the term 'informed consent' is used constantly you need to be able to articulate just what this means. While one client may need to be given extensive, intensive and repeated information another may not. How do you know when you have provided sufficient information?

In *Ellis v. Wallsend District Hospital* (1989) the judge stated, 'It is difficult to understand how the plaintiff may make a final decision whether to undergo an operation on his own body, if the information upon which the decision is to be taken is distilled by a doctor in discussing the operation with the patient' (Aust. Torts Reports 80-259, cited in Macfarlane and Reid, 2003).

As a result of a number of cases in negligence that addressed the issue of how much information is sufficient, the medical profession has guidelines published through the Royal Australian College of Physicians and the National Health and Medical Research Council (NHMRC). A key case, *Rogers v. Whitaker* (1992), dealt with this. In this case an ophthalmologist (Rogers) did not explain that a very rare complication was possible as a result of proposed surgery. Post-operatively Mrs Whitaker suffered this complication, resulting in total blindness. The court disregarded the defence of Dr Rogers that he had acted within established and normal parameters in his advice and care to the patient. The standard expected was to be determined with careful consideration of a number of factors.

- The nature of the information to be disclosed.
- The nature of the treatment.
- The desire of the patient for information.
- The temperament and health of the patient.
- The general surrounding circumstances.

Another extract from this High Court judgment illustrates the importance of providing sufficient information: 'In legal terms, the patient's consent to the treatment may be valid once he or she is informed in broad terms of the nature of the procedure which is intended. But the choice is, in reality, meaningless unless it is made on the basis of relevant information and advice.'

APPLICATION to practice

Application to practice

The law does expect that there is a duty to warn a client of 'material risk' that exists for an intended treatment. The way to determine if something is a material risk in a particular situation is to ask yourself:

- Is this something that a reasonable person, in this patient's position, if warned of the risk, would attach significance to it?

or

- As a professional, do I know that this particular patient, if given information about the risks, would probably attach significance to it?

There are always circumstances that affect the decision making and opportunity to provide extensive, considered and timely discussion about a treatment.

- This is where professional judgment and policies come into play.

Consider the physical and mental status of the client. You cannot make an arbitrary decision about this. Suspecting a client will refuse treatment if you tell them it will hurt or withholding information 'because he won't understand it' should not be done without consultation with someone who can assess the true mental state.

What might be the effect of the disclosure or information on the client? Will it affect them negatively? Collaboration with relevant staff is necessary and adherence to policy is important. However, recall the *Rogers v. Whitaker* case where, just because the preoperative information and explanations given were current practice and what other doctors did, this was not sufficient for the court. In that case the client had been very particular and asked many questions. The doctor had even written in the notes that her questions about the procedure were extensive. He had noted that she had specified that any risks to her 'good eye' were important considerations before she would consent to an operation on her 'bad eye'. His failure to mention very rare complications in the face of her desire for information and her subsequent loss of sight opened the way for a finding against the doctor.

Each client has the right to seek as much information as they desire, and routine or current practice and policy is balanced against the needs of the individual.

- Consider the degree of risk involved. The more invasive a treatment the greater the risk.

Consider the circumstances; is it an emergency, can the patient actually understand this information? Do you need an interpreter, a parent or guardian? Is there any chance that medication such as sedation is affecting the client? Could the client feel coerced or pushed into consenting due to pressure from relatives, the power relationship between client and professionals, a fear that failure to agree might mean denial of any other support or treatment alternatives?

Capacity to consent

The concept of 'legal capacity' means that an adult of sound mind is competent to make decisions about their treatment and thus has the right to give or withhold consent to treatment. In our work we often deal with clients who are not of sound mind, who are not competent to make decisions about their treatment.

Legislation governs who has the authority to consent on behalf of people with reduced mental capacity. We will look at these issues in depth in relation to mental illness in a later chapter. In the matter of consent, however, the key factors are age and mental capacity. It is important to note that when a person cannot give valid consent, this does not automatically give the health professional freedom to proceed. The law does not condone or accept as a defence to assault the fact that a person was incompetent to consent.

A case where the client could not consent, so the surgeon relied on next of kin was: *Harvey v. Strickland*, 566 S.E.2d 529, 2002

A Jehovah's Witness explicitly rejected blood transfusions during surgery. However, while in surgery, the need arose. Since he was unconscious, the surgeon sought the consent of the patient's mother. He obtained the consent, claiming it to be an emergency. The Court disagreed because the wishes of the patient were well known.

Age

Legal capacity in Australia is 18 years of age; people under that age are referred to as minors. For a child under the age of 16 years a parent or legal guardian must consent to medical or dental treatment unless it is an emergency situation and they cannot be contacted.

In most states through legislation, a person 16 years or over can legally consent to medical or dental treatment if they are capable of understanding the nature and effect of the proposed treatment *and* can freely decide for themselves without unfair pressure or influence from other people. Consent must be informed and effective. If there is any doubt about the minor's level of understanding or comprehension the consent is neither informed nor effective. Simply nodding or answering yes or no to questions is insufficient; the young person must be able to demonstrate in their own words that they have a complete grasp of the situation. Should there be any doubts the parent, guardian or carer will need to be involved in the matter.

Where a minor is in conflict with a parent over proposed treatment the law is not rigid. Matters of contraception have been found to be within the capacity of 14 year olds to make an informed and effective decision about. The courts have the power to intervene in conflicts in relation to proposed treatments on the basis of deciding the best interests of the child. An example that has come to the courts on a number of occasions is the request by parents for sterilisation procedures to be carried out on their intellectually disabled children. The High Court has held that this cannot be done without a court order where the situation is one where either there is a risk a wrong decision will affect the future of the child or the consequences of such a decision are serious.

Legislation exempts health professionals from the obligation to seek consent from a parent or guardian in particular circumstances such as when there is suspected child abuse or if the client has a notifiable disease.

Intellectual disability

An adult who lacks the capacity to understand issues is not mentally ill but neither are they legally competent. At common law, consent by the family or a friend of an intellectually disabled adult is not sufficient to uphold a defence against an action of assault, therefore it is important to know legislative provisions. Some states have specific legislation to protect the rights and interests of persons with disabilities, while other states incorporate the issues of guardianship for persons with an intellectual disability within mental health provisions. Generally the focus of protection is to ensure that the welfare and rights of persons with intellectual disabilities are paramount and from the health professional's perspective it is important to recognise that those rights mean that the adult who is able to make decisions that are within their capacity is entitled to do so.

States and territories have set up boards or councils that are responsible for matters of guardianship. Some specifically appoint medical and financial guardians as well. Appointment of a guardian is not automatic for people with disabilities. Families frequently establish effective support or the individual has the resources to manage their affairs and can call upon someone who is their representative or, as it is referred to in many statutes, there is a 'person responsible'. This may be a husband or wife or *de facto* spouse or the person who has the care of the individual on a permanent basis. This person is still the responsible person even if the individual has been admitted to short- or long-term institutional care.

Figure 4.1 Summary of characteristics of capacity to consent

- There is no requirement for consent if the client is unconscious or so seriously ill that intervention is necessary to save life. The duty of care that arises in this situation overrides any requirement for consent.
- Minors and persons with intellectual disabilities are entitled to make decisions within their capacity and understanding of what is intended but generally for consent to treatment a parent or guardian must provide consent.

- Should there be serious consequences to proposed treatments or conflicts between the client, parent/guardian or professional the courts will intervene to ensure the welfare and rights of the child/client are protected.
- Involuntary patients, diagnosed as mentally ill, are protected by legislation and this legislation recognises circumstances where consent is not necessary for treatment to be carried out.

Application to practice

APPLICATION to practice

A clinical reality is dealing with a client who may experience differing levels of comprehension at different times. Some clients are lucid during the day but become confused at night. Some clients insist they have capacity to make decisions but staff members may have grave reservations about that capacity. In these situations, particularly where there is no nominated guardian or next of kin who can take responsibility, the first step is to confirm whether or not the client does have that capacity. This is often a clinical decision based on status at assessment. An elderly client suffering acute trauma may not, at the time of assessment, be lucid. Here duty of care overrides the obligation to gain consent for life-saving measures. In reality, particularly in aged-care settings, this rarely has serious consequences but staff are frustrated or anxious about the validity of consent.

On admission it is usual to identify who is the representative, next of kin or guardian, and this is the person who should be contacted in the first instance. If there are conflicts between next of kin or representatives and the client it is important to determine who is acting in the best interests of the client. This may require intervention by a social worker, psychologist or even a representative from the Public Guardians Office.

From the immediate clinical point of view, limiting treatment, postponing non-urgent interventions or working with a colleague who will provide objective and written assessment to support your planned intervention is reasonable.

Consent forms

Not every procedure requires written consent; recall that consent may be implied or verbal. It is not a legal requirement to have written consent, but institutions and practitioners use it as evidence should a dispute about the treatment given arise. The same principles apply to written consent as to any other form of consent.

The words used on the document must be understood, consent must be voluntary and the client must understand all material facts for it to be valid. It is best practice that the form be *explained and signed by the clinician doing the procedure*. Having a surrogate provide information, obtain a signature then leaving it to the doctor to sign later is not appropriate. Contemporaneous explanations, signatures and, if desired, witnesses' signatures should be aimed for.

It is common for clients planning elective surgery to sign consent forms well before admission, while they are consulting the doctor and planning admission. Such consent overlooks the possibility of changed circumstances, clients changing their minds or forgetting matters that were discussed. On admission the matter should be revisited; opportunity for questions and clarification and signing another form is often institutional policy prior to surgery.

Figure 4.2 Ensuring valid consent

- Ask the client or, if relevant, family/guardian what they understand to be involved to determine if there are misunderstandings or knowledge gaps. Use interpreters if necessary. Avoid jargon or complex medical language.
- Recognise that patients may be overwhelmed with information and that people forget what is said so provide brochures, a note, booklets or diagrams, even videos that are within the clients' literacy and language capacity.
- If you do not actually know the answer to a question find someone who does. One of the greatest complaints patients and families have is that 'everyone says something different'. This is often simply because of the way different staff members phrase or emphasise matters; among themselves staff are certain there is no inconsistency but clients hear the differences not the similarities. Misinformation, whether through staff ignorance or innocent misunderstanding, needs to be avoided.
- People need time to think about important matters and to discuss them with others. Provide time for them to ask questions and suggest they write down any questions they think of later to bring back and have answered. We all have experienced after a visit to a doctor the frustration of 'I forgot to ask . . .'.
- Restate or repeat information; good communication strategies reinforce information without being condescending.

Always make a note in the client file about your information session, what was covered and the level of understanding the client evidenced.

Refusal of treatment

A number of states now have legislation which gives statutory force to the common law principle that competent persons may refuse treatment. Treatment provided in knowledge of legally binding refusal of treatment is the offence of medical trespass.

Generally we rely on an advanced directive when a client refuses treatment. In some institutions a refusal of treatment certificate (or similar) is required to be completed by the person when competent. Treatment may be refused by the legal agent or guardian of an incompetent person.

However different state Acts use slightly different terminology. For example, in Victoria, refusal of treatment may be from a person given "Enduring Power of Attorney (medical treatment)" under the Medical Treatment Act 1988 (Vic) whereas in New South Wales refusal of treatment may be from a person given "Enduring Guardianship" under The Guardianship Act 1987 (NSW). (In NSW, "Enduring Power of Attorney" refers to a person appointed to manage financial affairs of an incompetent person under the Powers of Attorney Act 2003) (Australian Resuscitation Council, Guideline 10.5, 2012).

Most nurses raise the issue of Jehovah's Witnesses refusing blood transfusions but there are many circumstances where personal, religious or cultural beliefs underpin a refusal to give consent for treatment. Earlier the point was made that just because a client presents at hospital or consents to some treatments this cannot be taken as consent to all.

The courts will deny adults the right to refuse treatment if it risks the life or health of others. For example, caesarian section has been carried out under court order to save the baby, in spite of the mother's refusal for surgery on religious grounds. The courts have held that blood transfusion to save the life of a child despite opposition on religious grounds was lawful. In *Birkett v. Director-General of Family & Community Services & Others* (unreported 3161/91, February 1994) the Supreme Court Justice Bryson relied on the *Children (Care and Protection) Act 1987* (NSW) to support this judgment. However, this section of legislation replicates common law principles whereby in emergency situations consent is not necessary. There is also provision in the Motor Vehicles Acts of each state to allow blood to be taken with or without consent for analysis in the event of a motor vehicle accident.

Faced with refusal to consent to treatment, only the intervention of the state Supreme Court can override a competent adult. This situation has occurred in Australia in relation to blood transfusion but there is no certainty that the court will support the request to override the client. In fact there is a case where the client, a Jehovah's Witness, successfully sued her doctor as her express and stated wishes refusing a blood transfusion had been ignored (*Malette v. Shuman et al* (1991)).

The situation for children depends upon circumstances. While 18 years is the legal age of adulthood, the courts do recognise that capacity to give consent is valid for young people from 14 to 18 years old. Should parents refuse consent for treatment each state has legislation that identifies that if, in the opinion of the medical practitioner, the treatment is reasonable and essential to save the child's life then it can be carried out. This has happened where parental religious or cultural beliefs ran counter to recognised medical practice.

Children who are wards of the state are covered by state legislation. This legislation specifies which minister or government officer must provide consent for medical or surgical treatment. In addition, all states have some form of legislation to protect 'children at risk'. In Queensland this is the *Child Protection Act 1999,* in the ACT, *Children and Young People Act 2008 (ACT),* in NSW, the *Children and Young Persons (Care and Protection) Act 1998 (NSW),* in the NT, it is the *Care and Protection of Children Act 2007 (NT),* SA has the *Children's Protection Act 1993 (SA),* in Tasmania, the *Children, Young Persons and their Families Act 1997(Tas.),* WA has the *Children and Community Services Act 2004 (WA)* and Victoria, the *Children, Youth and Families Act 2005 (Vic.).* Many of the states have amended the original legislation and have in addition regulations governing these matters. Primarily aimed at ensuring children at risk from abuse or neglect are identified and removed from that risk, these Acts also spell out the obligations for notification of suspected or known neglect or abuse. All health and welfare professionals are obliged to notify the relevant government department responsible for investigating and, if necessary, removing the child and prosecuting the offenders. If a child who is in this category is admitted to hospital they can be treated without parental consent.

With a few special exceptions, there is no requirement in law for obtaining the consent of a spouse although there are institutions that have this policy – usually in relation to interventions affecting reproductive capacity or termination of pregnancy. Legislation does require the spouse or legal guardian to give consent in the following situations.

- Under mental health legislation where the client lacks capacity.
- Under the Human Tissue Acts, the nearest available next of kin must consent to removal of organs where the deceased person's wishes are unknown.
- For in-vitro fertilisation both husband and wife must consent to participate in the program.
- Intention to adopt a child requires consent by both partners.

Emergency situations

Under the common law doctrine of emergency, a doctor (and in particular circumstances trained health staff), may treat a patient if the doctor acts reasonably and honestly believes on reasonable grounds that the treatment is necessary to prevent a serious threat to the victim's life or health.

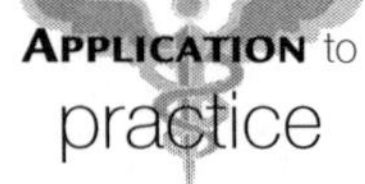

Application to practice

In effect this means that should you walk into a situation where the client is at risk or has collapsed, whether or not you *suspect* there are orders not to intervene you must take reasonable steps to save them. You cannot not be held liable for initiating steps, rather the risk would be *assuming* the client had refused consent to treatment; until you have proof that there are written 'not for resuscitation orders' you proceed to make every effort. Of course the circumstances and situation will govern the extent and duration of these lifesaving efforts.

The States of Tasmania, Victoria, New South Wales and Queensland have legislation allowing urgent treatment to be provided by the doctor or dentist of an incompetent person without consent. Urgent treatment is generally defined as that to save a person's life, to prevent serious damage to health or to prevent or treat suffering, pain or distress. Similar legislation in Western Australia states urgent treatment may be provided by "the health professional" (undefined) without consent. This Act defines urgent treatment as life-sustaining measure, palliative care or other health care. In Victoria and New South Wales, urgent treatment may be provided by other persons under a doctor's supervision.

Not for resuscitation and terminally ill clients

The dying and terminally ill client's right to refuse treatment is recognised as a particular situation requiring particular considerations. The focus of medical intervention is to save lives. Above we have explored the principles of consent and issues of what is legal should consent be withheld at a risk to one's own or another's life. However, the ethical aspects that Chapter 1 alerted you to come into play when we contemplate the right of an individual to choose to die or refuse life-prolonging, even life-saving, interventions. The common law and legislation uphold the rights of an individual to choose to give or withhold consent. Health professionals fear legal consequences if they withhold care that they know would alter the course of illness. Legislation does exist that protects the health practitioner and the terminally ill and their carers from civil and criminal liability . . . in particular circumstances.

There is recognition in most states of advance health directives whereby an individual may specify their wishes for current and future health interventions.

It has long been settled law that parents or guardians of minors, in conjunction with doctors, may make legal and ethical decisions on withholding and withdrawing life-sustaining treatment.

Queensland and Western Australia are the only States whose legislation specifically includes references to withholding or withdrawing (discontinuation) of treatment *without* consent. In Queensland under the *Guardianship and Administration Act 2000 s 63A* a life-sustaining measure may be withheld or withdrawn without consent as consistent with good medical practice. This however has caused some real world problems as there was a case where the family disputed the medical decision and would not have agreed to the not for resuscitation decision (Coronial inquest 2009 report of into the death of June Woo). The Coroner examined how Mrs Woo's daughters were involved in the NFR decision. The evidence indicated that when the NFR order was made in the emergency department, the treating emergency physician "did not consider the decision was one the relatives could consent or object to" as further intervention was medically futile. The Coroner found that the communication that occurred in the emergency department did not constitute consent by the daughters. The Coroner also reviewed the hospital's NFR policy and was critical that it did not require consent from the appropriate decision maker for an NFR order to be obtained. The result was Queensland Health developed an Acute Resuscitation Plan which directs assessments of futility should include appraisal of the quality of life to be pursued and, as such, are not the sole remit of clinicians. Conversations with family regarding the patient's quality of life are necessary to decide whether treatment is futile for that individual (Lawrence et al. 2012).

In Western Australia the *Guardianship and Administration Act 1990 s 110ZD* states a person responsible may refuse consent to commencement or continuation of any treatment.

The law recognises that an adult who is conscious and capable of making decisions has the right to refuse resuscitation (or as discussed above, any treatment).

In Queensland *The Powers of Attorney Act 1998* covers this situation. In Victoria, the *Medical Treatment Act 1988* requires a witnessed certificate, as does the ACT *Medical Treatment Act 1994*. The Northern Territory has the *Natural Death Act 1988*. South Australia, like Queensland, has more recent legislation that specifies the right of competent adults to make an advance directive through the *Consent to Medical Treatment and Palliative Care Act 1995*. Other states rely on the common law but Department of Health guidelines exist giving direction and definitions of palliative care.

- It should be clearly understood that no state or territory will accept active or deliberate acts to cause death. Just because an individual consents to their own death does not give another person the right to cause that death. Euthanasia is not the same as allowing someone to die with dignity. (This is revisited in Chaper 13.)

The concept of futility underpins a medical decision to not initiate life saving measures or withdraw life sustaining treatment. Even with Queensland legislation giving support to medical staff making a decision based on futility it was still deemed essential to communicate and gain consent from family. It is recognised that families may be unable to accept this medical assessment and legislation contains a mechanism to resolve intractable disagreement between clinicians and family by requesting the Adult Guardian, a statutory officer, to consent to the withholding or refusal of treatment.

No state or territory guidelines or legislation allows the withdrawal of palliative care measures aimed at ensuring comfort and alleviating suffering. The lines are often blurred between what constitutes active medical treatment to maintain life and what is in place to ensure comfort. Enteral and PEG feeding have been subject to court hearings where the issue of whether withholding feeding amounts to withholding the means of palliation. A competent adult can refuse oral feeding but an unconscious client or client in a vegetative state cannot refuse these interventions.

Such a situation was argued in *Gardner; re BWV* (2003) in the Victorian Supreme Court. Determining whether artificial feeding was a medical treatment or a palliative care was the issue. The patient's husband had sought the right to be her guardian as she had never made arrangements for an agent or guardian prior to suffering dementia. After seven years of constant deterioration, with only the PEG feeding keeping her alive, her husband wanted an end to her suffering. It was declared by the court that artificial feeding was in fact a medical treatment based on the need for interventions, prescribed formulae, protocols and procedures. Therefore artificial feeding could be withheld. If the court had found artificial feeding was a palliative measure it could not be withdrawn.

Optional reading

Ashby, M. & Mendelson, D. 2004, '*Gardner; re BWV*, Victorian Supreme Court makes landmark ruling on tube feeding', *Medical Journal of Australia*, 18(8), 442–445, <www.mja.com.au/public/issues> (accessed 6 July 2014).

Doctrine of double effect

It is obvious that some treatments that give relief and comfort can in fact hasten death and it is this intent to alleviate suffering that makes palliation different to assisting death. Often called the doctrine of double effect, 'was the intention to relieve pain or take the life' is the question that will be asked. Should the treatment fall outside the accepted best practice for palliation then doubts about intent would be raised.

The first time the concept was introduced into common law was in 1957 when the judge issued instructions to the jury in *R v Adams* in a case involving end of life care with opioid medications.

The fact that the law does not condone intentional death creates a real legal risk to medical practitioners. Criminal codes in many jurisdictions directly conflict with the ethical position of treating a client to alleviate suffering while conscious that the treatment will hasten death. Two prosecutions in Victoria under the *Victorian Crimes Act 1958* resulted in suspended sentences for the medical practitioners but the fact that there were prosecutions lies behind efforts to clarify the law through legislation (*R v Hood* 2002; *R v Maxwell* 2003).

For the double effect principle to be invoked to provide moral support for the taking of an action, there are four necessary conditions that are to be met. Firstly, the action under consideration must be either morally good or morally indifferent; secondly, that the negative result is not intended; thirdly, that the positive result not be a direct causal result of the negative result; and fourthly, that the positive result be in proportion to the negative result. It is argued that, if all these conditions are met, then it is morally permissible for the action to be taken despite the negative effect (Solomon, 2002). Confusing isn't it!

Remember, euthanasia a deliberate intentional taking of life is against the law. So the dilemma for end of life treatment or withholding of treatment that is predictably going to hasten death is both a legal risk as well as a moral issue. There have been attempts to legislate protections for medical staff caught in these situations. The *Consent to Medical Treatment and Palliative Care Act 1995* states there is: ... *no civil or criminal liability by administering treatment with the intention of relieving pain or distress ... even though an incidental effect of the treatment is to hasten the death of the patient.*

In Queensland a private members Bill was introduced in 2002. The rationale underlying the Care of Terminally-Ill Patients Bill 2002 was described in the following way:

> ...many Queensland doctors hold back from prescribing enough medication to effectively relieve pain in the terminally ill, because under present state law they could be prosecuted if their patient dies as a consequence of their action. This in turn causes many people with terminal illness to spend their final moments in acute agony and causes intense distress to their loved ones.

The problem between providing care that is life prolonging and withholding care such as life support or resuscitation is often solved with clear institutional policies and open communication with client and family. What is reasonable in the situation is often the test. If intervention is necessary to promote healing, recovery or ensure comfort and pain control it would be considered necessary. When it is obvious that in spite of the treatment there is no chance of healing or recovery then the treatment can have no therapeutic value; again the existence of an advance health directive may give direction to practitioners for making decisions. (These issues are revisited in Chapter 13).

Not for resuscitation: 'do not resuscitate' orders

Deciding whether or not to initiate life-saving measures for a client who has no possibility of a quality of life is a common experience and can cause great anxiety where there is no clear direction or policy. In these cases the right of the patient to refuse resuscitation attempts must be upheld. It is a refusal to consent to medical treatment. Policies should be in place to ensure any decision to refuse treatment is informed and unambiguous. This requires good communication and documentation.

The decision to withhold medical treatment should the patient or their family/guardian not have made their wishes known must be based on medical evidence. Experienced clinicians need to discuss and document the decision and justify that decision based on assessment and medical facts. The decision must be reviewed and if the client's condition improves or the client or their agent changes their mind and wants intervention, the order must reflect these changes.

Policies exist that specify procedures and documentation in most institutions for not for resuscitation decisions. Refusal of treatment, such as 'Do-Not-Attempt-Resuscitation' (DNAR) or 'Not for Resuscitation' (NFR) orders should be documented in case notes and signed. Instructions should be specific, detailed, transferable across health care settings, and easily understood.

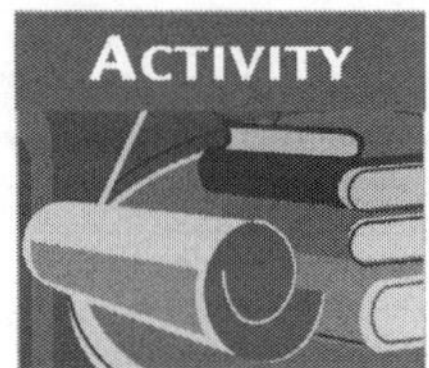

Activity

It is obvious that the common law does recognise the right of a competent individual to make decisions for themselves, that legislation exists to allow individuals to have agents or guardians appointed to protect their interests and in some states the right to make provisions and give directions for future circumstances.

- What might be the risk of accepting a written statement found in a client's wallet directing that 'should I be injured or impaired so seriously that I am unable to make decisions about my health care, I wish it to be known that I do not, in any circumstances, wish to be kept alive on life support or undergo treatments that prolong my life'.
- What are the professional issues?
- What do you think would be the legal considerations?

One way to look at a 'not for resuscitation' order is that it is a client's prerogative rather than a health professional's decision to withhold treatment.

- Do you feel this is a preferable stance to take on the issue?

Read the following case study and answer the questions below.

A 20-year-old woman has suffered irreversible and massive brain damage. The costs (in time, resources and money) to maintain her on mechanical life support systems are enormous; there is no chance of any recovery.

- Who has the legal right to decide to turn off the machines? Should it be the patient's next of kin? The attending doctors? The hospital authorities? The Court?

Although the Tort of Negligence, which will be addressed in following chapters, is mentioned frequently, at this point we will look at one Australian Law Reform report as this might give you a better understanding of just how the rules about consent and the concepts of informed consent have evolved from case law.

While the most significant Australian case *Rogers v. Whitaker* focused on issues of negligence, much of that case explored issues of consent. Below are some issues that were raised in The Legal Liability of Health Service Providers Final Report May 1997.

In Chapter 2, the report states clearly that in Australia when issues of conduct are questioned, it is not the professional opinion or habit of professional practice that sets the standard, the standard is determined by the court. The court will rely on evidence from medical practitioners as to whether the standard of care was breached. While the court recognises that such evidence will be highly persuasive in helping reach a decision, it is still the courts' decision.

The report is clear that findings in medical negligence cases are specific to the facts of each particular case. However using the example of *Rogers v. Whitaker* the facts of that case were examined. The report explains that Ms Whitaker had been referred to Dr Rogers, an ophthalmic surgeon, to determine if a penetrating injury to her blinded right eye could be treated. The injury had happened nearly forty years ago. Dr Rogers had advised her that an operation on her right eye would not only improve its appearance but would probably restore significant sight to that eye. The operation was carried out with the 'appropriate skill and care'. However the surgery did not restore sight in her right eye; sadly she developed sympathetic ophthalmia in her left eye, which resulted in a loss of sight in her left eye as well.

The court had heard from experts what a surgeon would typically provide a patient regarding information about the treatment, prognosis and standard of care. The issue was whether Ms Whitaker would have consented to the operation had she been told of this risk. The evidence was that the risk of developing sympathetic ophthalmia was approximately one in 14,000, although the risk of occurrence was slightly greater, where there had been an earlier penetrating injury to the eye operated upon (as was the case here).

The court also relied on Dr Rogers notes which identified that Ms Whitaker had 'incessantly' asked questions about possible complications and she had inquired as to whether something could have been put over her good eye during the operation. In the court's opinion it was the evidence that Ms Whitaker was extremely anxious about any risks to her remaining eye that raised the question of informed consent even though she was suing Dr Rogers for negligence.

The High Court judgment did not adhere to an established legal precedent known as the Bolam principle. That principle accepts that it is medical opinion that determines how much information about risks and complications are given by a health professional to a patient. If the Bolam principle were to be followed, the evidence of Ms Whittaker's anxiety and questions would have been disregarded.

The High Court used the approach adopted by King CJ in *F v. R* (1983) where a woman became pregnant following a tubal ligation and brought an action in negligence alleging that the medical practitioner had failed to warn her of the failure rate of the procedure. In that case the judge had stated that the amount of advice or information that a responsible doctor should disclose depends on five factors including 'the nature of the matter to be disclosed; the nature of the treatment; the desire of the patient for information; the temperament and health of the patient; and the general surrounding circumstances' (pp. 189).

- Think about your own practice, we know we must gain consent before initiating care but do we actually provide information based on our assessment of the patient's capacity and, after determining through questions, the significance each patient attaches to identified risks? Health professionals needing to demonstrate informed consent is now the standard upheld the High Court held.

This important move from past legal precedent that had guided health staff in gaining informed consent for decades has changed the relationship between doctor and patient and other health professionals. If the Bolam principle governs our approach, the patient's questions regarding complications or risks would be of no consequence: medical opinion would dictate whether the risk should have been disclosed.

In *Rogers v Whitaker* the High Court majority accepted Chief Justice Kings' five factors and stated:

> *The law should recognise that a doctor has a duty to warn a patient of a material risk inherent in the proposed treatment; a risk is material if, in the circumstances of the particular case, a reasonable person in the patient's position, if warned of the risk, would be likely to attach significance to it or if the medical practitioner is or should reasonably be aware that the particular patient, if warned of the risk, would be likely to attach significance to it. The duty is subject to the therapeutic privilege* (Rogers v. Whitaker 1992 p. 490).

APPLICATION to practice

Application to practice

The Legal Liability of Health Service Providers Final Report points out that every case is assessed on its own facts and the specific facts that influenced the High Court in Rogers were as discussed above; Ms Whitaker had been very anxious and questioned the surgeon at length about complications. The surgeon knew (or should have known) there was a remote risk of sympathetic opthalmia, a very serious complication but he failed to address this. The surgery was elective so Ms Whitaker could have chosen to proceed or not proceed without risk to her health when she had all the facts.

Often we withhold information based on not wanting to 'frighten the patient' or we don't want to cause patient 'confusion'. The court did recognise that professionals have to make judgments about patient capacity and what they can cope with. Here, disclosure would have caused no harm, inconvenience or damage. These factors outweighed the fact that the risk was statistically remote.

These findings do not set the precedent for medical practitioners and health professionals to disclose every extraordinary little risk. Instead, health professionals are expected to look at all the circumstances surrounding each patient in relation to the known risks and evaluate the effect of the patient's realisation of the risk.

For true informed consent, health professionals need to facilitate a patient's autonomy, provide opportunity for meaningful communication and provide information that meets the client need rather relying on our established habit of practice or personal opinion.

Adequate disclosure by a health service provider: post-Rogers

The majority opinion in *Rogers v. Whitaker* put the ethical principle of autonomy ahead of all other considerations. There have been a number of cases since this landmark decision that have refined and applied the principle in relation to patient consent and patient information. The pre admission habit of giving a patient a pamphlet full of medical jargon to explain procedures was not recommended by the authors of the report.

Soon after the High Court *Rogers v. Whitaker* judgment the New South Wales Supreme Court heard *Karpati v. Spira & Ors* (unreported 1995) and held that when discussing risks with patients, subjective terms such as 'rare', 'unlikely' and 'likely' should not be used. The Judge in that case, Spender J, proposed that serious risks should be explained as percentages (if known). In that case the surgeon was not found negligent for not informing the patient there was a 5% risk of a stroke for stereotactic thalamotomy surgery to treat a Parkinsonian tremor in the plaintiff's right arm. In that case there was substantial evidence that the plaintiff was prepared to accept the risk of stroke in view of the operation's high success rate and the discomfort associated with his condition.

In *Teik Huat Tai v. Saxon*, (1995) the Full Court of the Supreme Court of Western Australia upheld the trial judge's findings that the doctor had negligently failed to inform the patient of the risks associated with hysterectomy and vaginal repair. The patient suffered severe complications and the court, using the *Rogers v. Whitaker* reasoning, felt the risks of this type of surgery were material and there was evidence the patient was an anxious person. Therefore the doctor should have been aware that the patient would attach significance to the risk.

In *Tekanawa v. Millican* (1994) the Court held that where the surgery is purely elective or cosmetic, there is a higher standard of disclosure. It was found that the plaintiff's doctor had failed to tell a patient of the potential for scarring following a 'tummy tuck' operation. It is worth noting that while the doctor had given the patient an information pamphlet about the procedure, the court found it was insufficient and misleading in terms of likely scarring that the patient eventually suffered. Accordingly, it failed to protect the medical practitioner from liability.

On 19 September 2013, the New South Wales Court of Appeal in *Paul v Cooke* [2013] NSWCA 311 confirmed that a radiologist was not liable where a patient suffered permanent disablement after the materialisation of an inherent risk.

Dr Cooke, a radiologist, negligently failed to diagnose a berry aneurysm in 2003. Surgery was performed on Mrs Paul in 2006 by another doctor. During the surgery, the aneurysm ruptured and Mrs Paul suffered permanent disablement. Mrs Paul sued Dr Cooke for damages resulting from the injuries she suffered after the surgery in 2006, alleging that Dr Cooke's negligence in 2003 was the cause of the injuries.

The NSW Court of Appeal held that the rupturing of the aneurysm was an inherent risk that pre-dated, and was neither created nor increased by, the radiologist's negligent failure to diagnose. The Court of Appeal said that:

> even if the radiologist had diagnosed the berry aneurysm, Mrs Paul would still have faced the risks of a procedure *that she willingly chose to undergo*; and those risks could only have been avoided had the decision to undergo surgery not been made.

The Court decided that the radiologist was not liable for the materialisation of an inherent risk. The case naturally focuses on the causation principles in the context of a medical negligence case. But it also notes that Mrs Paul willingly chose to undergo the treatment. This serves as a reminder that a patient should be fully informed of all material risks before deciding whether to receive any form of medical treatment (Mountford & Scanlan, 2013).

Summary

The existence of policies and protocols as well as codes of practice for obtaining consent should mean that there would be no risk that a client could feel their right to consent has been overridden. The routine nature of pre-procedure consent may in fact be a cause of problems as health professionals may fail to treat clients as individuals and be so focused upon the task that they forget the patients. Recognising that some clients may refuse or withhold consent and others may lack the capacity to consent does not mean health professionals are helpless or freed of professional responsibility. If a client makes a decision that health staff members believe is based on unsound judgment or one that puts the client at risk, where treatment has benefits, there are procedures to follow. As long as the rights of the patient, not the preference of the service provider, take precedence it is unlikely to be an issue. There are regular media reports about cases exploring the right of client or family to refuse treatments or to withdraw life-saving technology. Sometimes these cases get to court in order to clarify the law and to protect all parties from a fear of consequences; often they are ethical dilemmas. It is not just one nurse's responsibility to deal with difficult issues, it is a system issue and getting advice and recommending institutions provide written policies or guidelines is a way to ensure obligations are met both ethically and legally.

Practice assignment question

These 2 scenarios are a continuation of the practice assignment in Chapter 1. Length for each answer is 400-500 words.

Scenario 3 Length 400-500 words

Apply the bioethical principle of autonomy to the scenario.

You identify to Kate that there might be issues with her using client records and initiating studies without approval. You raise the question of client consent to participate in these activities. Kate replies "it is diversional activity, they don't need to know I am keeping records and they will appreciate the extra attention and stimulation".

Scenario 4 Length 400-500 words

Refer to the ANMC codes to discuss the ethical issues in relation to Kate's plan.

Sources

Consumers Health Forum of Australia, (2013) Informed Consent in Healthcare: An Issues Paper. https://www.chf.org.au/pdfs/chf/Informed-Consent-Issues-Paper.pdf (accessed 7 August 2014).

Forrester, K. & Griffiths, D. (2005) *Essentials of Law*, 2nd edn, Harcourt, Sydney.
Forrester, K. & Griffiths, D. (2010) *Essentials of Law for Health Professionals*, 3rd edn, Elsevier, Chatswood, NSW.
Kennedy, R. & Richards, J. (2004) *Integrating Human Service Law and Practice*, Oxford University Press, Melbourne.
Lawrence, S., Willmott, L., Milligan, E., Winch, S., White, B. & Parker, M. (2012) Autonomy versus futility? Barriers to good clinical practice in end-of-life care: a Queensland case. *MJA* 196 (6) 404-405.
MacFarlane, P. (1995) *Health Law*, 2nd edn, The Federation Press, Sydney.
MacFarlane, P. J. & Reid, S. J. (2003) *Queensland Health Law Handbook*, Queensland Dept. of Health, Brisbane.
MacLean, A. (2013) *Autonomy, Informed Consent and Medical Law: A Relational Challenge*. Cambridge University Press. Cambridge.
McIlwraith, J. & Madden, B. (2014) *Health Care & the Law*, 6th ed. Lawbook Co., Australia.
Mathews, B.P. (2010) Children and consent to medical treatment. In White, Benjamin P., McDonald, Fiona, & Willmott, Lindy (Eds.) *Health Law in Australia*. Thomson Lawbook Co., Sydney, New South Wales, pp. 113-147.
Mountford, L. & Scanlan, T. (2013) A recent case against a radiologist underlines the need for fully informed consent from patients.
HG Alert: 3 October 2013. HopgoodGanim.
Scanlon, S. (1997) *The Legal Liability of Health Service Providers*, Final Report, Parliament of Victoria, Australia Law Reform Committee, Melbourne.
Skene, L. (2008) *Law and Medical Practice, Rights, duties, Claims and Defences*. 3rd edition, Australia, LexisNexus,
Solomon, W.D. (2002) The Encyclopedia of Ethics, www.saintmarys.edu/~incandel/doubleeffect.html (accessed 6 July 2014)
Staunton, P. & Chiarella, M. (2003) *Nursing and the Law*, 5th edn, Elsevier, Sydney.
Staunton, P. & Whyburn, B. (1997) *Nursing and the Law*, 4th edn, Harcourt Australia Pty Ltd, Sydney.
Wellington, P. MP, (2002) Care of Terminally-Ill Patients Bill 2002 (Qld), Second Reading Speech, Queensland Parliamentary Debates, 19 June 2002, p 1874.
White, B.P. Willmott, L. & Ashby, M. (2011) Palliative care, double effect and the law in Australia. *Internal Medicine Journal*,41(6), pp. 485-492.

Cases

Birkett v. Director-General of Family & Community Services & Others (unreported 3161/91), February 1994.
Cole v. Turner (1704) 6 Mod. 149; 87 E.R. 907.
Cardozo J in *Schleondorff v. Society of New York Hospitals* (1914).
Ellis v. Wallsend District Hospital (1989) *Aust. Torts Reports 80-259.*
F v. R (1983) SASR 189 *Gardner; re BWV* (2003) VSC 173.
Gardner; re BWV (2003) VSC 173.
Karpati v. Spira NSWSC, 6 June 1995.
Malette v. Shuman et al (1991) 2 Med LR.
Rogers v. Whitaker (1992) 175 CLR 479.

R v Adams (unreported, Central Criminal Court, Devlin J, 9 April 1957) reported at Palmer H. Dr Adams' Trial for Murder. Criminal Law Review 1957; 365–377.
R v Hood [2002] SC 123
R v Maxwell [2003] VSC 278
Schleondorff v. Society of New York Hospitals (1914) 211 NY 125.
Teik Huat Tai v. Saxon (1996) WASCA 113.
Tekanaw v. Millican (QDC, 11 February 1994).

Negligence

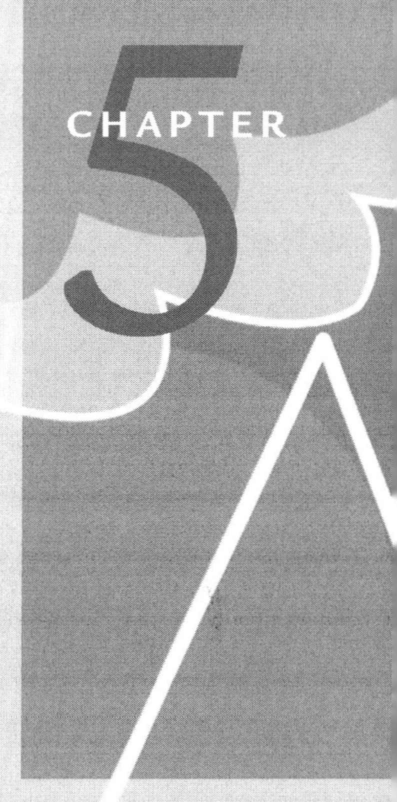

Learning outcomes

After studying this chapter you should be able to:

- Describe the role of the law in providing direction for health care practice.
- Apply legal and professional standards when assessing and responding to client needs, practice and policy situations, professional reporting and communication.
- Relate concepts of negligence law to clinical practice.
- Relate concepts of negligence law to policies governing medications.

Overview

You will note in any textbook relating to law and the health profession just how extensive the coverage for the tort of negligence is. This is the most common cause of action against health facilities and individuals. It is important to realise that there are many policies and legislation governing our lives that have evolved from actions in negligence.

Negligence is a tort and this area of civil law has grown over the past century. Negligence has evolved from an action to achieve adjustment of losses based on recognising liability if fault could be proved to an expanded, and still growing, concept that also recognises damage caused by omissions, that is, failure to act.

Trespass is now often seen as part of negligence. Think about issues of touching another person; this could be trespass on another person without consent, but today negligence captures this concept. Recall your readings on consent in Chapter 4. Negligence actions are often closely tied to the concept of consent.

You need to realise that negligence is not a state of mind. There are strict parameters and rules governing what could be identified as loss, harm or damage and equally strict rules about who can in fact be blamed for that damage.

A person can be found negligent even though they did not actually intend to harm another person.

- Negligent conduct is behaviour that results in unintended harm.

Consider this example. The case was about a woman residing in Florida who sued a nurse for negligence. During her pregnancy this woman attended a routine prenatal appointment at her hospital. While waiting she complained to the nurse of severe abdominal pain. Over the next hour and a half the mother complained of pain five times, and each time was told she would have to wait to be examined. When the mother was finally examined the foetal heart rate was only 60 to 70 beats per minute. An emergency caesarean was performed but the baby was born severely depressed and hypoxic and developed seizures within the first hour.

In this case the nurse did not intend to cause harm to the baby or the mother, but the nurse's failure to have the patient examined when she complained of severe abdominal pain and failure to recognise the onset of foetal distress was negligent.

A reasonably prudent and careful nurse would have had the patient examined by a doctor and recognised signs of foetal distress when the patient complained of acute abdominal pain.

The hospital settled this case for $2 million for severe brain injury to the newborn infant.

Another example:

Illinois Supreme Court's 1965 decision in *Darling v. Charleston Community Memorial Hospital*

The plaintiff in that case went to a hospital with a broken leg. After a cast was placed on it, he experienced great pain and his toes became swollen and dark, then cold and insensitive. Ultimately, his leg had to be amputated below the knee. He sued the hospital.

The jury found for the plaintiff.

Upholding that verdict, the Illinois High Court found that the jury could reasonably have concluded that skilled nurses would have recognized the dangerous circulation problems and informed hospital authorities if the attending physician failed to act.

Negligence: to deter and compensate

Fear of legal consequences can inhibit instead of giving guidance to health professionals. It is important to understand that a negligence action requires a number of elements to be satisfied before ever getting to court. The purpose is not to burden professionals or to control them through fear of legal consequences.

- A primary purpose of negligence law is to compensate those who have suffered harm and losses caused by others. Innocent victims are entitled to recompense for their injury, loss of work, financial expenses and other costs arising from the harm.

Liability, that is, holding the defendant responsible for their actions, is intended to deter the defendant from engaging in wrongful conduct in the future, and to send a message to society that there are consequences for negligent conduct that results in harm to others. Individuals and society benefit from the deterrence factor. The defendant will cease or reduce their unreasonably risky conduct in the future. In turn, society as a whole will benefit because the wrongdoer has been deterred from engaging in unsafe conduct.

Elements of negligence

Courts have developed concepts to explain these rules and identify what falls inside and outside of negligence. Each of the elements below must be satisfied before an action in negligence can be brought.

- There was a duty of care.
- The act or failure to act (omission) fell below the standard expected.
- The act or failure to act was the direct cause of damage.
- This damage was reasonably foreseeable.

Some of these concepts have become incorporated into our daily language; for example the idea of duty of care is familiar to health professionals. However, in a legal sense this term has a precise meaning and the way professionals use the term at times can be somewhat different from the legal meaning.

The courts have not only sought to set boundaries to what could be actionable in negligence but they have developed strategies to limit liability. By this they aimed to apportion blame, so if there was a claim that X did the harm, the liability of X is balanced against whether the plaintiff, the person seeking compensation (Y), actually contributed to their own harm.

- This is the idea of contributory negligence.

It is important to realise that a patient may be affected by anaesthetic, medications, fear and confusion so they would not be liable for 'contributing to their injury', such as if they got out of bed post operatively or failed to follow orders while under the influence of medications. There would need to be clear evidence for the patient comprehending risk and undertaking that risk. Staff can not displace responsibility back onto a patient if the patient is provoked or affected by something the medical staff did.

There are two other limitations:

1. Voluntary assumption of risk, where the person knowingly did something that resulted in damage.
2. When the claim is made for something that was in fact done a long time ago or the direct link between the damage and the cause is remote.

So it is not quite as easy as the public sometimes thinks simply to point to damage, point to a cause and get the court to award compensation. That said the risk of law suits being brought against health professionals is real. Litigation and its attendant costs to the health system is a genuine problem. Should an individual or an institution be sued there will be costs involved. Legal representation is not the least of these costs. The professional and personal costs can be severe. Just being required to be a witness in such an action can be a terrible experience for some people.

There are many hurdles to negotiate before a person can actually get a case to court in an action for negligence. Even when a case gets to court considerable time is spent establishing if all these hurdles have been satisfied.

The elements of a negligence action are critical guidelines for practice today. As we will see in Chapter 6, legislation and policies have been created to ensure the problems captured by any of these elements of negligence are avoided.

The language of negligence

Some of the common phrases that are linked to this area of the law have been used in earlier chapters. You are familiar with the concept of damage; this can be physical, financial or emotional harm. Liability is responsibility for the damage and compensation for that harm is generally called 'damages'; an award of damages to redress the harm can be made by the court to the plaintiff, against the defendant.

Negligence has some particular concepts, however. One of these is the *neighbour principle*, while others include duty of care, foreseeability and proximity.

Just as *Rogers v. Whitaker* is the key case for issues of consent, so the key case in negligence is *Donaghue v. Stevenson*. This was heard in 1932 by the House of Lords, which is the highest court of appeal in England. Lord Atkin stated many of the principles that today govern negligence issues in his findings of that case.

The case involved a woman who found the remains of a snail in her bottle of ginger beer and subsequently suffered a bout of gastroenteritis and nervous shock. Who could she sue for damages? The retailer? The manufacturer? Or the friend who bought her the drink? Until this case the law required that there had to be a clear relationship between the person who suffered damage and the person who caused that damage. Lord Atkin created a precedent by allowing her to sue the manufacturer and bottler of the drink. He said: 'The rule that you are to love your neighbour becomes in law, you must not injure your neighbour' (*Donaghue v. Stevenson* (1932)). This meant that Donaghue did not have to prove that there was a direct relationship between herself and the manufacturer (*proximity*). The court held that it was sufficient that the manufacturer could reasonably *foresee* that a defective product could harm users of that product. Further, the manufacturer had a *duty of care* to customers.

- So a neighbour is someone who can be reasonably foreseen as being affected by your actions, and there does not need to be immediate, direct physical proximity.
- Duty of care therefore captures those who delegate, those who have responsibility over their staff, students, volunteers and contractors, anyone whose actions could reasonably affect others by those actions.

Are you feeling overwhelmed and confused? Even if you grasped only some of the content it is obvious there are many issues to deal with. The basic issues are:

- In civil law the tort of negligence allows an individual (the plaintiff) to bring an action to claim for damages that have occurred as a result of an act or failure to act by the defendant.
- To bring an action the plaintiff must show that the defendant owed them a duty; this duty is one that is recognised by the law. For a health professional there is usually little room for argument about this element in most situations.

- The plaintiff must show that the defendant *breached* that duty, by falling below the required standard of care. As a professional the expected standard would be identified through reference to education, professional recognition, professional standards, experience and expertise. Codes of practice and scope of practice are sources of information the court will draw upon. The professional standard would be measured against 'what is reasonable in relation to the circumstances and other professionals who had the same background'; it would not be 'reasonable' to measure a student against a new graduate or a new graduate against a specialist nurse. *But* should there be evidence that the nurse deliberately worked outside of their level of knowledge and skill, or flouted policy or directives to remain within safe practice limits, this safety net would be lost.
- There must be 'actual' damage to the plaintiff.
- The damage must be attributable, have a reasonable connection to, the actions of the defendant.
- The plaintiff must not have contributed to this damage by their own behaviour.

Every element has case law exploring and arguing the concepts.

Activity

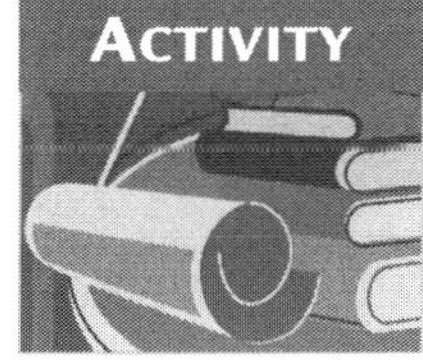

- Can a health professional provide more care for one individual than another or is there a minimum standard of care?
- How does the health professional know what are the parameters of care and what is their duty to the client?

Non-delegable duty: institutional liability

Not only individual practitioners can be found liable; a hospital owes a duty of care when a patient presents at the hospital. Among the many obligations is a safe environment for the client and visitors, competent staff, appropriate record keeping and appropriate and adequately maintained equipment.

Restriction on the activities of students, professional rules about delegation of duties and policies directing or limiting the actions of different classes of staff are the result of the risks of liability that an institution can incur.

Activity

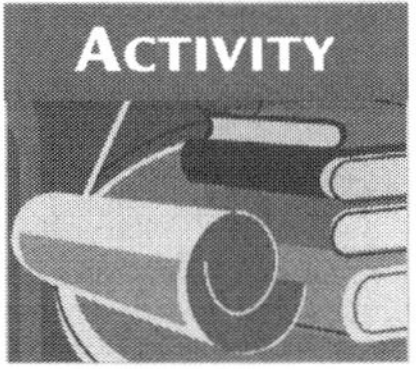

Read the extract below from *Health Business*, September 2003, and reflect on the content.

> Since the early 1980s, Australian courts have recognised a 'special duty' in some relationships such as those between a hospital and patients or a school authority and students. A health care institution owes a duty to ensure all reasonable care is taken in the performance of medical treatment it undertakes to provide.

This is known as a non-delegable duty of care and may apply where treatment and medical services are performed by visiting medical officers (VMOs), staff specialists, residents, nurses and others for private or public patients. Although the concepts of vicarious liability (where an employer may be liable for the negligence of its employee) and breach of a non-delegable duty of care appear similar they are very different.

Some features of a non-delegable duty of care:

- It cannot be delegated even to a suitably qualified doctor under a contract for services or to an independent contractor such as a VMO;
- It is not merely a duty to take reasonable care but a duty to ensure that reasonable care is taken;
- Breach of the duty by a health care institution will not arise because of breach by its agents or employees of their duties of care but because the institution itself breached its personal duty of care;
- Even where there is delegation of performance (for example, to a staff specialist) or a systemic failure, the health care institution will remain directly liable, rather than vicariously liable for negligent performance by the delegate.

When will the duty arise?

Where a health care provider has undertaken to provide care, supervision or control of the patient or where it has assumed responsibility for the management of the patient's care and safety. The scope of a health care provider's duty is determined by the services it has undertaken to provide.

A look at the cases

Albrighton v RPAH (1980) – The patient was treated by staff chosen by the hospital. The hospital was found to owe a non-delegable duty of care to the patient in respect of treatment provided by all of its 'staff' including surgeons and consultants.

Ellis v Wallsend District Hospital (1989) – The hospital was found not to owe a non-delegable duty of care to a patient in respect of treatment provided to the patient in the hospital by a neurosurgeon engaged directly by the patient.

Ren v Mukerjee (1997) – A hospital failed to provide adequate obstetric services over a long weekend causing a delay in performing a caesarean section to deliver the plaintiff resulting in his cerebral palsy. As it was the hospital which provided the negligent service due to an inadequate system, the doctor was not at fault.

Elliott v Bickerstaff (1999) – A surgeon sued for leaving a surgical sponge in the plaintiff's abdominal cavity was entitled to rely on theatre staff to count the sponges used during the procedure.

Conclusion

Hospitals, medical centres, pathology providers, nursing homes, other health care institutions and professionals owe a non-delegable duty of care to patients the extent of which depends upon the services the institution or professional has undertaken to provide.

(Tress Cox Lawyers Health Law Division)

Breach of duty

Breach of duty is the failure to meet the standard of care the law requires. The court will take into consideration all of the relevant circumstances. Where a child or client with a known disability or mental illness is involved there is no doubt that a higher level of care would be expected. The more risk there is involved in a procedure the more precautions should be taken. The law does recognise that situations occur where an error of judgment, a wrong diagnosis or a mistake can be the cause of the damage. If such a thing were equally as likely to happen to someone with ordinary levels of competence, who was of the same professional level as the defendant, it is unlikely to become a successful action in negligence.

So your responsibility will be to ask yourself some critical questions whenever you are working in a professional capacity.

- Do I have all the facts and do I know what I am doing and why I am doing it?
- Is there a policy or procedure that specifies whether I can do this? Does it specify how it should be done? Are there any limitations on my doing this?
- Is there someone more competent, more experienced or safer than I am in this particular circumstance who would be more appropriate to do this?
- Can I point to evidence that shows that this is within my level of competence?
- Have I documented my actions, my findings and my professional assessment of the outcome of my action?
- A definition of nursing negligence is when *a nurse who is fully capable to care does not use such care as a reasonably prudent nurse would use, and as a result the patient suffers in some untoward way.*
- It is not carelessness but can be generally defined as conduct that is culpable because it falls short of what a reasonable person would do to protect another individual from a foreseeable risks of harm.
- It could be such negligent behavior that it is categorized as a crime: Gross negligence means conduct or a failure to act that is so reckless that it demonstrates a substantial lack of concern for whether an injury will result.

Legislation in a number of states actually gives direction to limit the liability of persons who have been sued for a negligent act by specifying that if the person had taken all reasonable precautions for any foreseeable risks and was working within established professional and institutional guidelines, they satisfy the required standard.

These Civil Liability Acts have been passed in each state since 2002. In four States, the legislation took the form of Civil Liability Acts (New South Wales, Queensland, Tasmania and Western Australia), in South Australia the legislation took the form of an amendment to an existing Act Civil Liability Act 1936 (SA) and in Victoria the legislation took the form of amendments to the

Wrongs Act 1958 (Vic). The Australian Capital Territory enacted the Civil Law (Wrongs) Act 2002, and in the Northern Territory the reforms were made in the Personal Injuries (Liabilities and Damages) Act 2002. There have been reviews and amendments made to some state Acts. For example Queensland introduced amendments to Queensland's Civil Liability Act, there has been an increase in the amount of payments to victims.

This has not solved all the problems related to clarifying the many issues involved in negligence claims, every Act uses different terms and rules. However although there are some differences between the jurisdictions, these Acts do deal with issues arising from the provision of professional services and confirm that the standard expected will be considered to have been met if there is agreement among the profession that the actions were accepted professional practice.

As long as there is agreement about what is the professional standard and the staff member can show they did conform to the standard of care, this can be a defence to a claim of negligence. The standard expected of an experienced clinician will be higher than that expected of a novice. The court will use various means to determine the standard expected. Documents from the institution such as policy and procedure manuals, institutional and professional organisations' practice guidelines, peers and experts can be called upon.

In chapter 1, there was a discussion about the way the law changes in response to society's expectations and new ways of looking at things. Negligence actions have received great media coverage. Many actions have been an attempt to gain enormous compensation for injuries that were, perhaps caused by the plaintiff failing to take reasonable care. Other cases where medical staff were held liable for claims impacted on insurance premiums and willingness of practitioners to work in particular areas. An example of recent limitation to court actions created by both courts and legislation is the issue of "wrongful life" cases. These are situations when a child brings an action against a doctor who the child claims failed or negligently diagnosed, a critical condition in the mother. A number of cases related to failure to diagnose rubella during the first trimester as the cause of disability and it was usually argued that would have been grounds for the mother to seek abortion. In May 2006, the majority of the High Court of Australia rejected wrongful life, refusing to accept that life can be considered a compensable harm. This means that children who are born disabled as a result of a doctor's (admitted) negligence cannot claim damages. Parents are able to pursue 'wrongful birth' claims if the child (disabled or not) is the outcome of a negligently performed sterilisation procedure (*Cattanach v Melchior*, (2003) 199 ALR 131).

It is important to note that here the issue is professional practice in relation to work, not the provision of information subsequent to obtaining consent. The courts have been quite clear about the need to provide information about the risks and benefits of a procedure having to be more than generally accepted practice; for consent the particular needs of the individual, in every particular circumstance, must be met (see Chapter 4).

Claiming against your employer

If you or another employee chose to sue an employer for negligence, even if there is evidence of damage and all the elements of negligence are satisfied there are, particularly in relation to situations where a worker sues an employer, established defences. These are in relation to 'contributory negligence'. As an employee you work within a number of regulations and contractual obligations that will be explored later. There is legislation in most states which directs the court when making an award for compensation to reduce the amount of compensation if the plaintiff (employee) contributed to their own injury.

For example, the *Queensland Work Cover Act 1996* specifies that contributory negligence can be found if the injured employee:

- failed to comply with the employer's workplace health and safety instructions;
- failed to use protective clothing and equipment provided;
- failed to use anything provided to reduce the risk of injury;
- interfered with or misused something provided to reduce the risk of injury;
- was adversely affected by the intentional consumption of a substance that induces impairment;
- failed, without reasonable excuse, to attend any relevant safety training organised by the employer during work hours.

At this point recall your experiences with 'no lift' and 'manual handling' education. At the time you may have found the theory addressing policy, legislation and responsibilities a bit boring or irrelevant to your need to master the techniques of patient transfer. Now, looking at the list above, it should be clear just how similar to the common law principles of negligence and the legislation that theory is. For anyone wishing to look at occupational health and safety legislation further, a national index can be found at <http://australia.gov.au/topics/health-and-safety/occupational-health-and-safety>.

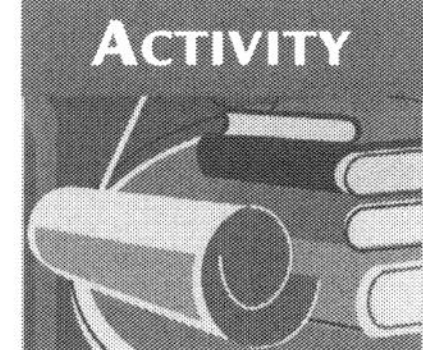

Activity

Read the scenario below and answer the questions following. Answers have been provided for the purposes of broadening understanding of various interpretations, legal reasoning and relevant issues.

> Student Karla, while participating in clinical experience, assisted Mr Green to transfer from his bed to the chair. While supporting this very tall, overweight and fearful client, Karla stepped backwards and tripped over the bag left by Mrs Green, which had fresh clothes and magazines for Mr Green. Karla did manage to sit Mr Green in the chair without his suffering any ill effects, but she suffered a severe lower back injury. She wants to seek compensation for her financial losses as she had to drop all subjects, was unable to keep her part-time job and had considerable medical and rehabilitation expenses.

Apply the principles of negligence and answers the following questions.

- Who has a duty of care to Karla?
- Was the duty of care breached?

- Was there conduct on the part of the person who had a duty of care to Karla the cause of her injury?
- Was it reasonably foreseeable that Karla could be injured in the course of her activities?

Answers and discussion

The university and the institution have a duty towards Karla. This is recognised by the fact that both facilities carry insurance and, in fact, for student placement the hospital requires considerable documentation and evidence from the university to support appropriate placement.

However, the question cannot be resolved by this first element alone. The issue that now arises is whether there is evidence that either or both the university or institution failed to ensure Karla was safe, and was in a position where her education, capabilities and the environment were sufficient to allow her to carry out this duty.

- Has Karla been taught, practised and assessed in the techniques of safe client transfer? If yes, did this situation fall within the level of her skill and practice? If no, did the situation 'coerce' Karla or did she choose to do something beyond her level of expertise and knowledge?
- Was there something in the environment or in the expectation of providing care for Mr Green that was the responsibility of the institution that could not reasonably be within Karla's knowledge or abilities?
- Has Karla the skill to assess client mobility status and/or is there documentation that could be relied on to give her direction as to client mobility needs?
- Has Karla been taught to do a risk assessment of the environment and to take steps to create a hazard-free transfer?
- Did Karla actually assess the client in relation to her own skills, ability and the circumstances?

So the many and various considerations could come down to: was Karla and any other student with the same level of skill and knowledge able to make an informed decision based on education and experience about the client, herself and the situation in relation to carrying out this transfer?

If there is proof Karla has had education in relation to client assessment, risk assessment and practised safe transfer, what gap, if any, might exist that would enable the court to see the institutions as being liable instead of Karla as being the cause of her injury for failing to adhere to policy?

If there is no proof Karla had sufficient education to perform this task safely, is there any proof to show that Karla has knowingly gone outside of her scope of practice and chosen to put herself and the client at risk?

Instead of asking 'Can I do this, is it legal?' the professional is expected to use education and judgment to answer the questions 'Is this within my role and function? Do I have sufficient knowledge and skill to carry this out safely?'

No one would wish to deny Karla financial support and help; accidents do happen and uncontrolled, unexpected situations occur every day. The court does consider all the circumstances but will be constrained and limited by competing evidence. Just because Karla had been taught to assess and take precautions and did not, her inexperience could be seen as a balance to that.

Scope of practice and negligence

With a moments reflection it should be obvious that an accountable nurse would apply thought and care to their decisions in practice if they wanted to avoid harm or disciplinary action. We will investigate matters of governance in a later chapter but here in relation to the concept of negligence it is worth noting that the concepts of boundaries of practice or scope of practice would apply to the individual nurse seeking to justify their actions and defend against a claim of failing in their duty of care, failing to adhere to standards of practice or failing to take steps to prevent foreseeable/predictable harm.

The term "scope of practice" is used to define the actions, procedures, activities that are permitted by law for a specific profession. It outlines restrictions to what the law permits, based on specific experience and educational qualifications.

In the real world, experience and continuing education increase the nurse's knowledge beyond what was documented as in their formal education. Therefore some formal and approved decision making process should be implemented to ensure not only the action taken was justified but to provide a defence for any questions raised.

The Nursing and Midwifery Board of Australia has published a fact sheet:

Scope of practice for registered nurses and midwives, February 2013; go to NMBA publications and guidelines. This clarifies roles and identifies a range of skills and expertise held by the professions.

Another publication is the national framework for the development of decision-making tools for nursing and midwifery practice (2007). The stated rational:

Decisions about nursing or midwifery practice in response to the rapid and dynamic changes that are occurring within nursing, midwifery and the environment of practice need to be planned rather than ad hoc. Unplanned responses could result in wide variation in practice between individuals of similar background and experience and between similar settings. Effective decision-making tools provide a framework where quality and safety are central considerations in decisions about nursing or midwifery practice allowing:

- new services/practices to be introduced safely and in an orderly way
- everyday practice to be undertaken confidently and competently
- delegation decisions to be safe

This document provides a template for both the profession and the public and should the worst happen the courts, to determine if the nurse or midwife did adhere to expected standards of best practice. There is also a flowchart available from the same site to give direction for decisions. Nursing-practice-decision-flowchart-2013.PDF

Activity

Download the document and peruse the content comparing what you now know are the elements of negligence to identify how following such a framework would avoid getting into a situation that might have legal consequences.

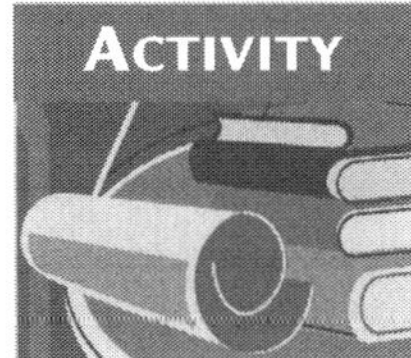

Case relating to scope of practice

Specialist doctor criticized – nurse deregistered for botox injections 13 June 2014

A TRIBUNAL has cancelled the registration of a Sydney cosmetic medicine nurse, stressing the need to deter others from overstepping the bounds in injecting patients with restricted drugs such as Botox without adequate supervision.

NCAT expressed some sympathy for the registered nurse, Rosalie Piper, and was critical of her employer, the burns expert and plastic surgeon Dr Peter Haertsch. During 2009–2011, it said RN Piper worked one day per week as a nurse injector at Dr Haertsch's Epping clinic using cosmetic injectable medicines supplied by the doctor. She also supplied and administered the drugs to clients at a day spa in Collaroy. The seven medications contained botulinum toxins and hyaluronic acid, used in tissue augmentation. All were restricted substances under Schedule 4 of the Poisons List.

The Tribunal noted evidence from Dr Haertsch that when RN Piper commenced work at his clinic she adopted a system that had been in place for 18 years, and that most clients had been treated by the previous nurse injector.

The nurse said she had presumed, in taking over from the previous nurse, that the practice was appropriate and that she had professional indemnity insurance for her work as a nurse injector. But in acting without the direct supervision of a medical practitioner and without authorised prescriptions, RN Piper breached a 2005 protocol governing the use of S4 drugs for cosmetic procedures by nurses (See http://www0.health.nsw.gov.au/policies/pd/2013/pdf/PD2013_043.pdf). She supplied and administered the medications obtained by Dr Haertsch to 29 patients at his practice, and on more than 230 occasions involving 97 patients at the day spa, between mid 2009 and late 2011.

"The nurse reimbursed Dr Haertsch for the medications with a sizeable share of the fee she received from the patients receiving the injections from her," the Tribunal said. While the nurse would not have engaged in such conduct without the supply of restricted substances by Dr Haertsch, she did not take sufficient responsibility to ensure she was within the law, the Tribunal said.

It found RN Piper guilty of professional misconduct, cancelled her registration for three months and ordered her to pay costs.

"The Tribunal hopes the orders will remind and deter all nurses working in this field of cosmetic medicine to ensure they are practising within the law. The administration of Botox and dermal fillers is a medical procedure that must be medically supervised," it said. Dr Peter Haertsch is scheduled to attend a Professional Standards Committee Hearing on 30 July 2014 (Medical Error Action Group, 2014).

Medical negligence: medical malpractice

This is no different legally from any other action in negligence but when the damage is caused by a health professional it has become usual to use this label. Medical malpractice can occur when a health care professional fails to exercise the degree of care that a reasonable health care professional would exercise under the same or similar circumstances. Medical malpractice is the area of law that deals with negligence claims against health care professionals. Although medical malpractice is frequently perceived as conduct that is somehow worse than mere negligence, this perception is wrong because medical malpractice is simply ordinary negligence by a health care provider that causes some injury to the client.

In past years nurses were unlikely to be sued in a negligence action. However, as nurses exercise more autonomy, their legal liability has changed.

Doctors, like nurses, paramedical and allied health staff, have a duty of care. Most medical cases revolve around misdiagnosis or a failure to diagnose a problem, but, as discussed in *Rogers v. Whitaker,* findings of negligence in relation to failing to provide adequate, appropriate or timely information to a client nullified the client's consent and opened the way for a compensation award.

Prior to *Rogers v. Whitaker* the standard expected had been articulated in an earlier English case where a patient sued the doctor after sustaining pelvic fractures while undergoing ECT (*Bolam v. Friern Hospital Management Committee* (1957)). The client claimed the doctor had failed to administer relaxant medication, failed to appropriately restrain the client during the treatment and had not given the client any warning of the risks of the treatment before obtaining consent.

- That case established the Bolam Test: a doctor was not in breach of their duty of care if they practised to the standard accepted by responsible peers. The courts would accept medical opinion as to what the standard should be.

Now the courts will not only ask what is the practice of the medical profession but look at what standard conforms to what the law expects.

Application to practice

APPLICATION to practice

Duty of care arises where, through our relationship, proximity, professional responsibility or contract of work, it is foreseeable that our actions or failure to act will affect others. The standard of that care, what is expected of us, is determined by what is reasonable in the circumstances, what would be expected from another professional with the same experience and education and what is best practice of the profession at large. Further, the court will expect the professional to be able to identify and meet the specific needs of a client.

It is important to note that there are standards that are not negotiable. For example, legislation sets out absolute requirements for drug storage, labelling and administration. Failure to adhere to these is evidence of a breach of duty, failure to satisfy standards.

Institutional policies and professional standards and guidelines are more than simple procedural recommendations. If these are aimed at ensuring safety, providing client protection from high-risk procedures and protecting the public from unsafe or unqualified staff, failure to adhere to these will provide evidence that standards were not met. As a result of cases such as *Rogers v. Whitaker* the National Health and Medical Research Council (NHMRC) established guidelines that make very clear the obligations for disclosure and information to clients. These guidelines will be used by the court as evidence of standards expected by the profession. The NHMRC guidelines can be found at <www.cqu.edu.au/research/research_services/nhmrcstatement.htm>.

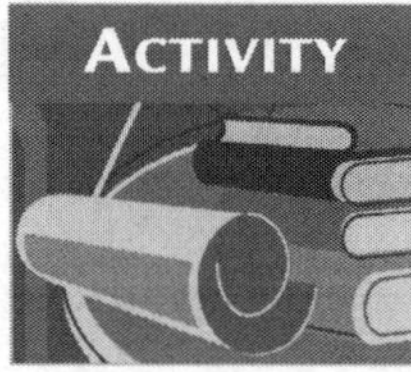

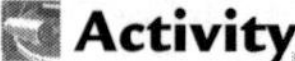

Activity

Before moving on to the next concepts take a moment to reflect and apply concepts to a scenario.

Scenario

During handover the night staff reported everything was satisfactory with one of your allocated patients, Mr G who is a diabetic going for a CAT scan today at 9 am. He had been given his insulin as ordered. You proceed between 7–8.30 am to work with clients in another room intending to check Mr G is ready for transfer and gather his paperwork before 9 am. When you get to his room he is confused, sweating, his IV drip has run out and the fluid balance indicates he has had no oral intake or IV fluids for 5 hours. No observations have been carried out since yesterday.

Questions

Can you identify where the duty of care lies in the scenario?
What elements of negligence would apply to this situation?
What standards have been failed?
Was the outcome predictable?

Reflection

Most nurses wonder if it wasn't the night staff who failed the duty of care. The problem is the day nurse did not check the patient, did not confirm his status and thus failed to see the inevitable consequences of an IV running out plus the effects of insulin.

While the night staff might be questioned about the IV it is policy and competencies that direct the nurse to check all patients on accepting them as their assigned responsibility. The lack of observations would also be a matter of questioning all staff but again responsibility for checking status will still lie with the day nurse.

The cause of the clients change and risk to his health are predictable.

Failure to monitor and the known effects of insulin post administration would be considered knowledge the day staff nurse must have.

The client suffered a predictable consequence of failures of staff to satisfy standards of care. Most situations are the result of oversights and missed care by a series of staff, rather than one person. However in this scenario, the day nurse would be the most likely to suffer investigation leading to severe sanctions. The other staff may well be disciplined for their failures, but the day nurse, IF they had worked to policies and standards could have prevented the harm to the client.

Defences to claims of negligence

In a claim of negligence the plaintiff must prove the following:

- The plaintiff must prove on the balance of probabilities (civil standard of proof) that the health professional had a duty of care.

- We have looked at the standards expected, how these are established and legislation that provides a defence; however, in every case the plaintiff must prove that the care or actions of the health professional fell below the standard expected.
- The plaintiff must prove that there was damage *and* that the damage was a direct result of the actions of the defendant *and* that the damage suffered was reasonably foreseeable.

Mention has already been made of contributory negligence, assumption of risk and the need to establish a link between the plaintiff and the damage being claimed. These issues will be revisited now.

Cause of damage, who is at fault?

The legal concept is *causation*. The person claiming that damage occurred must prove that damage was a direct cause of the act or failure to act of the health professional.

- Contributory negligence is where the client has or has not done something and as a result the damage is, to some extent, their fault.

This is not always easy to prove. If a client were to worsen their condition by refusing to remain on bed rest it might indicate a failure of the health professional to educate, inform or provide safety rails. If a client were to fail to adhere to a medication regime and suffered complications is it because the health professional did not provide adequate information or did not identify client reluctance and find a better alternative?

Before you get too anxious remember that the courts apply 'reasonable in the circumstances' tests. Individuals are expected to avoid injuring themselves. Denning J explains it thus:

> Contributory negligence is a man's carelessness in looking after his own safety. He is guilty of contributory negligence if he ought reasonably to have foreseen that, if he did not act as a reasonable prudent man, he might hurt himself (*Froom v. Butcher* (1976).

Here is a case that provides a good example. A client did not mention to his doctor he had experienced rectal bleeding, a significant symptom of bowel cancer. As a result bowel cancer was not diagnosed until too late. The court held that the client's failure to report contributed to his situation (*Lochner v. Turner* (1995)).

Another defence that today has little relevance to areas outside of sport is that of voluntary assumption of risk. The plaintiff chose to do something that had known risks of injury.

Delay in bringing an action can provide a defence. Legislation and the courts have limitations on how much time can elapse between the damage and initiating an action. In some situations this is a year and a day; for personal injury claims it is three or six years depending on the jurisdiction. Damage as a child can be brought as an action when they are an adult.

A defendant to a case can in some circumstances point to another who was involved to share the burden of defending an action. This joint liability has been used where the harm has been attributed to a junior doctor but the doctor can show that the institution created the risk in requiring that doctor to act outside of their level of expertise (*Jones v. Manchester Corporation* (1954)).

Vicarious liability

This doctrine shifts the responsibility for financial compensation from a negligent employee to the institution. Hospitals and other services have a responsibility to their clients. This is referred to as a non-delegable duty of care.

The health care institution is responsible for ensuring staff, equipment and the environment are appropriate to the needs of the client. The education and qualifications of the staff, the adequacy of staff numbers and appropriate skill mix of staff in all circumstances is the institution's responsibility.

The doctrine of vicarious liability brings this non-delegable duty into play. Although innocent of causing the harm, when it can be shown that an employee has been the cause of negligent damage, if the employee had acted within the scope of their employment the facility can be liable for the compensation. The negligent actions of an employee or contractor remain the personal responsibility of that employee *but* when it comes to paying damages (financial compensation) the facility takes that burden.

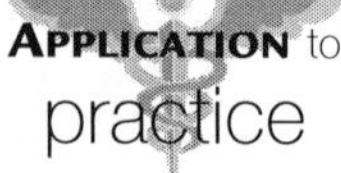

Application to practice

As long as a person is under the 'control' of an employer, that is, the employer in spite of the level of expertise or specialised skill or form of contract, has the right to direct that health professional or employee, the doctrine of vicarious liability can apply. The institution can be relieved of financial liability, in part or for the whole amount, if it can show that the employee was not acting within the scope of their employment. If the institution seeks to recover all the money this is called 'indemnity from the employee'; partial recovery is called a 'contribution from the employee'.

The facility has to prove that the negligent action was caused by an employee who, as Parke J has put it, 'is off on a frolic of their own' (*Joel v. Morison* (1834)). What this means is if the employee has deviated from the normal and expected route when driving for their work to carry on some personal business it would be difficult to shift liability to the employer should that deviation lead to an accident. If an employee chose to do something normal, say, taking a coffee break, but decided to go to the roof and dropped the cup on a pedestrian's head while they were sitting in a forbidden or restricted area, again the employer would seek to recover from the employee what was paid in damages.

The key once the tests for employee status have been satisfied is whether the negligent employee was working within authorised boundaries or had chosen to do something that was expressly forbidden.

Working for an agency; independent contracts

The common law recognises the right of an employer found to be vicariously liable, as a result of an employee's negligent action, to seek compensation from that employee. This is not common, however; the risk of industrial action and the fact that insurers for the employer cover the payout means that employers tend to leave the matter there. Legislation in a number of states has been passed to prevent employers taking such action but where the employee can be shown to have acted outside the course of their duties and the actions can be defined as serious and wilful misconduct, the door remains open for the employer to seek contribution to the costs awarded.

Private-duty or agency nurses are not employed by the agency; they pay the agency a fee for finding them work. This fee might be paid direct to the agency by the institution or service or the nurse themselves. While the doctrine of vicarious liability might come into play should the nurse be working in an institution where there is 'control' over the nurse's actions such as policies, procedures and guidelines, in a private home or similar circumstance the nurse will be personally liable.

Direct employment by a client for nurses' services is relatively common. Home birth midwives are an example. For agency or privately hired nurses or health staff, having indemnity insurance would be an important consideration. However, the cost of indemnity insurance for all Australians has risen enormously. Media coverage of this issue has been extensive. The costs of and numbers of large awards have meant availability of insurance or the costs of premiums has led many health professionals to withdraw from private practice.

Recommended reading

Nelson, T. 2003, 'Pressure ulcers in Australia: patterns of litigation and risk management issues', *Primary Intention*; 11(4); 183-184, 186-187 at <www.awma.com.au/journal/library/1104_02.pdf> (accessed 9 July 2014)

An article proposing that pressure ulcers are grounds for an action in negligence makes interesting reading. The issues in relation to just how the tort law is applied are discussed.

Activity

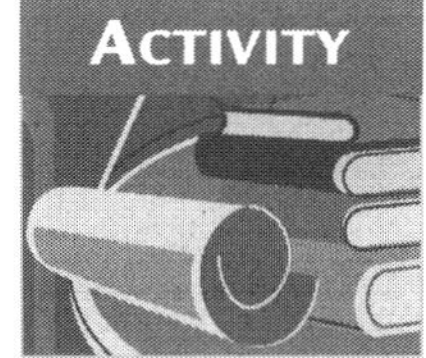

For information on medical indemnity, go to the Centre of Independent Studies, <www.cis.org.au/publications/.../2460-feature-insuring-against-negligence> (accessed 9 July 2014), and search for 'Insuring against Negligence: Medical Indemnity in Australia' by Julian Morris. This article, published in 2002, looked at the relationship between negligence and how courts have dealt with the issues that claims have raised compared with insurance and costs that cannot be predicted accurately in the environment where each case is treated differently. This set the background for Australian parliaments developing legislation that limited compensation claims.

Another idea the article explores is the way a negligence claim is seen by the health practitioner (personally and professionally devastating to their reputation and skills), and the perceptions of both the individual and legal representatives (a way to compensate for errors or problems that arise in the course of a treatment).

Morris explores concepts of negligence in relation to medical practice and argues that the High Court's dismissal of the Bolam Test (*Rogers v Whitaker*) to determine a practitioners actions created great uncertainty. The Bolam Test only required evidence that the practitioner abided by standards of practice accepted by the profession. The need to individualise and cover all potential issues had led to very defensive practices and increased vulnerability.

The issue that was spread nationally made practitioners vulnerable as well as the burden of the costs of legal actions and the volume of compensation payments. A number of inquiries were held due to pressure by Members of Parliament, community groups and commentators such as Morris. At the time it was clear that the costs to practitioners for adequate insurance were spiralling up as the number of compensation payments increased. The number of legal actions relating to public liability and actions in negligence were escalating every year. The Insurance Council of Australia had reported that from 55,000 claims in 1998 there had been an increase of 33,000 by 2000 (Lozusic, 2002).

- What effect do you think a claim of negligence would have onyou?
- In light of these numbers, how likely is it that you or a colleague might find themselves involved in litigation?

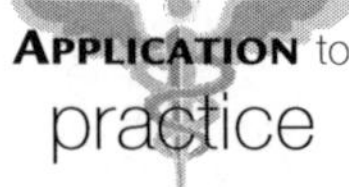

Application to practice

While most nurses are fully aware of their personal and professional accountability, they tend to believe that if a claim was made against them, the doctrine of vicarious liability will ensure the facility they work for, not them individually, will be responsible for paying compensation costs. This may not be the case. Midwives who practice independently and nurses who contract their services independently must have medical indemnity against claims, that is, insurance. The growth in the volume of claims in Australia indicates social change. Patients are aware of their rights. The existence of legislation to limit the amounts of awards and impose restrictions on when and why a claim can be made does not remove the chance of having a claim made against an individual or a facility.

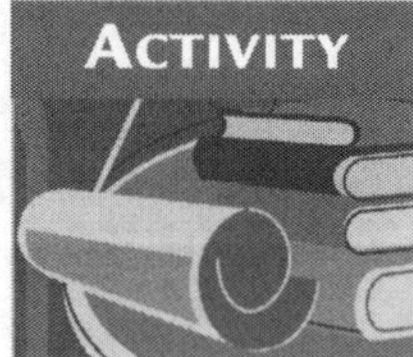

Activity

Prior to the transfer from State regulation of nursing and midwifery to a National Health Practitioner Registration and Accreditation, many nursing boards and councils had developed publications giving guidance about scope of practice and other issues as well as accepting the Australian Nurse and Midwifery Accreditation Council (ANMAC) standards and codes. In preparation for the national changes the ANMAC undertook the development of a number of coordinated activities to ensure national consistency for nurses and midwives.

One of these publications is: A National Framework for Decision Making by Nurses and Midwives on Scopes of Practice: (National DMF) (2009). If you did not undertake the activity noted earlier in the chapter, take time now to find and download the National Decision making framework.

No matter where you study and practise the concepts in this document will have relevance; however, at this time, in relation to the issue of an action for negligence, read Pages 9–11 which gives guidelines about delegation: ask yourself how you might be vulnerable to a claim if you were a registered nurse who delegated responsibility for care to an enrolled nurse. (*Hint*: Read the section on accountability.)

Summary

This chapter brought to your attention some very complex terms in relation to the tort of negligence. There have been many cases exploring every concept discussed and with subtle differences in interpretations of each element, each context and each legal concept it is easy to be overwhelmed. Health professionals are not the only group who are anxious about the risks and liabilities of their actions should damage occur to another person. Over the past decade the complexities of this law, the costs to the individual and community in legal actions and the perception that there have been 'frivolous claims' upheld by courts have brought legislators into the picture. A desire to take control over extraordinary payments (compensation) – where judges/juries awarded costs that could be seen as punitive (punishment) rather than simply compensating the particular damage – was evident in most common law jurisdictions. The public's perception that 'acting' as hurt was going to get you a huge court settlement was another issue. The tendency to seek compensation for what in other times were 'accidents' plus the massive growth in insurance premiums to cover the costs have in fact led to considerable control over the area. However, the concepts embedded in and resulting from these common law cases are still valid and still give direction to health professional practice.

Practice assignment question

In April of 2014 RN White was employed by the Christian Nursing Home Group and was based at the "Victory Unit" of the Residences as a Registered Nurse and nurse in-charge of the Unit.

1. On 1st May she witnessed Hilda, a care provider drag Mr Brown by his ankles along a cement path into the Unit.
2. She failed to record or report the incident.
3. Ms White in her role as RN soon assessed the client Mr Brown and applied clean dry dressings to abrasions on both elbows, helped the client change out of torn clothes and saw bruising on ankles, buttocks and scalp.
4. Ms White also failed to record any injuries sustained by Mr Brown as a result of being dragged along the path.
5. Mr Brown's daughter saw the injuries, heard about what had happened from another client and intends to see a lawyer.

Discuss relevant issues in relation to the elements of negligence. Length 1500 words

Sources

Commonwealth Treasury (Ipp Report) (2002) *Review of the Law of Negligence*, <http://revofneg.treasury.gov.au/content/review2.asp.> (accessed June 2006).

Fleming, J.G. (1987) *The Law of Torts*, 7th edn, The Law Book Company Ltd, NSW.

Forrester, K. & Griffiths, D. (2005) *Essentials of Law*, 2nd edn, Harcourt, Sydney.

Forrester, K. & Griffiths, D. (2010) *Essentials of Law for Health Professionals*, 3rd edn, Elsevier, Chatswood, NSW.

Health Business, 2003, September, Health Law Division of Tress Cocks & Maddox.

Kennedy, R. & Richards, J. (2004) *Integrating Human Service Law and Practice*, Oxford University Press, Melbourne.

Lozusic, R. (2002) Public Liability. Briefing Paper No 7/02. New South Wales Parliamentary Library. Available at <www.parliament.nsw.gov.au/ WEB_FEED/PHWebContent.nsf/PHPages/LibraryPublications> (accessed 7 July 2014).

MacFarlane, P. (1995) *Health Law*, 2nd edn, The Federation Press, Sydney.

MacFarlane, P. J. & Reid, S. J. (2003) *Queensland Health Law Handbook*, Queensland Dept of Health, Brisbane.

Morris, G., Cook, C., Creyke, R. & Geddes, R. (2001) *Laying Down the Law*, 5th edn, Butterworths, Sydney.

Morris, J. (2000) 'Insuring against negligence: medical indemnity in Australia', *Policy*, Vol. 18, no. 3, 10–15, <www.cis.org.au/policy/Spring02/polspring02-2.htm> (accessed 7 July 2014).

Nursing and Midwifery Board Australia (2013) Guidelines and Publications National Framework for Decision Making <http://www.nursingmidwiferyboard.gov.au/Codes-Guidelines-Statements/FAQ/Scope-of-practice-for-registered-nurses-and-midwives.aspx> (accessed 7 July 2014)

Queensland Health Law Handbook, Queensland Dept of Health, Brisbane.

Richards, B., de Zwart, M. & Ludlow, K. (2012) *Tort Law Principles*, Thomson Reuters, Australia.

Staunton, P. & Chiarella, M. (2003) *Nursing and the Law*, 5th edn, Elsevier, Sydney.

Staunton, P. & Whyburn, B. (1997) *Nursing and the Law*, 4th edn, Harcourt Australia Pty Ltd, Sydney.

White, B., Wilmott, L. & McDonald, F. (2014) *Health Law in Australia*, 2nd edn, Thomson Reuters, Australia.

Cases

Bolam v. Friern Hospital Management Committee (1957) 1WLR 582.

Cattanach v Melchior [2003] HCA 38; (2003) 215 CLR 1

Donaghue v. Stevenson (1932) AC 562 per Lord Atkin at 580.

Froom v. Butcher (1976) QB 291.

Joel v. Morison (1834) 6 C. & P. 501.

Jones v. Manchester Corporation (1954) 2 QB 852.

Lochner v. Turner (1995) Court of Appeal Qld, unreported.

Rogers v Whitaker (1992) 175 CLR 479.

Negligence: relationship to institutional policies

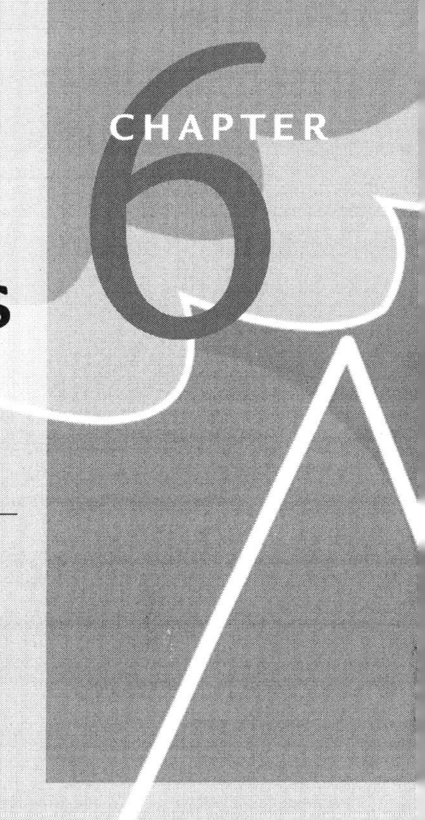

Learning outcomes

After studying this chapter you should be able to:

- Show an understanding of practices and procedures in clinical settings that reflect policies.
- Apply legal and professional standards when assessing and responding to client needs, practice and policy situations, professional reporting and communication.
- Discuss guidelines for effective recording that meets legal requirements.
- Demonstrate an understanding of the legal ramifications for incident reporting, report writing and documentation.

Overview

Chapter 5 introduced the tort of negligence and the components of a civil law action in negligence. The principles of negligence and the elements that must be satisfied to initiate an action to gain compensation for damages were covered. As you have seen, these principles have been taken up in professional standards and provide the basis for guidelines for professionals.

The element or principle in an action for negligence that the defendant owed the plaintiff a duty of care was discussed. This principle raises the idea that in general people must consider those who could be affected by their actions. In law this is often referred to as the 'neighbour principle'. It is obvious that the health professional has a duty of care and, unlike a manufacturer or retail business, it isn't hard to identify the relationship and obligations that exist between health professionals and the public.

The issue is more likely to be 'Was it reasonably foreseeable that the act or failure to act would cause damage?' It is just as likely that doing something badly can cause as much damage as not doing something, so avoidance of responsibility is not an option where there is a professional relationship. This level of responsibility does not usually extend beyond the work environment. However, if your position and knowledge gives someone a belief in you, such that they act on your comments even outside of work, and it is predictable that your actions or comments are relied upon, the issue of duty of care would come into play.

In order to extend your clinical knowledge and introduce legal and policy requirements into your knowledge base, this chapter provides clinical practice guidelines that address many of the legal risks nurses face.

The aim is to help you see how legal theory which is nebulous and sometimes difficult to grasp becomes policies that ensure legal risks and of course, risks to the client are minimised.

Delegation: who is responsible?

- Delegation by a supervisor or manager does not devolve their duty of care in all situations. As a representative of the institution managers are responsible for setting up safe systems of work.

The role of the manager is to:

- identify resource requirements;
- ensure that the skill mix of staff and client to staff ratios match the need;
- determine priorities;
- notify shortages with senior staff and work to ensure clinical supervision is in place;
- document fully.

Note that if a manager delegates to another professional who has proven experience, knowledge, training and education and competence to fulfil the duties delegated, if that professional is functioning within safe systems, the manager (or person who has the right to delegate) is not liable for the actions of the professional who has taken on those duties.

What this means is that when duties are delegated by a supervisor or person who has the right to delegate, they have an obligation to ensure that the person is capable of functioning in that role. Once that is established the supervisor has grounds to expect the duties to be carried out to the standard expected.

It is common to hear registered nurses (RNs) claim that they will be liable for the actions of students, enrolled nurses or nurses' aides/assistants in nursing so they can't delegate or they feel they have to be responsible for every action taken by these staff. This is incorrect. When delegating duties it is imperative that the RN assess the situation and establish the level of competence of the other staff. Then that individual who takes on the job becomes personally liable for their own professional actions. If they fail to admit that they do not know what they are doing, if they do not identify that the duty is outside of their competence and if they proceed to work outside best practice guidelines then they will be personally and professionally liable for their own actions; it will not be the RN who delegated who is liable.

Students frequently complain about how often they are asked 'can you do . . .?' Every colleague has an obligation to establish competence before expecting another to assist. If the student or assistant fails to admit that the task is outside their scope or education they are failing in their duty. A professional has the right to rely on the word of a colleague.

A second element/principle covered in Chapter 5 was standard of care. Professional standards and education standards provide guidance here. Judging another professional is done by reference to what is expected of someone of similar experience and education. The risk here is when a professional goes beyond the level or scope of practice defined by role or education or experience.

The roles and functions of nurses and the rules governing delegation of duties are defined by the Nursing and Midwifery Board of Australia. The final activity in Chapter 5 directed you to the relevant publication.

Examples of failures that led to claims of nurse malpractice: i.e., nursing negligence

1. Failure to assess patient's condition such as blood pressure, vital signs, or blood glucose levels on time and failure to document or report changes that indicate risks to the client.
2. Failure to administer correct medication and/or report and documentation of medication errors.
3. Misusing a medical device or gadget for example infrared lamps have caused burns, drainage tubes have been left clamped.
4. Failure to perform a procedure; this could include hygiene cares displaced due to short staffing, forgetting to attend a dressing, not preparing client for surgery as directed.

Proper demonstration of standards of care means absence of malpractice in the work place.

It is important to recognise no one rule, guideline or policy can capture every situation, every day in clinical environments as circumstances are always different. Should there be an investigation of these circumstances, everything becomes relevant.

Later we will explore coronial investigations in depth but it is important to note here that civil actions may arise out of coronial findings as to the cause of death. The findings of a coroner's inquest can lead to professional disciplinary actions, civil actions or even criminal prosecution if there is sufficient and relevant evidence of failure on the part of the system or individuals.

The coronial inquiry into the death of Tracey Baxter in 1979 led to extensive changes in procedures and policies throughout the health system. This six-year-old girl died post-tonsillectomy. The coroner was very critical of the care given by nursing staff: The fluid intake (IV) and fluid balance record showed excessive input. The staff had responded to the recovery nurse's verbal comment to push fluids as the child had bled. The way the court looked at the situation was to ask 'what would an ordinary reasonable registered nurse be expected to know or do in relation to a child's fluid requirements'?

Further, not only did the court want to establish what was reasonable to know in relation to this situation but what was reasonable to expect was done such as assessment, evaluation, documentation and clarification of fluid orders.

Another area of failure by the staff was the fact the observations indicated a definite change in status yet there was no record of action taken in response to these indicators.

So it is not enough that professionals can perform tasks, take observations, record and document information. From this we can see that what is essential is *the ability to interpret and act upon data in an appropriate manner.*

Policies and procedures directing routine and special interventions and care exist, and policies for notification and procedures for contacting key staff are now common. Written directions rather than word of mouth explicitly show lines of communication and actions to be taken.

Another case that underpinned policy and procedure changes was *McCabe v. Auburn District Hospital (*1989). Here a 21-year-old male's post-operative status after an appendicectomy was all downhill. He died from peritonitis leading to renal failure. The inquiry reviewed the history and documentation.

Routine and special tests had been done but the results had simply been filed without comment or notification to medical staff of the presence of a significantly raised white cell count, indicating infection. The medical officer on call did not visit or phone in, nor did the nursing staff notify medical staff about the deteriorating condition of the patient. Nursing notes were separate from medical notes and there were no references to each by different staff.

Negative findings about the accuracy and reliability of written notes were a major factor in the case's outcome, finding the hospital and staff negligent.

Integrated patient notes were one solution to the many failures this case documented. Policies and protocols to ensure timely notification of pathology results have been another. The quality of and standard of written notes also led to many hospitals providing specific education about documentation. Over time this has become a normal area of learning and study but until this case most nurses learnt to write their notes by simply copying the style and content of the nurse who wrote the notes on the previous shift.

Accountability for the standard of care

All health professionals are expected to know what the generally accepted standard of care entails and to follow that general standard in practice. The institution's policy and procedure manual is where to find nursing care guidelines. However, if the facility you are working in does not adhere to or comply with the generally accepted standard of nursing care, then following the facility's policies and procedures will not protect you from a charge of malpractice. This is because all nurses are accountable for the nurse's standard of care.

- If you are aware that your facility's policies and procedures are below the generally accepted standard of care, then you should notify your nurse-manager or the health and safety committee of your concerns.

Medication and drug policies

The existence of legislation governing all aspects of medication administration has been mentioned. The fact that medication errors underpin many actions in negligence was also raised in Chapter 5. These issues will be revisited in relation to professional governance (Chapter 7) but here we will look at policies and procedures that reflect legislative requirements and institutional strategies for protection of clients.

The Therapeutic Goods Administration (TGA) is part of the Commonwealth Department of Health and Ageing. Created by the *Therapeutic Goods Act 1989* (Cwlth) the TGA has extensive legislative obligations in relation to therapeutic goods and devices.

Every state and territory has legislation governing all aspects of legal and illegal substances that in health care jargon tend to fall within the general label of 'drugs or medications'. Each state and territory has its own laws that determine where consumers can buy a particular drug or poison, and how it is to be packaged and labelled. However, state and territory governments classify the vast majority of drugs and poisons in accordance with the *Standard for the Uniform Scheduling of Drugs and Poisons* (SUSDP) to achieve a uniform national approach to the scheduling of substances and uniform labelling and packaging requirements. The SUSDP contains the decisions of the National Drugs and Poisons Schedule Committee (NDPSC) regarding the classification of drugs and poisons into schedules.

The implementation of the SUSDP, as it affects access to and supply of drugs and poisons, is given legal effect through relevant state and territory drugs, poisons and controlled substances legislation. Examples of such legislation are:

Poisons Act 1966 (New South Wales)
Drugs Poisons and Controlled Substances Act 1981 (Victoria)
Poisons Regulations 1973 under the *Health Act 1937* (Queensland)
Controlled Substances Act 1984 (South Australia)
Poisons Act 1964 (Western Australia)
Poisons Act 1971 (Tasmania)
Poisons and Dangerous Drugs Act (Northern Territory)
Poisons and Drugs Act 1978 (Australian Capital Territory)

Under the *Therapeutic Goods Act*, NDPSC determines what schedule a substance should be placed in. Adoption of the NDPSC decisions by the states and territories then determines the controls that apply to any given substance and the products containing that substance.

> *Schedule 1* covers dangerous poisons.
>
> *Schedules 2* and *3* are for human non-prescription medicinal substances.
>
> *Schedule 4* is for prescription human and animal medicinal substances.
>
> *Schedules 5* and *6* are for domestic, agricultural and veterinary substances ranked lower to higher risk.
>
> *Schedule 7* contains dangerous poisons requiring special precautions.
>
> *Schedule 8* contains medicinal substances requiring stricter controls.
>
> *Schedule 9* substances are prohibited for manufacture, possession, sale or use.
>
> (Galbally, 2000, p. 31)

Legislative requirements are reflected in education relating to medications and administration and institutional policies. For example:

- A person must have sufficient information, understanding and skill to select and use a product safely and effectively.
- Access is restricted where general knowledge and label information are not sufficient to overcome the consumer's lack of knowledge. Generally the level of restriction increases with the level of knowledge and expertise required for safe and effective use of the product.
- Additional restrictions are imposed where the substance is likely to be diverted for abuse or manufacture of illicit drugs.
- The controls specify who may sell or supply, which customer may have access, and the amount and form of the product supplied – all based on the level of risk potentially associated with use of the product.

Advice on the interpretation of the SUSDP and/or the legal requirements in a particular state or territory may be obtained from <http://www.tga.gov.au/industry/scheduling-st-contacts.htm#.U7oCQvmSzD8>.

Education for health staff is also available. See: <http://www.tga.gov.au/hp/education-hp.htm#.U7oBRfmSzD8> (accessed 9 July 2014).

The community setting

The policies governing safe storage and accounting for medications in an institutional setting do not extend into a private home. Staff working in community settings will frequently see 'dangerous drugs' left on the kitchen table. There is no legal requirement for the homeowner to adhere to the measures taken in a service environment but client education about best practice for storage and use is a good practice. The requirement to adhere to best medication administration and documentation standards does not lessen in the non-institutional setting, however.

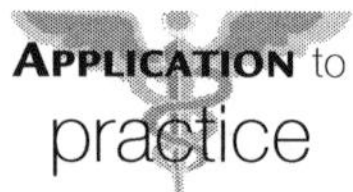

Application to practice

A number of reviews of policies and practices in relation to drug administration issues were undertaken in Victoria after an inquiry into two deaths attributed to drug administration errors in 2004. For a good summary of best practice (recommendations) see *Recommendations on the Security and Custody of Schedule 8 and Schedule 4 Drugs within Hospitals*, Victorian Therapeutics Advisory Group (VicTAG) (formerly Melbourne Teaching Hospitals' Drug Usage Group), October 2002 (revised December 2003), <http://www.victag.org.au/wp-content-/plugins/pv_security> (accessed 9 July 2014).

Who can administer medications?

Chapter 5 made reference to the National Decision Making framework and scope of practice documents that direct practice. Prior to the move to a national authority, some State regulatory authorities had published regulations specific to which drugs each class of nurses could administer. The Nurse Practitioner role in relation to medication prescriptions and drug administration is a difficult area due to State legislation however institutional practices adhere to a requirement that endorsement for proven capacity is necessary through competency assessment. Each state and territory Department of Health has guidelines that are entrenched into institutional policies. A web seach for your own state's guidelines would be a worthwhile exercise.

An example

A **Registered Nurse** may only delegate the administration of medicines to someone appropriately qualified to administer medicines. This means that **Registered Nurses** may use their professional judgement about whether to administer medicines themselves or whether to delegate the administration to someone with appropriate qualifications or scope of practice to administer medicines by the specified route.

Enrolled Nurses (who do not hold a Nursing and Midwifery Board of Australia approved qualification in medicines administration) and personal care workers (with appropriate medicines administration training) may, in some circumstances, be competent to administer medicines under the delegation of a Registered Nurse. If a Registered Nurse judges that an Enrolled Nurse or personal care worker is not appropriately qualified to administer to a 'high care' resident they should administer the medicines themselves or delegate to appropriately qualified personnel. Appropriate supervision must be provided (Department of Health Victoria 2005).

A good resource particularly for those working in aged care is: Australian Nursing and Midwifery Federation (ANMF) Nursing Guidelines: Management of Medicines in Aged Care 2013.

The Nursing and Midwifery Board of Australia has published guidelines; *Explanatory note (2010) Enrolled nurses and medicine administration.* <http://www.nursingmidwiferyboard.gov.au/Search.aspx?q=Explanatory%20note:%20> (accessed 14 July 2014)

An area that is frequently a source of anxiety is whether only qualified, endorsed or specific staff can administer medications and what rules govern these. Institutions often have policies that create further limits on their staff. Requirements may exist for further education, competency assessment in relation to all or particular types of medications in a particular facility.

Below are extracts from the Queensland Department of Health's extensive guidelines.

- The Health (Drugs and Poisons) Regulation 1996 grants different authorities to different classes of health professionals. For example a doctor has greater authority to obtain and administer medication than a dentist. Similarly, a nurse's authority would be more extensive than a podiatrist's authority.
- Registered nurses working in 'rural hospitals', 'isolated practice areas' or island resorts have been given an additional authority to supply medication under certain conditions (Queensland Health, 2000, Environmental Health Unit, The Health (Drugs and Poisons) Regulation 1996, What Nurses Need to Know, p. 4).
- Oral instructions in institutions (hospitals, nursing homes etc) Section 97 A doctor may issue an oral instruction to a midwife or registered nurse to administer or, in certain circumstances specified in the Regulation and in

other sections of this booklet, supply a controlled drug or a restricted drug to a patient.

- The doctor must reduce an oral instruction for a controlled drug to writing and supply it to the midwife or registered nurse within 24 hours. The doctor sending a written instruction by post can meet this obligation, which meets the requirements of the Regulation. If the doctor fails to comply with this requirement, then the registered nurse must report the matter to the Director of Nursing. If the doctor does not meet this obligation within 48 hours of the Director of Nursing becoming aware of the contravention, the Director of Nursing or the Medical Superintendent of the institution must report the matter to the Chief Executive, Queensland Health.
- A written instruction is not required under the Regulation for the supply or administration of a restricted drug or Schedule 2 or 3 poison, as such matters are usually dealt with through internal organisational policies (Queensland Health, 2000, Environmental Health Unit, The Health (Drugs and Poisons) Regulation 1996, What Nurses Need to Know, p. 6).

- There is no requirement in the Health (Drugs and Poisons) Regulation 1996 for a registered nurse to have a witness when administering or recording controlled drugs. These requirements are in addition to current legislative requirements and are usually addressed through internal organisational policies.

- Requirements for checking, recording the use and witnessing the administration of a controlled or regulated restricted drug by a second person, do have the potential to improve the security of these drugs and to prevent misuse.

  However if the person who is designated as the 'unit storer', that is the person who is in charge of the controlled drugs in a unit at a particular time, is a different person from the one who is obtaining the drug to administer it, then the unit storer is to enter the transaction and the registered nurse or doctor who is to administer the drug signs the record (Section 103) (Queensland Health, 2000, Environmental Health Unit, The Health (Drugs and Poisons) Regulation 1996, What Nurses Need to Know, p. 8).

The extract below from the (pre-July 2010) Nurses Board of Victoria should help you understand the policies that are in place throughout Australia governing students and drug administration. (Note that in Victoria enrolled nurses are called division 2 registered nurses; division 1 nurses are what most other states refer to as registered nurses.)

- Registered nurses division 2 and undergraduate students
  - unless registered as a division 2 nurse endorsed to administer medication, division 2 nurses and division 2 undergraduate students **cannot** administer medications in the course of their employment or studies.

- Division 1 undergraduate students
  - division 1 undergraduate students can administer medication **provided** it is within the scope of the Bachelor of Nursing course under the direct

supervision of a registered nurse division 1, 3 or 4 according to the curriculum.

- Student nurses employed as unregulated health care workers
  - an undergraduate student nurse employed as an unregulated health care worker should not administer medication. [Unregulated health care worker in other states may be an assistant nurse or personal carer.]

(*Guidelines for Registered Nurses, Student Nurses and Pharmacists Regarding the Use of Dose Administration Aids (DAA) for Clients in Care in Victoria*, jointly developed by the Nurses Board of Victoria and the Pharmacy Board of Victoria 2004, pp. 1–2.)

Understanding the limits and responsibilities of staff that have different levels of education is the responsibility of the supervisor. However, working with staff who have different qualifications means that colleagues should be aware of the role and role limitations that are created by legislation and the State Registering Authority.

Under the previous system of state nurse regulation most state boards published guidelines for enrolled nurses and medication administration. With the changes to those authorities the guidelines now available tend to be published by each state health department. Each state and territory may be slightly different, and vaccinations and Schedule 4 medication administration may be specifically prohibited in some jurisdictions. However, a review of the Act Medication Administration by Enrolled Nurses or other policy documents is worthwhile <http://www.health.act.gov.au/c/health?a=dlpubpoldoc&document=2206> (accessed 7 August 2014).

Duty to report a breach in the standard of care

Every nurse has an ethical obligation to serve as a patient advocate. Therefore nurses are obliged to report when another health care professional breaches a standard of care. For example, if you observe a co-worker working while under the influence of alcohol, or you see them falsify a medical record, you have a duty to act promptly to protect the patient's welfare if necessary and then to report your observations.

- Always check the institution's policy and procedure manual regarding how to address a reportable situation. Usually hospital policies recommend making a report to an immediate supervisor or nursing administration. It is unlikely that policies will direct you to report to the National Regulatory Authority but in some circumstances this may be necessary.

Damages

Once damage has been proven and it has been shown that the damage the plaintiff is complaining about was a 'reasonably foreseeable consequence of the defendant's negligent act' it comes to the point where the question is 'who pays?'.

The court determines the amount of damages by reference to two concepts:

1. Specific damages are compensation for proven financial losses.
2. General damages are governed by previous court awards and the individual situation and these are often referred to as compensation for pain and suffering.

The courts are not required to establish if the plaintiff can actually find the sum of money the court awards. The defendant has to get this money from the plaintiff or the plaintiff's insurance company. This can lead to further legal actions.

This area has been the focus of considerable legislation. Governments have passed Acts to control and limit the amounts and circumstances that allow for compensation payments. These are discussed below.

Expert witnesses

An expert witness is a person who has special skill or knowledge in a particular field. In a medical malpractice case an expert nurse may be hired to explain the appropriate standard of nursing care to the jury, and to help establish whether or not the defendant deviated from the acceptable standard of care. The nurse expert will be specialised in the same area of nursing practice as the defendant.

In order to avoid potential bias or partiality, the nurse expert should not have a prior, or existing, relationship with the defendant or plaintiff and cannot be personally involved in the lawsuit. Experts are often hired by both the plaintiff and the defendant in cases involving complex medical issues that are not within the comprehension of an average layperson and are thus outside the jury's common knowledge.

Medications: One of the most common causes of negligence actions

In Chapter 1 a case study drawn from a real situation was presented to highlight just how hard it might be to get a hearing when there are doubts about medication and how intimidation led to an RN administering medication in spite of her doubts about the safety of the dosage.

Medication errors have led to serious injury. Most institutions have policies and procedures for notification of errors; these are called incident reports. There have been instances where the staff member who reported the medication error was dealt with so harshly that other staff members soon learnt to avoid the risk of being chastised, humiliated or having a negative report on their employment record and they hid their mistakes. Sometimes the matter reported was never followed up by checking the client's status, and all the attention was centred on the person who made the error.

The advent of quality assurance processes and research into the issue has led to a revision of this type of management of medication errors. Now every incident report is reviewed and instead of simply 're-educating' or reporting the staff member who admitted the error, an analysis of contributing factors is required involving questions about whether there were trends or the frequency of errors.

While every individual involved in the steps of prescribing, ordering, packing, labelling, storing, supplying, administering and documenting medications is personally responsible for following standards of practice and demonstrating competence, the issues of short staffing, workloads and other circumstances that may contribute to a mistake are investigated. Here is an example of such an investigation.

On Monday mornings on a busy surgical ward preoperative preparations concurrent with other patient care put extreme pressure on nursing staff. It was always hectic and pre-medication orders were often fulfilled on call from theatre. On a particular Monday the RN gave the wrong pre-med injection to a client at 7.30 am and another RN administered the wrong dose of Pethidine at 7.45 am. Both RNs wrote out incident reports and notified theatre staff and their supervisors. Both were interviewed by a panel of senior staff at the end of the shift.

Instead of being severely reprimanded and put on restricted duties as they expected, both RNs were surprised to find the panel was interested in *all* the circumstances that were relevant. Both staff members were assessed by clinical educators and their knowledge and competence was confirmed by assessment; however, as a result of their information the quality assurance committee observed and monitored the ward.

Changes to the level of staffing occurred. Two RNs responsible for preoperative patients only were routinely rostered not just for Monday mornings but for every day there was a heavy theatre list. New policies about 'on-call' medications, new policies for drug checks and support and education to all staff members about medication management and reporting of errors were implemented.

Medication Errors

The World Health Organisation defined the term, 'adverse drug reaction' (ADR) as 'noxious and unintended, and which occurs at doses used in man for prophylaxis, diagnosis, and therapy'. Another definition is: 'An appreciably harmful or unpleasant reaction, resulting from an intervention related to the use of a medicinal product, which predicts hazard from future administration and warrants prevention or specific treatment, or alteration of the dosage regimen, or withdrawal of the product' (Edwards & Aronson, 2000, p.1255).

Incidence of Medication Errors

There have been many local, national and international audits and research into types and causes of medication errors. Every large study has identified there are many thousands of errors and resulting deaths. The terms describing a medication error vary among authors. The WHO term Adverse Drug Reaction (ADR) is common, but you may see Adverse Drug Error (ADE), or the same acronym could mean Adverse Drug Event, another frequently used term is Medication Error (ME). Irrespective of the terminology chosen just a glance at some of the statistics will tell you how serious the problem is. Below are findings from a number of studies that have been undertaken. It is worth reflecting that, in spite of earlier findings, more recent studies continue to report enormous numbers of drug errors.

Bates et al (1998) reviewed 4031 adult admissions to 11 medical and surgical units at 2 tertiary-care hospitals and extrapolated an ADE rate of 6.5% for non-obstetrical admissions. Twenty-eight percent of ADEs were deemed preventable. In a study of patients admitted to coronary intensive care, medical, and obstetrical units (Barker et al., 2002), the researchers found the rate of drug-related incidents was 73 in 2967 patient days. Of the 73 drug-related incidents, 27 were defined as ADEs, and 56% were judged as preventable. Barker reported that across 36 hospitals in two states in the US his team had identified that 19% of every ordered dose was an error of either time, dose, omission or authorisation (2002).

In the US, the Institute of Medicine reported in 2006 that at least 1.5 million residents were harmed or killed due to medication errors. In 2010 Wilmer et al. reported their review of studies of ICU adverse drug events (ADEs) and medication errors (MEs) identifying that occurrences were both common and under-reported. An Australian study observed nurses in two hospitals and reported an 80.2% medication error rate (Westbrook et al. 2010).

The Australian Government Department of Health and Aging funded the National Prescribing Service Ltd. to undertake a major review of published studies for their report: Medication Safety in the Community (2009). Their findings reflect the incidences cited above.

- In Australia they found that approximately 6% of hospital admissions are associated with adverse drug events.
- Almost one third of admissions for the elderly are associated with adverse events.
- Consistently high error rates occurred during transfer of care between hospital and community settings.
- Ten percent of general practice patients reported experiencing an adverse drug event.
- Twenty-five percent of high risk patients reported adverse events associated with medicines.
- Documentation errors that occurred during transfer of care had consistently high error rates, with 52% to 88% of transfer documents containing an error.

The latest review, Australian Commission on Safety and Quality in Health Care (2013) makes depressing reading:

Administration Errors

The new studies provide further support for a clinical error rate for medicine administration in the hospital setting of between 5% and 10% of medicine administrations. Interruptions of the nurse during administration were associated with increased risk of error. Factors found to contribute to administration errors included interruptions or distraction of nurses during medicine administration.

Interruptions were common, occurring on 58% of occasions when nurses were administering medicines to patients.

One study demonstrated that there was a 13% increased chance of error with each interruption. Error-prone abbreviations, which may also contribute to administration error, were also found to be frequently used, occurring on 8.4% of all medicine orders in one study undertaken across three hospital sites.

One new study provides evidence of the high rates of error with intravenous medication administration of any type. It found clinical errors occurred in 70% of administrations.

Factors that Contribute to Medication Errors

Every student and registered nurse is aware that the whole process of medicating a patient is a complex and demanding aspect of nursing care. Researchers have tried to identify causative factors and there are a number of ways to describe these but generally findings show that there are system problems and individual or staff problems.

While an individual may make mistakes, there is an awareness that the system itself is frequently the root cause of drug errors. That does not lessen the responsibility on the professional for their actions. Rather it should make the professional very careful and alert to these system factors.

Activity

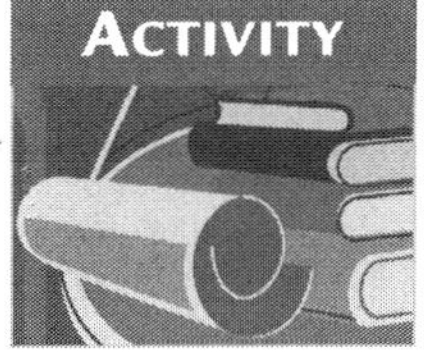

Can you identify some system issues?

If you thought of staffing shortages, patient status, lack of time or lack of resource information to check drugs, pressure of routines, habits and policies you would be correct.

Can you list some professional issues?

Some of the identified, individual mistakes are: inadequate knowledge about the individual patient and the medication; failure to follow policies or best practice rules; and poor numeracy leading to incorrect drug calculations.

Some other causes that have been identified could be either personal failures or system issues. Workloads and distractions are an example.

The US Institute of Medicine (IOM) has published a series of nine recommendations that would reduce the risks and remove the causes. While these have not been entrenched in Australian legislation, it should be possible for you to recognise these as policies in place in the clinical area.

Read Recommendations for Reducing Medication Errors: Implementing Processes, Policies, and Rules. Go to: http://www.medscape.com/viewarticle/408566_3 (Accessed 7 July 2014)

Legislation and reforms that affect health professionals

Negligence issues are complex. Attempts to keep things simple inevitably overlook the many cases and subtle differences in interpretation of the principles discussed in every case. A variety of legislation that attempts to balance issues of liability and costs of compensation and insurance now creates statutory liability for actions that once had to be argued by every plaintiff. Some legislation goes as far as creating criminal liability for actions once considered negligent.

As you have been working through this chapter you have no doubt found yourself wondering 'what about if . . .' or recalling someone's experience or a media report about health professionals and actions in negligence.

- It is essential for you to keep in mind that every case is decided on the facts and evidence of that case. While general principles and rules can be identified these are not static and one case appealed to the High Court can overturn decades of precedents, just as new legislation can change or limit access to compensation.

It has often been mentioned that there are differences between jurisdictions, the desire for harmony between state, territory and Commonwealth laws was recognised in the Ipp Report (*Review of the Law of Negligence*, 2002). This review headed by Justice Ipp was tabled in July 2002. Recommendations were aimed at ensuring consistency in the area, lessening or reducing the need for interpretation of the elements of negligence in relation to an action and setting limits on compensation. A number of the report's recommendations for legislative development are extracted here to assist you to summarise the many issues we have discussed, see what has been proposed for the future through legislative controls and increase your grasp of the jargon of law.

Recommendations for inclusion in legislation covering negligence

The following are adapted from Doepel (2005) Tort law reform throughout Australia. A brief review of recent amendments, Minter Ellison.

Negligence – duty and standard of care

A person is not negligent for failing to take precautions against a foreseeable risk unless:

- the risk is 'not insignificant'; and
- a reasonable person in the same position would have taken precautions (taking into consideration the probability, likely seriousness, the burden of taking risks and the social utility of the risk-creating activity).

Defence – assumption of risk

There may be no finding of negligence where the risk or kind of risk in question was obvious to a reasonable person. An obvious risk includes risks that are patent or matters of common knowledge. A risk may be obvious even though it is of low probability.

Standard of care – professionals

In cases involving an allegation of negligence on the part of a person professing themselves to possess a particular skill, the standard of care should be determined by reference to what could reasonably be expected of a person professing that skill at the date of the alleged negligence, unless the court considers that the opinion is 'irrational'. Professional opinion does not have to be universally accepted to be considered widely accepted.

Recreational services

The professional should not be liable for personal injury or death that resulted from a person taking an obvious risk.

Negligence of medical practitioners

A medical practitioner will not be negligent if the treatment provided was in accordance with an opinion widely held by a significant number of respected practitioners in the field.

Medical practitioner's duty to inform

Medical practitioners should be subject to a legislatively prescribed duty to inform, both proactively and reactively, on the basis that they must take reasonable care to provide such information as to enable the patient to make a decision as to whether or not to undergo treatment (referred to as the 'Bolam test'), unless the opinion is irrational.

Contributory negligence

The test should be whether a reasonable person in the plaintiff's position would have taken precautions against the risk of harm, having regard to what the plaintiff knew or ought reasonably to have known, taking into consideration:

- probability of harm
- seriousness of harm
- burden of taking precautions
- social utility of activity

Under apportionment legislation, a court should be entitled to reduce a plaintiff's damages by 100% where it is just and equitable to do so.

Causation

The plaintiff bears burden of proof to establish both:

- factual causation; and
- scope of liability – normative issue of the appropriate scope of the negligent person's liability (encompasses legal causation, foreseeability, remoteness, commonsense causation).

Proportionate liability

In relation to claims for negligently caused personal injury and death, the doctrine of solidary liability (where multiple wrongdoers are severally liable and can be held liable for the full amount of any damages awarded to the plaintiff) should be retained and not replaced with a system of proportionate liability.

Liability for mental harm

A health professional is not liable if there is no recognised psychiatric illness, should an individual claim for mental harm. The action would need to be a predictable cause of psychiatric harm in a person of normal fortitude. Relevant factors include:

- whether the injury arose from the plaintiff witnessing a sudden shock or its aftermath;
- whether there was a pre-existing relationship between the plaintiff and the defendant;

- the nature of relationship between the plaintiff and any person killed, injured or put in peril.

Limitation of actions

Commencing from the date when the plaintiff knew, or ought to have known an injury had occurred an action must be initiated within 3 years. There is discretion to extend this period to 12 years and in the case of minors who wish to bring an action if the cause of damage is attributable to the defendant, the delay can be even longer.

Non-economic loss/general damages – thresholds

The minimum threshold for non-economic loss is that a threshold for general damages would be based on 15% of a most extreme case (assessed as a percentage of the capped maximum to be awarded).

Non-economic loss – caps

A cap on maximum damages for non-economic loss recoverable of $250,000.

Loss of earning capacity

A cap on maximum loss of earning capacity at calculations based on twice the average full time adult ordinary earnings.

Protection to rescuers/good samaritans/not-for-profit organisations

A rescuer/good samaritan is a person acting without expectation of payment or other consideration who comes to the aid of a person (and usually includes a medical practitioner). A rescuer/good samaritan should not be liable for assisting in an emergency if the rescuer/good samaritan was exercising all reasonable care and skill.

Not-for-profit organisations should not be liable for personal injury or death of a voluntary participant in recreational activity as a result of an obvious risk.

There should be no provision regarding the liability of not-for-profit organisations for personal injury and death caused by negligence in the provision of emergency services.

Review of recommendations

Recommendation 1 of the Ipp Report suggested a national response whereby tort law reform should occur by the enactment of a single statute styled the Civil Liability (Personal Injury and Death) Act in each jurisdiction. This unifying recommendation was not adopted and the states, territories and the Commonwealth each introduced their own separate legislation to give effect to some or all of the Ipp recommendations.

For example, the Commonwealth enacted the *Medical Indemnity Act 2003*. This Act established a scheme to fund the costs of medical indemnity insurance payouts and subsidise insurance premiums for those medical practitioners working in very high risk specialties.

In New South Wales the *Civil Liability Amendment (Personal Responsibility) Act 2002* has changed some common law principles and created clarity on areas that might otherwise need to be argued in court:

For example

- an injured person is presumed to have been aware of an obvious risk associated with undertaking a particular activity, and there is no duty of care to warn participants of such obvious risks (*except in certain situations, such as the provision of professional, including health, services*);
- a professional is not liable in negligence if the professional acts in a manner that is widely accepted in Australia by peer professional opinion as competent professional practice (with the exception of any duty to warn of the risk of personal injury or death associated with the provision of a professional service);
- there is no liability for pure mental harm resulting from negligence unless the harm consists of a recognised psychiatric illness;
- a 'good Samaritan' who, in an emergency, comes to the assistance of an injured person, is protected from all civil liability for acts or omissions done in good faith (unless performed while under the influence of alcohol or drugs); and
- an apology by or on behalf of a person alleged to have caused another injury or damage, does not constitute an admission of fault or liability.

In South Australia the *Wrongs (Liability and Damages for Personal Injury) Amendment Act 2002* creates a presumption of contributory negligence in the case of intoxication, provides immunity to 'good Samaritans' and allows an apology to be made without it constituting an admission. Limits on the amount of damages have been included in the Act.

The *Civil Liability Act 2002* in Tasmania, the *Wrongs and Other Acts (Public Liability Insurance Reform) Act 2002* in Victoria and the *Civil Liability Act 2002* in Western Australia are similar to the South Australian legislation. All involve less sweeping changes than New South Wales while still dealing with issues of contributory negligence (intoxication), immunity to good Samaritans (discussed in Chapter 8) and limitations to the amount of damages.

Queensland's parliament rejected the first Bill addressing these issues, and since 2002 the various recommendations have been included in the *Civil Liability Act 2003*.

The new provisions of the *Professional Standards Act 2004* apply to claims for economic loss or damage to property in an action for damages arising from a breach of a duty of care.

Vicarious liability

The financial responsibility if an employee is liable for damage can, in particular circumstances, be shifted to the employer. The doctrine of vicarious liability has relevance to nurses and other institutional employees as it provides a defence to an action in negligence as discussed in Chapter 5. The independent practitioner may be required to insure (indemnify themselves) against this possibility by law or by the recommendation of their professional body. The legislation limiting liability is aimed to reduce the risks of liability and costs of indemnity.

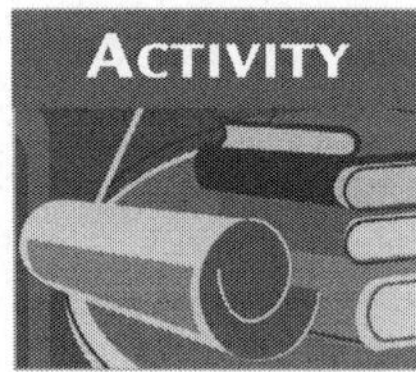

Activity

Read the scenarios below and identify the legal issues. The answers and discussion have been provided to ensure that you have grasped the essentials.

You are working in your first graduate job as a Community Health Worker based at a remote clinic where the clients are a mix of indigenous people, tourists and mine workers and their families. Your role involves educating community groups and school children about health issues. On one of your school visits, Tracey, a 14-year-old child of Fred who works in the mines and Sue who is a school teachers aide, tells you she thinks she is pregnant. She suspects things are going wrong as she is bleeding, but begs you not to tell anyone. Tracey wants you to help her go with the older school children on a visit to the regional centre where she intends to see a doctor and work out what to do. You agree in the face of her anxiety and she joins you and the others for the trip. During the trip Tracey has severe pain, extensive bleeding and loses the baby. She is admitted in a very serious condition to the regional hospital and you notify her parents.

- Put yourself in the parents' position; they are furious with you and threaten to sue you. Apply the elements of negligence to this situation. Identify issues in relation to each element and identify relevant principles that would apply to this situation.

Consider the following scenario.

An elderly, frail and deteriorating resident in a nursing home appeared to be dying. The RN on duty called an ambulance to transfer the patient to the local hospital. The patient was extremely distressed by this and she died on arrival at casualty.

The RN claims that the transfer was carried out on the basis of her duty of care to ensure the patient received the best possible medical attention. The RN admitted she was also concerned about her own situation; she had told a colleague she was 'covering herself' by transferring the patient.

- Her family wishes to sue the RN for hastening the patient's death and causing her distress. There is an ethical dimension in this situation. Issues of being the patient's advocate and working to ensure the needs of the patient could substantiate the RN's claim of meeting the standard of care. From a legal perspective how do you fit the elements of negligence to this scenario?

Answers and discussion

The elements of negligence include the following.

- There is a duty of care.
- The act or failure to act (omission) fell below the standard expected.
- The act or failure to act was the direct cause of damage.
- This damage was reasonably foreseeable.

Consider whether there might be grounds for an action in negligence against the RNs. If there was a finding of negligence, how would the doctrine of vicarious liability affect the situation?

The RN who failed to refer the pregnant adolescent might be found to have fallen below the standard of care expected. While adopting an advocate role and accommodating the young woman's request, the RN did not assess and care for a medical condition.

The RN who chose to transfer the client could be found to have failed to meet standards of care. This RN would have been more responsible if they had assessed the client, sought a second opinion about the likely risks and benefits to the patient and then initiated discussion of options with the family. Consequently the distress of the patient which could lead to legal action might have been avoided.

Recommended reading

The article below from the *Medical Journal of Australia* will give you an insight into how, from a doctor's perspective, the issues in the activity above are considered. The strategies recommended to limit or reduce complaints will give direction to your own practice. Go to the homepage of the *Medical Journal of Australia* at

<www.mja.com.au/public/issues/contents.html>. Scroll down to 1999, Jun 21 issue. There you will find: Angered patients and the medical profession. Paul Nisselle (MJA 1999; 170: 576-577)

Looking out for yourself

There is no question that there are risks and burdens in practice. Sometimes it seems overwhelming trying to learn everything you need to know while recognising how much can go wrong. However, if you know where these risks lie you can be confident in your own assessment of situations. After making constant reference to the known and high risks of drug administration and medication management it is important for you also to know you have rights and defences as a professional functioning in this area. An article that explains these rights is by Michelle Colleran Cook, and is entitled 'Six rights for safe medication administration' Massachusetts Nurses Board at <www.mass nurses.org/nursing-resources/nursing-practice/articles/six-rights> (accessed 9 July 2014).

Defending against allegations

Documentation can save you...

You know already the importance of written documentation. Clinical environments depend on accurate and timely documentation. Failure to maintain accurate records, signed proof of jobs completed and reports and evaluations of client status is professional malpractice it will be used as evidence of negligence.

Education focuses upon developing an awareness of this need and provides experiences to develop these skills. From a legal perspective it is the facility reliance on this documentation that lies behind the massively increased demands on nurses to undertake the duty. Documentation is a defence against claims made against health professionals. Time and again in court hearings or coronial investigations in the past, nurse documentation was found inadequate.

The formulaic, routine daily nurse notes were often incorrect. The lack of objective and critical information was often a problem. The poor literacy and grammar gave the impression of poor education and capacity. Observations were documented on forms that had printed times, rather than space for the nurse to record the correct times.

It is true, "if it was not written, it did not happen" in law. However investigations, court hearings and reviews are not unrealistic in their expectations. It is appreciated that situations arise that cause delay and memories are unreliable. Mistakes and oversights happen.

It is the commitment to standards, the correction of mistakes and honest reporting that will provide the nurse with a defence. It is not a case of how much is written. The clear and lucid report that tells the reader facts is more valuable than pages of justifications. We all need to "cover our butt" and documentation achieves that.

Optional reading

For information on protection from negligence lawsuits read *Nursing Management*, 1999 by Jennifer Lee Showers available through library on PubMed or to subscribers via <http://journals.lww.com/nursingmanagement/abstract/1999/09000/protection_from_negligence_lawsuits.10.aspx> (accessed 9 July 2014).

A possible assignment question

RN Jane is on her second post graduate rotation in a large general medical ward.

One of Jane's assigned patients is Mr G who is 80 years of age; he requires 6pm IV antibiotics but Jane needs to get this re ordered as the medication chart shows the old order has run out and at handover it was confirmed he is to continue these. Mr G is one of two of Jane's patients going to X-ray at 4pm.

At 3.30 X-ray phones and asks for the two clients to be transported. Jane attends to this getting an orderly for both transfers.

Jane placed a call for the medical officer to update Mr G meds and also to get an order for pain med's for Mrs Y as she had not responded to simple analgesic. The Dr returned the call and said he will order Pethidine 50 mgs for Mrs Y and renew the antibiotic order as soon as he can.

At 5.55pm Mrs Y is very distressed, Jane went another RN and ask her to check Pethidine 50mg out with her, stating the Dr has given a verbal order and will write it up soon, they do this together and administer the drug per protocols.

Jane went to tea, Mr G was still at X-ray, the other patient had been transferred back and had dinner. Later when Jane attended observations she noticed Mr G was not yet back, Jane intended to call X-ray but was called to Mrs Y who was confused, sweating and agitated at 7.15pm.

Mr G's son visited and he went to x-ray to find his father, he found Mr G on a trolley in the corridor and returned Mr G to the ward stating 'dad was left and everyone in x-ray had gone'. The son is furious, Jane immediately assessed Mr G and he was so unstable she initiated a MET call.

1. Apply the elements of negligence to the situation of Mr G, discuss for each element how you would analyse the actions of RN Jane and other staff.

2. Consider in light of professional governance the activities in relation to the administration of the Pethidine. How would investigators analyse these activities?

Summary

Much of this chapter is revision and application of content from Chapter 5. The legislative changes to the common law approaches to the tort of negligence will no doubt continue, so you will need to keep abreast of these as you progress through your career. As many of the guidelines and policies that direct our practice have grown out of this area it is worth being able to articulate the concepts and have sufficient understanding of these to be able to draw upon them in active practice. Being fearful of legal consequences should become 'being aware of and thus guided by legal reasoning' in relation to practice.

Should someone say to a nurse she has been negligent, that the nurse failed in their duty of care, that they created a legal liability, you can imagine it would be devastating to that nurse.

You will often hear nurses talking about someone's duty of care, failure of standards of care when they are finding fault or believe that nurse has been "slack". This use of legal terminology can be very confusing. It is easy to snap at someone and tell them they are guilty of malpractice when a mistake occurs. It is a cultural thing, a form of fear and discipline to keep us all on the straight and narrow in the risky, high pressure situations we work within. There is a need to ensure nurses do adhere to standards of behaviour and care that they adopt the professional way of functioning and bandying about legal terms is as good a way as any to get us to shape up.

However, it is important you do know where to get guidance and direction for decisions and care when you are under pressure. You need to be able to point to your actions and behaviours and show these clearly demonstrate professional standards.

This is the point of understanding the elements of negligence.

- Do you have a duty? Is this patient one for whom you have responsibility? Did you take all steps to ensure the patient was properly cared for – while you were being called away or caught up with a crisis?
- Meeting the standard: Did you know what you were doing with the intervention that might have gone wrong?
- Did you seek help before doing something you were unfamiliar with or frightened about?

Sources

Australian Commission on Safety and Quality in Health Care (2013), *Literature Review: Medication Safety in Australia*. ACSQHC, Sydney.

Australian Pharmaceutical Advisory Council, (APAC) (2006) *Guiding principles for medication management in the community*, 2nd edn, Commonwealth of Australia. <http://www.health.gov.au/internet/main/publishing.nsf/> Content/apac-publications-guiding (accessed 9 July 2014)

Barker, K., Flynn, E., Pepper, G., Bates, D. & Mikeal, R. (2002) 'Medication Errors Observed in 36 Health Care Facilities'. *Arch Intern Med*. 162:1897–1903.

Bates D et al (1998) 'Effect of Computerized Physician Order Entry and a Team Intervention on Prevention of Serious Medication Errors', *JAMA* 280(15): 1311–1316.

Clancy, T. R. (2004) 'Medication error prevention: progress of initiatives', *JONA's Healthcare Law, Ethics, and Regulation*, **6**(1): 3–12.

Colleran Cook, M. (2006) 'Six rights for safe medication administration', *Nursing Practice*, Massachusetts Nurses Board, Mass. at <www.massnurses.org/ nurse_practice/sixrights.htm> (formerly accessed 28 June 2006).

Commonwealth Treasury (Ipp Report) (2002) *Review of the Law of Negligence*, <http://revofnet.treasury.gov.au/content/review2.asp> (formerly accessed 9 July 2014).

Department of Health Victoria, (2005) *Key requirements for nurses in residential aged care services*, <http://www.health.vic.gov.au/dpcs/agedcare-requirements.htm> (accessed 9 July 2014)

Doepel, M. (2005) 'A brief review of recent amendments', Tort Law Newsletter, Minter Ellison Lawyers, www.minterellison.com/public/connect/Internet/Home/Legal+Insights/Newsletters> (accessed 5 December 2005).

Easton K., Morgan T. & Williamson M. (2009) 'Medication Safety in the Community: a review of the literature'. National Prescribing Service. Sydney.

Edwards, R. & Aronson, Y. (2000) 'Adverse Drug Reactions: definitions, diagnosis, and management' *The Lancet*, 356: 1255–1259.

Fleming, J. G. (2011) *The Law of Torts*, 10th edn, The Law Book Company Ltd, NSW.

Forrester, K. & Griffiths, D. (2009) *Essentials of Law*, 3rd edn, Harcourt, Sydney.

Galbally, R. (2000) *National Competition Review of Drugs, Poisons and Controlled Substances Legislation*, Final Report Part B, Council of Australian Governments, Canberra.

Kennedy, R. & Richards, J. (2004) *Integrating Human Service Law and Practice*, Oxford University Press, Melbourne.

MacFarlane, P. J. & Reid, S. J. (2006) *Queensland Health Law Handbook*, GoPrint Brisbane.

McIlwraith, J. & Madden, B. (2014) *Health Care & the Law*, 6th edn, Lawbook Co., Australia.

Morris, G., Cook, C., Creyke, R. & Geddes, R., *Laying Down the Law*, 12th edn, Butterworths, Sydney.

Morris, J. (2000), 'Insuring against negligence: medical indemnity in Australia', *Policy*, Spring, <www.cis.org.au/policy/Spring02/polspring02-2.htm> (formerly accessed 9 June 2005).

Nursing and Midwifery Board of Australia (NMBA). 2010. Explanatory note: Enrolled nurses and medicine administration. <http://www.nursingmidwiferyboard.gov.au/Search.aspx?q=Explanatory%20note:%20Enrolled%20nurses%20and%20medicine%20administration> (accessed 9 July 2014)

Queensland Government (2000) Environmental Health Unit, The Health (Drugs and Poisons) Regulation 1996, What Nurses Need to Know.

Reid, A. J., n.d. *Law All Nurses Should Know*, <www.continuingeducation.com/nursing/lawstoknow/lawstoknow.pdf> (formerly accessed 28 June 2006).

Richards, B., de Zwart, M. & Ludlow, K. (2012) *Tort Law Principles*. Thomson Reuters, Australia.

Stith, K 2007, *Nursing Malpractice*, Ezine Articles http://EzineArticles.com/?expert=Kevin_Stith (Accessed 9 July 2014)

Staunton, P. & Chiarella, M. (2003) *Nursing and the Law*, 5th edn, Elsevier, Sydney.

Staunton, P. & Whyburn, B. (1997) *Nursing and the Law*, 4th edn, Harcourt Australia Pty Ltd, Sydney.

Westbrook, J. et al. (2010) 'Association of Interruptions With an Increased Risk and Severity of Medication Administration Errors'. *Arch Intern Med*. 170(8):683–690.

White, B., Wilmott, L. & McDonald, F. (2014) *Health Law in Australia*, 2nd edn, Thomson Reuters, Australia.

Williams, G. (1982) *Learning the Law*, 11th edn, Stevens and Sons, London.

Wilmer, A., et al. (2010) 'Incidence of Medication Errors and Adverse Drug Events in the ICU: a systematic review'. *Quality and Safety in Health Care* 19, p. 1–9.

Victorian Therapeutics Advisory Group (2003) *Recommendations on the Security and Custody of Schedule 8 and Schedule 4 Drugs within Hospitals*, <www.health.vic.gov.au/vmac/downloads/custody1.pdf> (accessed 1 April 2011).

Cases

McCabe v. Auburn District Hospital (1989) Supreme Court (NSW) No. 11551 of 1982, unreported.

The extracts from the health (drugs and poisons) regulation 1996 were used with permission of © State of Queensland (Queensland Health) Further information at <http://www.health.qld.gov.au/phs/documents/ehu/9101.pdf>.

CHAPTER 7

Professional governance

Learning outcomes

After studying this chapter you should be able to:

- Demonstrate a knowledge of procedures and policies for investigation of health matters, professional and legal hearings and sanctions for failure to meet standards.
- Show an understanding of practices and procedures in clinical settings that reflect these policies.
- Apply legal and professional standards when assessing and responding to client needs, practice and policy situations, professional reporting and communication.

Overview

In Chapter 2 you were introduced to the Australian legal system – the hierarchy of Australian courts, sources of legislation and delegated authority to statutory, regulatory bodies. This chapter examines the regulation of nursing in Australia under legislation.

Until July 2010 each state had legislation that delegated responsibility for monitoring a particular group of professionals to a registering body. Since 2010 there are now 10 National Boards instead of the various State and Territory professional registration authorities for each health profession. Western Australia remains the only state that has not adopted the national legislation and continues to have its own Nurses and Midwife Registration authority. The creation of the Australian Health Practitioner Regulation Agency (AHPRA) has superseded State legislation for health professional regulation. AHPRA's operations are governed by the *Health Practitioner Regulation National Law Act 2009*, AHPRA role and limits on its powers is governed by this legislation.

Go to: http://www.ahpra.gov.au/About-AHPRA/What-We-Do.aspx (accessed 28 July 2014)

For those of you who are familiar with your former State Nursing Regulatory Boards of Councils, the activities AHPRA has been legislated to undertake are quite similar.

First and foremost the aim is to protect the public, and the Boards of each health-professional group have been given powers to undertake investigations of complaints or notifications submitted by members of the public. The AHPRA Board has power to investigate complaints of registered professionals and students. The registration functions provide a national database that anyone can check for proof that an individual is a registered health practitioner.

AHPRA is the source of guidelines, standards and codes governing the role and functions of each category of health professionals. These were formerly produced by State Boards and of course, the Australian Nursing and Midwifery Council. Many of these published guidelines and codes have been taken up and published by AHPRA.

Prior to 2010, the peak body for nursing and midwifery responsible for setting standards and developing professional guidelines was the Australian Nursing and Midwifery Council (ANMC). These codes were taken up by every State and Territory nursing and midwifery authority. These Codes and guidelines have been accepted by AHPRA and gradually they have been republished under that organisation's banner. The role of the ANMAC has been revised and this organisation will continue to monitor and promote nursing and midwifery through accreditation of programs.

There will remain at state level, professional representatives of the National Boards who have delegated responsibilities and are accountable to the National Authority. Complaints to state authorities such as the Health Commission or Ombudsman will continue to be referred to state representatives or directly to AHPRA. Investigations of incidents and decisions about practitioners may be resolved at state level but registration and professional recognition is under AHPRA control.

The health professions take their self-regulatory and disciplinary roles seriously, as members appreciate that to allow poor practice or inappropriate professional behaviour by one practitioner inevitably reflects on all members of that profession.

Each nurse is personally responsible for maintaining current registration or enrolment. It is an offence for a person to work as a registered or enrolled nurse if they are not in fact registered or enrolled. Whether they were never registered or their registration has lapsed it is still an offence. Your name will not usually be removed from the register if you fail to pay the annual fee; removal from the register is a very formal process and strictly governed by the legislation.

Professional skill is not the only criterion that must be met to remain on the professional register. Moral character and fitness to practice issues extend beyond the clinical setting. There is a requirement to notify your professional registering body of circumstances that may or may not relate to your work that can reflect on the profession. Under the national legislation there are now also mandatory requirements to report to the Board notifiable conduct. Specifically S. 140 of the National Law defines what 'notifiable conduct' of a practitioner is, and this conduct includes practicing while intoxicated, sexual misconduct, risking the public's safety by being impaired to practice or when a practitioner

deviates from professional standard. The definitions of notifiable conduct are outlined on this website:
<www.nursingmidwiferyboard.gov.au/Codes-and-Guidelines.aspx> (accessed 28 July 2014)

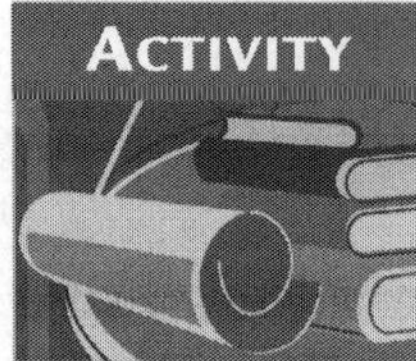

Activity

Spend time exploring this website; you will need to know it when you apply for registration. At this stage, go to tabs along the top of the page and click on Legislation and Publications. There you will see the student registration fact sheet. This is a new concept in Australia, and while the commencement dates for the processes have been delayed, it is another professional standard that has been introduced. As you will see from the fact sheet there is only one key aspect that would affect the right of a student to maintain registration as a student nurse.

The Nursing and Midwifery Board has published professional standards that are variously referred to as codes, guidelines and policies. These provide the public with clear statements of what they should expect from a professional. It is these publications that are used to measure complaints against a practitioner should an investigation and hearing be carried out in response to a complaint.

- Codes
- Codes of ethics
- Codes of professional conduct
- Guidelines
- Competency standards
- Decision making framework
- Guidelines for registration standards
- Professional boundaries
- Professional practice guidelines
- Re-entry to practice
- Policies
- Social media

It is all very well having these documents but the question you might ask is how can these standards be imposed? Think about professional competencies. Unless the individual practitioner takes responsibility for their own professional behavior and their colleagues and employers all accept these standards and monitor themselves and others they could be irrelevant. Until you remember that the public and the courts can refer to them to make judgments about the practitioner.

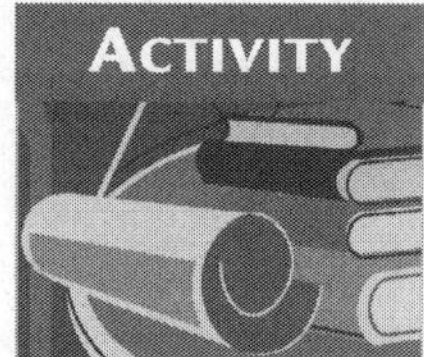

Activity

Go to <www.nursingmidwiferyboard.gov.au/Codes-and-Guidelines.aspx>. By following the links, you will see each publication's original dates and the date of effect by the Board that ensures these remain relevant to practice.

Competency Standards

- RN Competency Standards August 2008
- EN Competency Standards August 2002
- Midwifery Competency Standards August 2008
- Competency Standards for the Nurse Practitioner

Code of Ethics and Professional Conduct

- New Code of Ethics for Nurses August 2008
- New Code of Professional Conduct for Nurses August 2008
- New Code of Ethics for Midwives August 2008
- New Code of Professional Conduct for Midwives August 2008

Now have a look at: A nurse's guide to professional boundaries. This document gives direction for professional boundaries. Unlike the codes and standards that govern practice by providing a framework for legally, professionally accountable and responsible nursing practice in all clinical, management education and research domains, in Australia and New Zealand this publication drills down to specific situations and considerations. It aims to give nurses certainty in their practice. Risky behaviours are described and consideration of many "what if" situations is covered. Understanding these will provide you with a personal, professional decision making framework.

The codes and guidelines, standards of practice and regulation of education all combine to provide a benchmark against which the professional is measured. You have already seen in your readings about the tort of negligence that courts will use these documents to identify what the profession believes is a standard against which they can measure the behaviour of an individual nurse.

Professional discipline

- The regulating body has powers to investigate, discipline and deregister a nurse.

Legislation specifies that AHPRA can initiate an investigation if it receives notification/complaint electronically, hardcopy letter or telephone call and it is the legislation that identifies the types of behaviour that falls within AHPRA's obligation to investigate and take action. Complaints can be referred from State Health Complaints entities and the State's Ombudsman. For both Queensland and NSW the rules are slightly different than for the other states and territories.

While AHPRA manages notifications in most states and territories, different arrangements are in place in NSW and Queensland. (Source: AHPRA About Notifications <http://www.ahpra.gov.au/Notifications/About-notifications.aspx#how> (accessed 28 July 2014)

In NSW, the entire notifications process is managed by the Health Care Complaints Commission (HCCC) and health professions councils, meaning that the National Boards and AHPRA are not involved. In Queensland, complaints were received by the Office of the Health Ombudsman (OHO) who assessed their severity and determined which complaints go to the National Boards, and which were managed by the OHO. Since July 2014 a new health complaints agency; the Office of the Health Ombudsman (OHO) will commence operations as Queensland's independent health complaints agency, replacing the Health Quality and Complaints Commission which closed on 30 June 2014.

Below are examples that would justify complaint, investigation or discipline.

- Failure to hold (or loss of) relevant qualifications.
- Making false or fraudulent statements to obtain registration.
- Failure to comply with a lawful board requirement.
- Breach of the legislation governing that profession.
- Alcohol or drug abuse.
- Serious criminal conviction.
- Professional misconduct. (Professional misconduct means the same as infamous conduct, serious professional misconduct, misconduct in a professional respect, disgraceful conduct. At common law the case of *Qidwai v. Brown* (1984) settled these terms.)

When a matter is raised, unless the Board decides the matter should not be referred to a State Health Authority the steps are usually:

A preliminary assessment

The outcome of the preliminary assessment may be for the Board to decide if further action is required, such as health assessment of the health practitioner, student or assessing the performance of the practitioner. This is where the matter is judged whether it should be escalated through the next levels of enquiry, whether an investigation needs to take place or whether the matter is resolved at this first point of consideration.

Investigation

An investigation may need to be conducted to determine the appropriate course of action, which may refer the matter to a performance panel hearing or whether the matter required notifying another body, whether a caution needs to be issued, whether the professional concerned needs to have their actions monitored to make sure they are complying to the appropriate professional standards, or if conditions need to be imposed. The matter may also be deemed to have been resolved at this step in the process, and no further action is required.

Panel hearing

A panel hearing will be conducted to determine the appropriate course of action, which may be to refer to a tribunal or suspend a professional via a health panel or whether the matter does not need to escalate beyond this panel hearing.

Tribunal hearing

A tribunal hearing will be conducted to determine the appropriate course of action, which may be to suspend registration or cover the previous actions raised in the former steps in the process. Check the website to see the full list of actions for each level of the process <www.ahpra.gov.au/Notifications-and-Outcomes/Notification-Process.aspx> (accessed 28 July 2014). Tribunal hearing outcomes are made available to the public.

Published hearing decisions from adjudication bodies (other than panels_ relating to complaints and notifications made about health practitioners or students are available on the Austlii website.

As you can readily see there is a progress through increasingly formal structures. As discussed earlier, these formal structures must adhere to rules of both common law and administrative justice. They must demonstrate they follow the principles of natural justice and there are rights of appeal.

Example: A nurse reported a criminal conviction and subsequent two month imprisonment for fraud when renewing their licence to practise. An investigation confirmed the conviction and a tribunal found this nurse guilty of discreditable conduct, cancelled the licence to practise for 18 months and ordered that if this nurse were to reapply for registration both counselling and an appearance before the tribunal would be required.

This reapplication hearing was to allow the tribunal to determine whether the nurse was now a fit and proper person to hold a licence to practise (Queensland Nurses Council, 2005).

Penalties

As a result of investigation and findings that support disciplinary proceedings, under delegated powers given by legislation there are various penalties available to the disciplinary tribunal.

- Removal or suspension from the register.
- Reprimand or a caution.
- A financial penalty, a fine.
- Good behaviour bonds (the nurse provides a written guarantee for good behaviour).
- Re-education, skill updates and assessment of relevant skills.
- Practice limitations, restriction on certain professional activities.

Three published tribunal cases have been extracted below. The first deals with questions about nursing competence, the second is an example of a hearing as a consequence of a criminal conviction and the third is a salutary example for all nurses being responsible to work within boundaries of practice.

Example 1: A tribunal hearing (at which the RN pleaded guilty) was held after an investigation into facts that this RN had failed to give medication as ordered, had pre-signed that those medications were given, had failed to give adequate handover to the following shift. The RN was reprimanded for *breaching fundamental nursing ethics* of entering true and faithful client records. The finding was the RN's behaviour was incompetent and unprofessional. The RN's licence was suspended for three months and following this suspension conditions were placed on the nurse's licence. These included requirements for future employer reports about the RN's record keeping and further study by the RN in medication administration and nursing ethics (Queensland Nurses Council, 2005). (Italics inserted)

Tribunals have discretion about costs of hearings. A guilty party can be charged for the costs of a hearing and this can amount to many thousands of dollars being owed to the tribunal. The example above did not attract costs as the RN's cooperation and guilty plea mitigated against further penalty.

Example 2: A tribunal hearing about an RN charged and who pleaded guilty to 19 charges of using the internet to access pornographic material and 1 charge of possessing child pornography. Although it did not occur in a work context, the tribunal stated the RN's conduct "reveals character failings that impact on his own reputation and that of his profession". He was also convicted on his plea of guilty to one charge of an offence commonly referred to as upskirting. This involved the RN visually recording the genital area of a female nurse colleague, without her knowledge or consent, while they were both on duty. This offence occurred whilst the RN was working as a nurse. The image was discovered when police accessed his computer when investigating the child pornography offences.

"Conduct does not need to occur at work to be considered misconduct in a professional sense, if the conduct calls into question the character of the practitioner". The Tribunal found RN's conduct was:

Conduct of a lesser standard than might reasonably be expected of him by his professional peers and the public;

Infamous conduct in a professional respect;

Misconduct in a professional respect; and

Conduct discreditable to the nursing profession.

In considering sanctions the Tribunal considered the criminal penalties and time served in goal and probation. "The purpose of disciplinary sanction is different to criminal sentencing. The objects of disciplinary proceedings are to maintain professional standards and confidence in the profession and to protect the public". He was reprimanded for his conduct. "That is not a trivial sanction. It is a public denunciation of his conduct that is recorded on the public register". (Nursing & Midwifery Board of Australia v Brearley [2012] QCAT 323 (20 July 2012).

Example 3: Ms X had been an enrolled nurse since March 1978. Between January 2000 and May 2004 and then again between November 2004 and July 2009, she administered medication without holding the necessary endorsement. She also practised unlicensed for a period in 2004/2005, having failed to renew her enrolment during a period she was ill.

Ms X was trained in New Zealand, where endorsement was not required to administer medication. She maintains she completed a course in Queensland which entitled her to apply for endorsement several years ago. She said she assumed her employer would take any necessary action after the training.

Ms X presented to the officer who investigated the matter for her employer as cooperative, honest and forthcoming. She freely offered what little information she had and did what she could to assist the investigation. She immediately and willingly ceased administering medication when she was informed it was outside the scope of her authorisation.

The organisation involved in offering the nominated course has no record of her participation, nor does her employer who appears, also, to have played a role in organising and offering it to its employees. Ms X appears to have a detailed and accurate recollection of the course, how and by whom it was delivered, what she had to do to complete it and the names of some other participants. One of them does recall Ms X doing the course, others could not say.

The Board has not alleged Ms X was deceptive in her dealings with either the Board or her employer. The system of registration and endorsement is intended to ensure that only those who are trained and educated perform specific duties, in this case administering medication. It is not merely a matter of form. It is a strategy to protect patients and due regard must be paid to the requirements.

It is of concern to the Tribunal that the hospital did not pick this issue up for a very lengthy period; some 9 years. During that time a nurse not endorsed to do so was administering medication without authorisation. This indicates a serious flaw in the hospital's procedures for checking registration status.

Although the documentation is lacking, the Tribunal has proceeded on the basis that Ms X is appropriately trained to secure endorsement.

This is consistent with the Board's acceptance that her competence to perform the duties of an endorsed enrolled nurse is not in question. Ms X provided the Board with references from a number of her professional colleagues who paint a consistent picture of a nurse who is positive, diligent in the care she provides and patient focused. This case does not raise any concerns about patient safety. However, steps should be taken to assess and endorse this nurse so patients may receive the services she is competent to offer.

Regardless of any lack in the hospital's process, it is a nurse's responsibility to understand the scope of their authorisation to practice and to remain within its bounds. Ms X cannot shift that responsibility to her employer. She renewed her enrolment on numerous occasions during the charged period. It might be expected that she would have noticed her enrolment details did not contain the necessary endorsement. The importance of attention to her registration status was specifically brought to her attention by the then Queensland Nursing Council who wrote to her during the period her registration lapsed. (Italics inserted)

The Tribunal regards this as a case of unsatisfactory professional conduct. Ms X has neglected to give proper attention to her enrolment status. It is not a case of deliberate disregard for professional requirements.

The parties have jointly proposed a sanction which, with some variation, the Tribunal has accepted as adequate and appropriate. Ms X will be publicly reprimanded and fined. The parties proposed a fine of $1,500, which the Tribunal considers excessive in light of the other penalties that it will impose and given the view it has taken of Ms X conduct. The purpose of these proceedings is not punitive. A fine of $500 is a significant penalty for someone on a nurse's salary.

Ms X's enrolment will be subject to a 3 month suspension. That penalty will be wholly suspended for 1 year, provided she does not face any disciplinary proceedings during the year. The suspension serves to deter others from flagrantly disregarding registration requirements. The suspension of that penalty reflects the Tribunal's view that Ms X neglected this issue, albeit for a lengthy period, rather than deliberately disregarded the requirements.

Ms X must also pay the Board's costs of the proceedings, fixed at $2,000. The Board brought these proceedings in fulfilment of its statutory function. Their costs are funded by fees paid by members of the profession. In most cases, those against whom disciplinary grounds are established will bear the Board's costs of the proceedings. Ms X cooperation in the proceedings has ensured that the costs have been kept to a minimum in this case.

The sanctions described above are appropriate to maintain professional standards and public confidence in the profession. *They will reinforce to Ms X and to other nurses the importance of being aware of and observing the limits on their scope of practice*. (Italics inserted). (*Nursing and Midwifery Board of Australia v Collins* [2011] QCAT 270 (3 June 2011)

Appeal of board decisions

Should the professional disagree with a decision of the Board, the legislation allows them to make an appeal against the decision. The legislation will also set time limits within which any appeal must be lodged. For any professional who has a complaint lodged against them, their rights of notification, right to legal representation and right to fair procedures and time to prepare their defense is upheld by both legislation and the common law. It is usual for a professional to seek advice and assistance from their union or professional organisation when notified about a complaint against them. Each stage of the procedure is governed by strict rules. Legislation is clear as to the limits of the registration board's authority and to the processes and procedures that can be utilised.

Look again at the list of potential issues that fall within disciplinary responsibilities. Can you see that these types of situations are not the same as civil law? There is no damage or a plaintiff and a defendant so tort law is irrelevant; nor might there be a criminal aspect as the nurse may have caused no harm or committed a crime. So where does this 'law' fit?

Administrative law

Administrative law is another specialised branch of law where there are particular rules and limits to authority. Administrative law is the body of law regulating both the executive branch of government and the interaction of tribunals and courts. Professional disciplinary committees and tribunals exist through delegated legislation and must adhere to the rules governing all tribunals.

Tribunals operate at both state and federal level. There are two main components of administrative law:

1. judicial review, which is concerned with the proper exercise of power and evolved through the common law but is now governed by codes of practice and regulations; and
2. merits review, which is concerned with whether the decision was correct or preferable. Merits review is solely statute based.

One administrative law rule relates to who must prove the issue. In civil law the plaintiff must prove that their facts are true 'on the balance of probabilities'; for a crime, the prosecution is required to prove that the facts are true 'beyond reasonable doubt'. In administrative law, the burden of proof falls between the two and every individual is entitled to defend any claims made against them.

In administrative law, where people's careers are on the line, there is a need to be more certain of the facts than concluding that 'well, weighing it all up and looking at all the arguments it seems probable that this person did this thing'. However, unlike a criminal case where 'you need to as certain and as positive as it is possible to be, before making a decision as to guilt or innocence' here the burden of proof is somewhat less.

Disciplinary process

As the point of having a regulatory body is to protect the public, you can see why there is a responsibility imposed on professional regulatory bodies, created by statute to set standards, monitor and take action against members who fail to adhere to professional standards.

Regulations in each state direct what steps are to be taken and what departments must be notified, no matter what the source of the complaint.

In some jurisdictions, for matters assessed as 'less serious' the board can initiate informal or 'without prejudice' meetings to discuss and explore the claims against a professional. These might be convened for matters where there are concerns about a practitioner's health, conduct or competence.

Professional boards can make decisions within their delegated powers about issues brought to their attention, even before any formal hearings. Even if it is evident that all procedures leading up to a tribunal hearing have met legal requirements, the findings and procedures of a tribunal can be reviewed.

Where the matter is serious, that is, the penalty could involve deregistration, formal tribunal proceedings are initiated. The rules of evidence follow the civil system of law but a tribunal can call upon any relevant witness or documentation in order to investigate and come to a decision.

The process involves:

- Notifying the subject of the complaint, nurse or midwife, about the specific complaint.
- The nurse or midwife is usually invited to address the issues through both interview and written responses.
- The investigators are obliged to seek out and interview the person who has made the complaint and any witnesses and review documentation.
- Both the tribunal investigators and the person who is the subject of the complaint need legal advice. All registration authorities have access to solicitors who provide legal advice in response to a 'brief' or a report by the investigator/s.
- The nurse or midwife is entitled to a copy of this report.

Natural justice

Administrative law procedures dictate the rules for tribunal hearings and procedures. One of the most important ideals in common law is natural justice. Most successful appeals from tribunals tend to be the result of a denial of natural justice (Forbes, 2002).

Every effort must be made to ensure that the person about whom a complaint is made has timely and full notification of that complaint. The right to know about the accusation, and be given time to respond and to seek appropriate legal advice and support is part of the ideal. A case which clarified this was *Ping v. Medical Board of Queensland* (2004).

> The Medical Board of Queensland had a statutory power to choose between a disciplinary hearing conducted by correspondence or an oral hearing in the presence of the respondent. The Board initially decided to proceed by correspondence, but later required the defendant to appear in person. It was held on review that once the Board elected to proceed in writing it could not lawfully take another course. (in <http.www.federationpress.com.au.pdf/Tribunals%20UPDATE%203.pdf> accessed 26 July 2014).

The tribunal is expected to be independent and to act in 'good faith'. Evidence used and witnesses called must be fair to both parties. A tribunal cannot refuse information that provides facts or sheds light on the situation.

> When there is a 'prosecutor' as well as a defendant the tribunal's duty to act according to natural justice is owed to each party (*Dental Board of Queensland v. B.* (2003)).

Protecting the public

While some state legislation goes as far as including codes and standards, generally the right of the profession to monitor and manage its members is left up to the registering body.

The responsibility to inform and protect the public can be evidenced by publications that describe what the public should expect in their dealings with a professional. Most advisory documents are called guidelines but all can provide outsiders, such as the court, with benchmarks against which individuals are measured.

These, as you have found above, are all available on the Nursing and Midwifery Board web site.

The National Competency Standards give direction for education and practice, and thus exams. Conferring registration is recognition that this standard is achieved. Ongoing professional practice will also be measured against competencies. AHPRA has a requirement that for re-registration or renewal of the annual practising certificate proof of recent practice and continuing education is necessary.

Below is an extract from the then Nurses Registration Board of New South Wales publication of the (then) ANCI national competencies.

> **The significance of the competency standards.**
>
> 1. For the public, employers and others.
>   These core competency standards are designed to encourage understanding of their purpose in the community as well as by others involved in providing health and related services.
>   They contribute to positive health outcomes because registered nurses are equipped to provide safe and effective nursing care.
>   Nurses who are registered are required to demonstrate competence. They are accountable for their actions and they take responsibility for the supervision of enrolled nurses. In addition, they have a professional responsibility to maintain the standards in order to renew their licence.
>   Education courses leading to registration are accredited by nurse regulatory authorities. These programs require graduates to demonstrate

the competency standards. This assists in ensuring that registered nurses are fit to provide safe, competent care in a variety of settings.

2. For nurses.
The standards take account of the contemporary role of the registered nurse which covers clinical practice, management of care, counselling, health promotion, client advocacy, facilitation of change, clinical teaching, supervising, mentoring and research. They provide a benchmark for nurses in daily practice.
They may be used for academic assessment, workplace performance review and for measuring continuing fitness to practice.
The competency standards reflect the unique characteristics of nursing as well as broader attributes nurses have in common with other professions and occupations. In addition, they identify the knowledge, skills and attitudes required by nurses and reflect the complex nature of nursing activities.

Purposes of the ANMAC National Nursing Competency Standards

The ANMAC competency standards for Registered Nurses and Enrolled Nurses are core competency standards and have the following specific purposes:

- to provide a means of communicating to consumers the expected competency standards of nurses;
- to determine the eligibility for initial registration or enrolment of persons who have undertaken nursing courses in Australia;
- to determine the eligibility of nurses who have undertaken nursing courses outside Australia and who wish to practice in this country;
- to provide the basis for assessing nurses who wish to re-enter the work force after a period of absence defined by the registering authority;
- to assess qualified nurses who are required to show that they can demonstrate the minimum level of competence for continuing practice. (NSW, NRB, Boardworks May 2001 B1–B8)

Reproduced with the permission of NSW Department of Health 2001.

Professional misconduct

This term is used with some abandon and often the label is applied with little thought. Conduct that falls outside of another person's 'opinion' or expectation is not professional misconduct. The term has been used to describe various behaviours in various circumstances in both court and disciplinary hearings, so it is not surprising that it is open to interpretation.

In relation to professional governance, however, the point made above still holds. The conduct need not be criminal or provide grounds for an action in negligence to attract professional discipline. Unlike the general examples discussed in relation to discipline above, professional misconduct can be broken down to specific factors.

- Breach of a set of code of conduct.
- Departure from practice considered acceptable by competent practitioners of good repute.

- Conduct demonstrating a lack of knowledge, skill/care.
- Impropriety or unethical behaviour.
- Being convicted of a serious criminal offence (even if it is not directly related to the practice of the profession).

Establishing what is professional misconduct

Here is a case that clarifies how the court looked at a departure from practice considered acceptable by competent practitioners of good repute, and conduct demonstrating a lack of knowledge, skill/care. An appeal by Sophia Healthcote was lodged after a finding at first instance that she was guilty of misconduct in a professional respect which led to her being deregistered by the New South Wales Nurses' Registration Board in 1991. Sophia Healthcote was the only RN on night duty in Wilcannia on the night of the incident. A patient from an Aboriginal Mission was admitted with probable alcohol withdrawal. The patient's behaviour resulted in Healthcote contacting the Royal Flying Doctor Medical Officer and the police over the course of a few hours. The client was in fact taken into police custody in the early morning and was found dead in his cell some hours later.

The trial drew upon expert evidence describing the standards and skills that should have been implemented by an RN caring for such a client. It was a finding that her failure to demonstrate she had adhered to those standards that led to the guilty verdict in the first trial. At appeal the judge dismissed all of the allegations the Registration Board attributed to Heathcote. In assessing the evidence of the experts presented by the board the judge reported:

> In the light of my disagreeing with the decision of the Board, I record that it acted upon expert evidence which was largely cut down and exposed as based upon inadequate material or without appreciation of the relevance of other material facts (Ward J, *Healthcote v. Nurses Registration Board and Walton* (1991) p. 17).

The judge held that *all* the circumstances the nurse found herself in needed to be considered: *all* her actions and the fact of her inexperience, lack of support, need to take action to protect others from the client's behaviour were as important as any professionally identified 'best practice' text, guideline or witnesses.

This gives the profession clear direction in all disciplinary matters. All the issues, all the circumstances must be examined before applying the label professional misconduct. Practice guidelines and textbook recommendations are just part of the analysis in determining whether someone has fallen below standards and is guilty of professional misconduct.

Here is another example that illustrates the need to examine all the circumstances surrounding an incident. A doctor had been found guilty of professional misconduct and suspended from practice. The court in *Ex parte Meehan, The Medical Practitioners Act* (1965) found that the doctor had been 'ill-advised but neither reckless nor indifferent to the patient's welfare' for carrying out major elective surgery without another practitioner present. The terms reckless or indifferent to patient welfare have often been used synonymously with professional misconduct. In this case the suspension was reduced to a reprimand.

Sexual misconduct

An issue that is frequently grounds for a hearing by the professional regulating bodies representing various health workers is that of sexual misconduct. A case that identifies professional misconduct in relation to sexual activity is *Hoile v. Medical Board of South Australia* (1960). Here the hospital medical superintendent appealed to the High Court against a finding of misconduct by a medical board relating to a sexual relationship between the doctor and a nurse at his hospital. The court upheld a finding of misconduct as the sexual activity occurred on hospital premises *while the nurse was on duty* and, on at least one occasion, was the only nurse on duty.

The point here is that, from a court or professional governance standard, the question is generally whether the health worker was in breach of the written or unwritten rules, that is, whether their behaviour would be considered negatively by others of that profession.

Statutory definitions are somewhat unclear or vary in different states. Some state legislation actually opens the way for an act of negligence to be deemed 'professional misconduct'. However, to attract this degree of condemnation the act or behaviour has to have had *such a serious effect on the reputation of the relevant profession* that it is grounds for deregistration or, in the case of a medical practitioner, for being 'struck off'.

Cases where the health professional has been accused of improper conduct often hinge upon whether intimacy has occurred concurrently with the therapeutic relationship or the therapeutic relationship has been used by the practitioner to develop such a relationship.

Codes of ethics may not specifically say that a 'sexual relationship' is unethical conduct but the professional does need to ensure that their communication, interactions, proximity and post-discharge relationships are above reproach and not subject to misinterpretation. It is clear that should there be any sexual relationship with a patient it is considered a gross breach of the therapeutic relationship. The world has moved on and community attitudes to relationships are much less rigid than in times gone by, but the health professional (as we have discussed in earlier chapters) has an obligation to satisfy the highest standards. The risk in the therapeutic situation is that professionals may take advantage in their interactions or relationships and that these could be harmful to the client due to their vulnerability or because there are unequal power relationships between a professional and their client.

In another case demonstrating changing community attitudes a doctor had been convicted on two abortion charges and deregistered. On appeal, in *Skinner v. Beaumont* (1974), the court found that removal from the register was too harsh a punishment, but the judge still considered the convictions to constitute misconduct as 'the deliberate defiance, even with good motives, of a legal and professional responsibility, cannot be excused'. The court's finding that deregistration of this doctor was too harsh reflected changing community attitudes to abortion (as evidenced by the change in the law at the time).

- Community attitudes and perceptions will be important in consideration of whether a practitioner's behaviour has brought the profession 'into disrepute'.

Two summaries from hearings by a professional conduct committee may help you to see how professional behaviour can be found to be disreputable conduct.

1. A nurse pleaded guilty to the complaint that they had violated professional boundaries by taking advantage of their role in order to exploit a patient by engaging in a sexual relationship – after the discharge of that patient.
2. A nurse was found to have violated professional boundaries by engaging in a significant and emotionally intimate relationship – not just a sexual relationship. The issue here was that the relationship exploited the dependency created by the professional relationship.

Drugs and alcohol

A number of professional organisations specifically identify a person being drug or alcohol affected as one of the grounds for disciplinary action on the basis that this is a form of professional misconduct. Colleagues, employers and the professional body have an obligation to protect the public from a professional whose capacity to function and respond appropriately is impaired. Failing to take steps to report and remove the staff member from all situations that put clients, the profession or facility at risk is negligent.

One of the problems with drug and alcohol abuse is that it is less likely to be detected by senior management and co-workers and colleagues may doubt their own assessment or be afraid to jeopardise a friend or workmate's career. The user may rely on that ambivalence, deny that there is a problem or ask for some 'allowance' to be made for 'this one mistake'.

Should there be an incident or harm arising from the actions of the affected staff member there can be a claim of negligence. If you and other staff members suspect drug or alcohol abuse, it is likely that the clients can as well. If you take no action, other peoples' complaints, formal or informal, that arise from an incident will be investigated and your covering up will come to light. You will have failed on ethical and professional grounds to satisfy standards. Under the mandatory notification requirements all uncertainty has been removed. If the drug or alcohol affected person is on duty both the AHPRA notifiable responsibilities and the ANMAC Code of Conduct must be followed.

Gross misconduct

This is another term that nurses tend to use when they are in a stress situation and believe a colleague has failed to meet standards. The term is often used by employers as grounds for dismissal. There may be professional notifications arising out of such a finding but legally the term captures conduct serious enough to effectively break the contractual relationship between an employee and employer, resulting in dismissal.

Examples of gross misconduct:
dishonesty, theft or fraud;
malicious damage;
fighting or assault on another person;

serious incapability through alcohol or illegal drugs;
actions which endanger employees' safety;
falsification or unauthorised removal of company records or property;
a serious act of insubordination.

A recent case in the USA identified that an inflammatory post on facebook by a nurse which resulted in the employer dismissing her, was a valid ground for dismissal by the employer.

In *Guevarra v. Seton Medical Center*, No. C 13-2267 CW, 2013 WL 6235532 (N.D. Cal. Dec. 2, 2013), the plaintiff, a nurse at Seton Medical Center (Seton), posted on Facebook about her administrator. The content was abusive and threatening, written by an obviously furious nurse. The content was published to various "friends" and then forwarded to Seton. Seton called the police and ultimately terminated the plaintiff a day later. One of the many considerations the court explored that upheld the employer's right to terminate was: Facebook post undermined workforce morale and violated Seton's policy prohibiting harassment and the use of abusive language or behavior.

Complaints and investigations of professional misconduct

In practice most complaints go to the employer in the first instance, but there is also, in most states, a Health Rights Commission, that is, another statutory body created for the purpose of acting independently of the various professional bodies.

Every jurisdiction has systems for health complaints.

In addition, there are various routes available to the general public, such as a state or territory Health Commission, the ombudsman or state Health Departments. Most of these health complaints units are charged with the responsibility of investigating complaints and initiating conciliation procedures. In some states, for a serious matter, the health complaints unit can prosecute an offender, even before referring the matter to the relevant professional body; they can also hand over the matter to the police in certain circumstances.

There is no legislation directing a professional to lodge a complaint about a colleague unless they fall into the mandatory notifications. There are, however, powerful ethical pressures to ensure protection of clients and the profession as a whole from any aberrant colleagues. There are professional standards units that investigate most health professions other than nurses.

Above we discussed Boundaries of Practice, generally this relates to behaviours and interactions between professionals and clients.

The term Scope of practice indicates there are boundaries on practice. Violations can lead to disciplinary actions because there has been an undertaking of a role or an intervention that is beyond the proven competence and preparation through education and experience of that nurse. Thus the actions are considered unsafe.

Recall example 3 of the tribunal cases above. The EN was deemed to be working outside her scope of practice as she lacked proof of medication administration endorsement. The scope of practice of a student is very strictly monitored during their clinical placement. Unless evidence of education and supervised practice is in place, particular tasks and skills cannot be undertaken.

It is almost impossible to specify what is and what is not within an experienced nurses' scope in relation to skills. Further education, experience and circumstances all continue to add to the skills and knowledge of an individual. Guidelines cannot list every single skill or duty. Education programs cannot teach every single intervention. Skills transfer occurs with time and exposure so it is no wonder the concept is hard to grasp.

However functioning outside one's scope opens the way for disciplinary action. It should not be difficult for you to see that performing tasks or duties without adequate preparation and knowledge is going to put the client at risk of damage. Further, scope of practice is controlled by law. The range of duties that can be taken by different groups or levels of practitioners is specified by legislation (for example who can prescribe medication). Commonly violations occur as a result of "habits of practice, this is how we always have done things". Doing something because "everyone else is doing it", "prescribing and administering a medication because you think you can get a doctor to cover the order."

The governing standards, specifically the National Competency standards make clear the roles of nurses and midwives in Australia. There is a constant tension between the governing standards and legal controls exerted on health professionals and the realities of practice. Pressure to meet client needs in sometimes very difficult circumstances means nurses and midwives can find themselves undertaking roles that fall outside professional guidelines.

There are decision making frameworks to help us make rationale and safe judgments about what we will or will not undertake to do in practice.

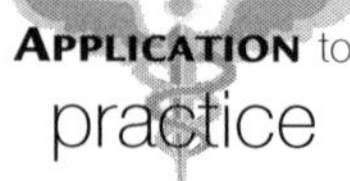

Application to practice

Below is an extract from an article in the *National Review of Nursing Education* (2000) by Francis, Bowman & Redgrave).

This article considers nursing issues from the perspective of the remote and rural nurse practice. It offers a good summary of the previous chapters, while highlighting the expansion in the role and functions of nurses. The article addresses many real-world issues that nurses must address.

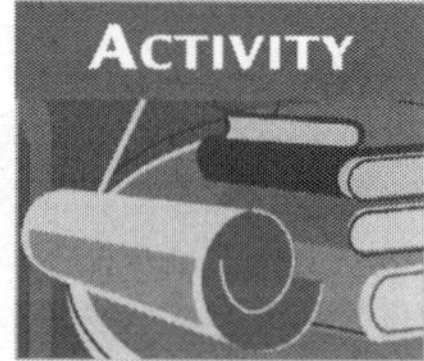

Activity

Read the summary below with a view to consolidating what you have learned, while asking yourself 'do the issues raised and the activities described leave these nurses vulnerable to sanctions?'.

Knowledge and skills required by rural nurses to meet the challenges of a changing work environment in the 21st century: a review of the literature

DEST, 2001 Copyright Ccommonwealth of Australia, reproduced by permission.

Introduction
Nursing in rural environments in the 21st century will pose many challenges. From the literature major issues facing rural nursing have been identified. These include recruitment and retention of rural nurses, practice issues such as legal issues, changing technology, and the work environment. It is recognised that the rural environment is responsive to extraneous factors such as national and international economies, political ideology, and climatic conditions. This section of the review will discuss these issues with reference to how they impact on nursing practice in rural areas. One way in which rural nursing practice has responded to these factors is the development of the philosophy of advanced practice and an investigation of skill mix issues. These aspects of rural nursing will also be examined in this section.

Educational providers, policy makers, the health service authorities and professional bodies must address the issues that are identified in this section.

Legal and ethical aspects of practice
Australia in the 21st Century will leave a legacy as an era of litigation. All health professionals practice within an environment in which autonomy of practice is demanded by practitioners, and responsibility and accountability for practice and improved health outcomes for actions implemented are expected by professional bodies, and the community (Mair, 2000).

Nursing practice in Australia is governed by the ANMAC competencies, which were developed to provide standards to regulate nursing practice. The ANMAC competencies communicate to consumers the competency standards that they can expect of nurses (Australian Nursing Council Inc., 2002). All registered and enrolled nurses are licensed to practice by the AHPRA Nursing and Midwifery Board.

Hegney et al (1997) point out nurses are concerned about negligence and breaching specific legislation in carrying out their duty of care. They assert that nurses should have a sound understanding of the law particularly common law and parliamentary or statute law and provide an overview of the legal requirements attached to the ordering and dispensing of Schedule 4 and 8 drugs. Mair (2000) argues that the very nature of nursing practice requires nurses to be vigilant about understanding the law. She cautions that nurses must recognise that if they claim to possess special skills they are required to exhibit higher standards of care and must be able to prove in court that care provided was to a standard expected if a case of negligence is bought against them. Hegney & Hobbs (1998) states nurses are concerned that they have become deskilled with the downgrading of health services in rural areas because they are unable to practise specialist skills routinely, eg midwifery. Conversely, the same situation has allowed some nurses to develop new skills and enhance their scope of practice (Mahnken et al 1997 in Hegney & Hobbs 1998). Plainly, the message that nurses must hear and respond to is that they must feel competent and have a knowledge base, which supports their practice. Many speciality organisations, mindful of the legal ramifications, are developing credentialling criteria as a benchmark for practice. For rural nurses this process is more difficult, given the multiplicity of roles expected in a multi-skilled nursing practitioner.

Several studies indicate that many rural nurses practise outside the legal parameters governing nursing practice (Kreger 1991; Hegney et al 1997; Handley

& Blue 1998; Spencer in Siegloff 1998). In a study by Cramar (2000) which investigated rural/remote nurses' practice she notes many of the nurses took on medical roles in the absence of medical practitioners, and practised in a manner which she deems did not meet the standards expected of either nursing or medicine. Hegney (1998) argues that many rural nurses are forced to practise outside the legal parameters governing nursing practice. Keyser (1997, p. 3) notes that '... rural nurses are often working well outside the legal parameters of nursing and providing services normally undertaken by a variety of healthcare workers'. Reasons nurses provided in Kreger's (1991, p. 22) study for undertaking practices which were outside legislation and standards of practice include:

- It is not realistically possible to cover all contingencies that arise in rural and remote health services with the human and material resources at present available;
- A medical practitioner is not always available on-site, or by telephone or radio, on all occasions advice or personal intervention is required for emergency or basic health care in rural and remote areas;
- Pharmacists, radiographers and other allied health and welfare professionals are not available on-site on all occasions required for basic care;
- Many rural medical practitioners, overtly and covertly, expect nurses to exercise their own discretion about the need for medical intervention or advice. The nurse is expected to determine whether he or she is competent to manage the presentation independently irrespective of the need for medical interventions. This perceived expectation can arise from open discussions between medical and nursing practitioners who trust each other, or as a result of nurses receiving professionally irresponsible responses when they do attempt to consult their distant medical colleagues on occasions legally requiring them to do so;
- The time involved in obtaining a medical practitioner's authorisation on every occasion it is legally required would render the remote area health service, in particular, dysfunctional in relation to the existing primary health care demands on the nurses;
- Some distant medical practitioners order nurses to undertake medical procedures and levels of care not appropriately performed at a remote location, or by a nurse;
- Cost factors associated with aerial evacuation are perceived by nurses to influence such expectations excessively, however reports on these matters are not confined to locations dependent on aerial evacuation of patients. The consumer's right to safe and appropriate health care, and the nurse's competence and capacity to fulfil extraordinary expectations within a remote community are often ill-considered;
- Consumers exert pressure on nurses to adhere to a standard of service based on previous fulfilment of medical, pharmaceutical and radiographic functions. Pressure occurs, particularly, when the alternative for the consumer involves returning for an investigation or therapeutic intervention at a later

time or date, a significantly increased waiting time, time consuming travel to another centre or an additional financial outlay;

- Nurses attempt to ensure ease of access to health services, and cooperation with consumer and colleague demands, needs and expectations. Nurses' moral and professional obligation to ease or prevent suffering is not related to the presence or absence of a medical practitioner, and frequently overrides the possibility of litigation;
- Nurses perceive tacit approval of their expanded practice. This is based on conclusions drawn from the inaction of others with responsibility in these matters. For example, the store or regional pharmacy continues to provide medical supplies and medications in the absence of prescriptions, licences to supply and accreditation certificates.
- The employer and medical, nursing and pharmaceutical responsibilities in the absence of written or verbal authorisation: The health service administration or regulatory authorities provide no practical alternatives or guidelines that are workable within the existing conditions.

Issues including the principles of ethics, professional responsibility and patient rights have become the focus of all health professionals' practice. Mair (2000, p. 124) warns that nursing practice involves touching health care consumers and in '... accordance with common law, all people have the right to determine what treatments or diagnostic tests they will be subjected to, unless there is some overriding law that allows treatment without consent.' Consent she claims must be informed consent, which involves the health care consumers' understanding of what is to be done and the risks involved.

In relation to your learning about professional governance, can you identify in this summary issues that could relate to all nurses and what, if any, might be the consequences for all nurses under current regulations should there be increasing discrepancies between real-world expectations and professional guidelines and education?

Application to practice

APPLICATION to practice

Formerly, every registering authority in Australia maintained records of complaints. There was a steady annual increase in every State and Territory about the number of complaints these boards received and dealt with. In the future this record will be kept by AHPRA, but it seems likely that there will continue to be increases in the volume of, and variety of complaints against nurses. In the past every registering authority published findings from tribunal cases. These publications identified categories of investigations, how many investigations there were, and some publications reported comparisons of numbers of similar complaints between years. For example, in 2005 the Nurses Board of Victoria reported that there had been more sexual misconduct cases reported, as well as those regarding failure to provide safe and competent care, unprofessional behavior and issues relating to the health of nurses, specifically matters relating to drugs and alcohol.

The Board identified that there had been nearly twice as many complaints from the aged care sector in 2004 compared with 2003, among those complaints were instances of verbal or physical abuse. Here is an example of an investigation into verbal abuse was reported. A nurse was before the Board in a formal hearing after a fellow nurse reported him for swearing at an elderly patient. The nurse under investigation had said he believed that his swearing was under his breath and it had not been directed at any patient in particular. However he accepted it was audible to patients in the ward.

At this hearing other complaints against this nurse were considered, and the tribunal held that his behaviour was found to have constituted unprofessional conduct of a serious nature. The Board placed conditions on his registration in spite of recognising the nurse did have a sound career in nursing (Nexus, 2006 p. 7). There were many reported complaints made to the Nurses Board of Victoria on a wide variety of issues, and what was worrying was the increased number of complaints over a one-year period. The trend was reflected in every state regulatory authority publication until the move to a National Authority occurred. APHRA will also be required to publish its decisions.

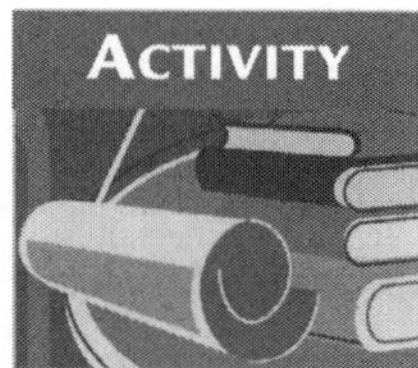

Activity

Since the move to national regulation, State Tribunals hear cases presented by each health practitioner, Board and Appeals against findings. Summaries of the Tribunal hearing are published. Full cases can be found for each Board by searching various State Tribunal publications. Just to get an idea of the number of cases one Tribunal deals with and to see the types of issues each regulating authority takes to a hearing, look at the published summaries.

Health Practitioner Tribunal case summaries 2012 go to: www.ahpra.gov.au/documents/default.aspx?record...dbid=AP

Health Practitioner Tribunal case summaries 2013 go to: www.ahpra.gov.au/documents/default.sapx?record...dbid=AP

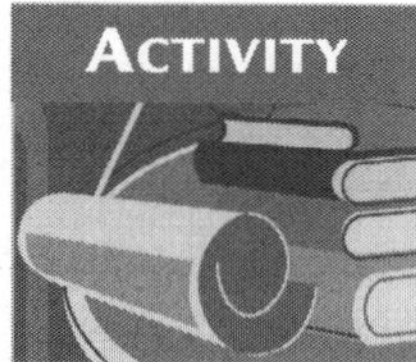

Activity

A colleague tells you at tea break: 'I am really worried, I was told to give Mrs G her meds; she isn't even my patient but the surgeon rang down the order as a pre-medication and I was the only one available to administer it. I've never given IV narcotics before but they were in such a rush waiting to transfer to theatre I went ahead. Before I came to tea I heard she was sent to intensive care; she collapsed before they even got her into theatre.'

- Explore this situation in relation to issues of professional governance.
- How might the professional registering body become involved in such a situation?
- What actions might arise from this situation, and what standards would be applied by the registering authority to any investigation or review of the situation?
- What guidelines or policies might have prevented this situation? What might be the findings of an investigation?

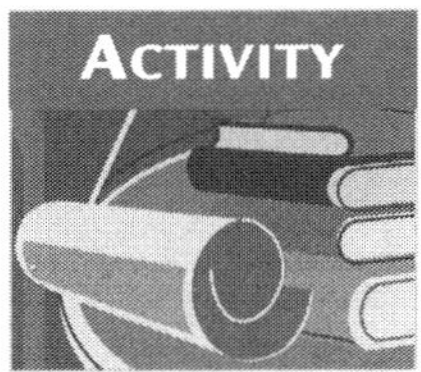

Activity

Carmel is a new graduate working as an RN in a medical unit. Her manager frequently corrects Carmel's work, finding fault with her documentation, the way Carmel manages her time and workload and in Carmel's opinion the manager is 'picking on her'.

This comes to a head when the manager chastises Carmel in front of other staff during handover. Carmel is angry and embarrassed and walks out of handover. Later Carmel tells her patients about how unfair the manager has been and feels comforted by their sympathy. At home Carmel tells her boyfriend and his mate (both are also nurses) about how terrible the manager is, what sort of person Carmel thinks she is and talks about how 'her patients' understood and discusses her patients at length to explain how their opinion was valid and how one had offered to report the manager to his son who was on the hospital board.

- Explore this situation in relation to issues of professional governance.
- How might the professional registering body become involved in such a situation?
- What actions might arise from this situation, and what standards would be applied by the registering authority to any investigation or review of the situation?
- What guidelines or policies might have prevented this situation?
- What might be the findings of an investigation?

A possible assignment question

Scenario 2 Length 1000-1200 words

Consider in light of legal requirements and nursing professional requirements, the issue below.

RN, Petra has 10 years of experience is a casual call nurse and has, over 2 years worked a few surgical shifts each month.

At 3pm she took handover for Holly Kinter 42 years post operative hysterectomy from recovery. Holly was alert but in mild discomfort, her observations stable, IV normal saline running and full post operative comfort and patient teaching measures were provided by Petra. Pain medication had been administered to Holly prior to her arrival on the ward.

At 4.30 pm Petra was required to go to x-ray and she delegated her 5 patients' care to EN George. At 5.30 she returned to the ward and sent George to tea. At six she went to tea.

At 7pm Holly's husband read the patient notes which had been left on her bed since return to the ward.

The husband was very agitated, he said Holly was in extreme pain, no one had done anything for her and she had been left without care for hours.

Her IV had just run out. Holly was so distressed she was demanding to be transferred to another facility by ambulance. Her husband said he would be going to see a lawyer about her care.

On investigation the observation chart showed these had been done by Petra at 3.45, by George at 5.15 and nothing was documented since.

Nothing was written in the patient progress notes. The IV was due to be changed at 8pm.

a) Apply the elements of negligence to this situation: to support your discussion refer to the ANMC competencies.
b) In reference to the issue of patient documentation what professional and/or legal standards were breached?

You are not expected to argue a legal case, you are required only to apply legal standards in negligence against the facts given.

Summary

Professional governance is a fact of the professional's life. Taking advantage of the knowledge and expertise embedded in professional boards is possible by utilising their guidelines, publications, websites and the information that accompanies annual registration applications. The point of having professional governing bodies is to protect the public and they do this by informing, monitoring and ensuring their professional members satisfy standards.

This chapter has also introduced a new area of law, Administrative Law and developed on some of the legal concepts that have been raised earlier. The notion of natural justice and the application of rules of law used to review investigations of complaints means that while frivolous, unfounded or malicious complaints will be investigated as rigorously as genuine complaints the professional under scrutiny can be confident that the procedures will be fair and open to review and their right to privacy and protection will be upheld by a tribunal.

Sources

Australian Health Practitioner Regulation Agency, 2010, About AHPRA at <http .ahpra.gov.au> (accessed 28 July 2014).

Colleran Cook, M. (2006) 'Six rights for safe medication administration', *Nursing Practice*, Massachusetts Nurses Board, Mass., at <www.massnurses.org/nurse_practice/sixrights.htm> (accessed 26 July 2014).

Forbes, J. R. S. (2002) *Justice in Tribunals*, Federation Press, Sydney.

Forrester, K. & Griffiths, D. (2005) *Essentials of Law*, 2nd edn, Harcourt, Sydney.

Forrester, K. & Griffiths, D. (2010) *Essentials of Law for Health Professionals*, 3rd edn, Elsevier, Chatswood, NSW.

Francis, K., Bowman, S. & Redgrave, M. (2002) 'Knowledge and skills required by rural nurses to meet the challenges of a changing work environment in the 21st Centry: a review of the literature', *National Review of Nursing Education*, Department of Education, Science and Training, Canberra, pp. 151–215.

Kennedy, R. & Richards, J. (2004) *Integrating Human Service Law and Practice*, Oxford University Press, Melbourne.

McCullough, S. (2002) 'Aged care: a Victorian perspective on complaints handling and the enforcement of consumer rights', *Alternative Law Journal*, **27**(2): 57–67.

MacFarlane, P. (1995) *Health Law*, 2nd edn, The Federation Press, Sydney.
MacFarlane, P. J. & Reid, S. J. (2003) *Queensland Health Law Handbook*, Queensland Dept of Health, Brisbane.
Morris, J. (2000) 'Insuring against negligence: medical indemnity in Australia', *Policy*, Spring, <www.cis.org.au/policy/Spring02/polspring02-2.htm> (formerly accessed 9 June 2005).
Nurses Board of Victoria (2006) 'How the Board Handles Complaints', *Nexus* **13**(2): 1–16.
Queensland Nursing Forum (2005) *Without Prejudice Meetings*, **13**(1): 27–28.
Sinclair, A. (1996) 'Codes in the workplace: organizational versus professional codes', in M. Coady & S. Bloch (eds), *Codes of Ethics and the Professions*, Melbourne University Press, Melbourne.
Staunton, P. & Chiarella, M. (2003) *Nursing and the Law*, 5th edn, Elsevier, Sydney.
Staunton, P. & Whyburn, B. (1997) *Nursing and the Law*, 4th edn, Harcourt Australia Pty Ltd, Sydney.
Stone, J. (2002) 'Evaluating the ethical and legal contents of professional codes of ethics', in, J. Allsop & M. Saks (eds), *Regulating the Health Professions*, Sage, London, pp. 62–75.
White, B., Wilmott, L. & McDonald, F. (2014) *Health Law in Australia*, 2nd edn, Thomson Reuters, Australia.

Cases

Amec Capital Projects Ltd. v. Whitefriars City Estates Ltd., The Times, 8 November 2004.
Dental Board of Queensland v. B. (2003) QLR 13 December.
Ex parte Meehan, The Medical Practitioners Act (1965).
Heathcote v. Nurses Registration Board and Walton (District Court of New South Wales, unreported, 12 April 1991).
Hoile v. Medical Board of South Australia (1960) 104 CLR 157.
Ping v. Medical Board of Queensland (2004) QLR 24 January.
Qidwai v. Brown (1984) NSWLR 100.
Skinner v. Beaumont (1974) 347 SW2d 950.

Legislation

Health Practitioner Regulation National Law Act (Cwth) 2009.

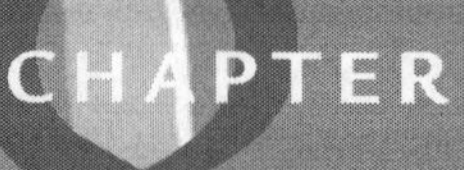

Nursing myths and facts

Learning outcomes

After studying this chapter you should be able to:

- Display an understanding of key legislation affecting health policies and procedures.
- Describe the role of the law in providing direction for health care practice.
- Demonstrate a knowledge of procedures and policies for investigation of health matters, professional and legal hearings and sanctions for failure to meet standards.
- Apply legal and professional standards when assessing and responding to client needs, practice and policy situations, professional reporting and communication.

Overview

It should be obvious by now that the law tends to be retrospective. It is usually after something has happened that investigation occurs and penalties are imposed. Recall that in Chapter 1 the difference between ethics and law was discussed. Ethical codes tend to direct people to review, analyse and assess their intentions before they proceed. The law tends to examine matters after they have occurred. Therefore, professional groups, parliamentarians, institutions and individuals will attempt to avoid repetition of circumstances or behaviours that caused problems by incorporating legal recommendations or findings into policy. They do this by implementing rules or directives, and putting legislation in place to change workplace conditions, for example making safety guards for machinery, first aid and fire warden training mandatory. Legislation requiring reviews of practices and equipment may involve creating new roles or delegating greater powers to those employed to monitor and ensure best practice is implemented. Think about environmental health issues, where the local council has powers to carry out health inspections and so on.

There are policies for so many things we may assume there is a policy for everything. As professionals, part of your education is to prepare you to be able to apply knowledge to specific situations, problem solve and make decisions after critically evaluating and assessing the situation. There are always going to be circumstances where there is no rule or procedure, the principle in law that keeps being repeated is that of 'what is reasonable', 'what would a reasonable person do in this situation'? Of course, the more education and experience you have, the higher the standard of 'reasonable' will be. Over time, as a result of media interpretation or highly publicised court cases (most often in the USA), there has been growing anxiety among health professionals as to their liability and responsibilities.

It is true, if someone has special skills, is a recognised authority or is employed on the basis of knowledge and competence, that expectations will be higher than for the 'ordinary man'. What is important is to recognise that as long as you perform within accepted professional standards, satisfy policy which reflects legislation and understand what and why you did something – and can provide a rationale for that choice – there is little reason to be anxious about your liability. Of course there may be questions and even investigations when an adverse outcome occurs, and this is where adequate, appropriate and accurate documentation comes into the picture.

Myths or facts?

There are many statements made throughout the health services. Some have a nugget of truth, some are just myths. Consider these.

- 'Don't ever stop at an accident; if the injured person dies you could be liable.'
- 'You must stop whenever you see an accident; you will be deregistered if they find out you didn't offer help.'
- 'Don't witness anything; you will end up in court.'
- 'Don't give information; if you say something different or explain it in another way you can get into trouble.'
- 'If something goes wrong, it will always be the nurse who ends up in court.'
- 'If a student or enrolled nurse does anything wrong, the registered nurse will be liable.'

So far you have seen that legislation and common law cases give direction for policies and direction for practice. Often there are no specific 'do's and don'ts' written in legislation or case law although there may well be directives in legislation that require institutions or individuals to implement procedures or policies to achieve standards.

One of the most common 'horror stories' bandied among nurses and doctors is the issue of failing to stop or, equally, stopping to help at the scene of an accident. In law this is often referred to as the 'good Samaritan' situation. Health staff fear that if they give aid at an accident an injured person might sue them directly if interventions or aid either worsened the condition or failed to resolve the problem. Recall from Chapter 7 that recent legislation changes specifically address and limit the liability of the good Samaritan.

Legislation does have specific requirements for rendering assistance in specific situations. Motor vehicle accidents are the most obvious. Drivers of vehicles involved in accidents are required to stop and provide assistance. There is no requirement for passengers or passers-by to do so.

Legislation imposes an obligation on medical practitioners to render professional services within a reasonable time *of being called* to do so. We will come back to this point below.

In emergency situations there *is* a legal duty to help where:

- the person requiring assistance is related; or
- the person requiring assistance is under the control of another who has a 'duty' towards them.

If you do stop to render aid, at that point the law will consider you have a duty of care. This is only the same duty that would be expected of anyone who stops and volunteers help (Commonwealth Treasury (IPP Report) 2002). What is important to understand is that the law expects only what is 'reasonable in the circumstances', so, whether you have extraordinary clinical expertise or not, at the scene all that can be expected is first aid. As long as the steps taken in a particular situation fall within what is reasonable, given the equipment, circumstances, knowledge and abilities of the person rendering aid, then history proves that no court will entertain a claim against that person by the injured party or their family. (*Lowry v Mayo Newhall Hospital* 64 ALR 4th 1191 (Cal 1986), 1196; *Vaughan v Webb* (1902) 2 SR(NSW) 293) (*Mid Density Developments Pty Ltd v Rockdale Municipal Council* (1993) 44 FCR 290).

The myth 'if you stop you could be liable for the outcome' is so pervasive that South Australia introduced legislation to ensure a victim cannot sue a good Samaritan. The parliamentarian who introduced the bill admitted that while there were no cases of such a thing happening the legislation was designed to overcome the fear of litigation, and get people to help. This logic explains why the Commonwealth and most states have taken up the issue in legislation relating to civil liability since the Ipp Report.

Below is the relevant legislation for each state.

ACT: Civil Law (wrongs) Act 2002
NSW: Civil Liability Act 2002
NT: Personal Injuries (Liabilities and Damages) Act 2003
QLD: Civil Liability Act 2003
SA: Civil Liability Act 1936
TAS: Civil Liability Act 2002
VIC: Wrongs Act 1958
WA: Civil Liability Act 2002
QLD: Law Reform Act 1995 Note: unlike other state's legislation the Queensland Act only provides protection from civil liability for doctors and nurses, and members or employees of listed organisations (such as the volunteer emergency services) (Law Reform Act 1995 (Qld) s 16).

In New South Wales the law specifically offers protection to health professionals who volunteer their help. The fact is there has never been a case where a volunteer who has acted in a reasonable manner, faced with the difficulties and pressures of such a situation, has been faced with litigation.

What is often discussed during tea break is the situation where a professional *chooses not* to attend and lend their expertise to an injured person. This *can* get a health professional into trouble. If someone has skill and acknowledged professional capacity, refusing to attend the injured could be construed as professional negligence. Avoiding or withholding your recognised skill goes against ethical codes and standards and these would be the standard used by a court to judge that behaviour.

In *Medical Board Of Australia v Dekker* [2013] WASAT 182 it was held that failing to at least go and see if people needed help when the doctor was aware that there had been a serious car accident (as she was nearly in the accident) constituted unsatisfactory professional conduct.

> "It matters not that there is no existing professional relationship between a medical practitioner and the persons involved in the accident. Because saving human life and healing sick and injured people is a core purpose and ethic of the medical profession, and because members of the profession have the knowledge and skills to do so, the failure by a medical practitioner to make an assessment and render assistance when he or she is aware that a motor vehicle accident has or may have occurred in their vicinity and that people have or may have been injured, when the practitioner is physically able to do so, would, notwithstanding that the practitioner reports the matter immediately to police or other emergency services, reasonably be regarded as improper by medical practitioners of good repute and competency, and there is a sufficiently close link or nexus with the profession of medicine"(page 39).

Fear of violence or alcohol and drug fueled reactions by the "victims" towards the rescuer may lie behind a decision to not stop and render assistance at an accident. This situation was proposed to the Tribunal in the *Dekker* case. While a Tribunal does not have the same standing as a court to set precedent this case does give direction to future hearings.

> "In any case, even if the practitioner had been thinking of these issues [alcoholism, drug use and violent behaviour], they would not have absolved her from her professional obligation to make an assessment and render assistance to the occupants of the second vehicle. Furthermore ... it was not reasonable to expect that the occupant or occupants of the second vehicle 'would have been agitated and might have posed a risk to the [practitioner's] personal safety', given that the practitioner was aware, by instinct as a doctor, that they had suffered 'a bad injury'. Of course, if the occupant or occupants of the second vehicle had threatened violence towards the practitioner, the practitioner would have discharged her professional obligation and could have driven to the police station" (page 44).

Most cases of professional negligence relate to situations occurring *after* injury when a medical officer has been called for assistance. Failure to attend in a timely manner, failure to provide care that reflects expected standards, failure to assess and diagnose patients appropriately have led to findings of professional negligence. So this is not a myth.

- There is a possibility of being accused of professional negligence should you fail to provide aid; this risk does not exist for the public at large.

Here again, though, the expected standard of care rendered would only be measured against what could be reasonably done in the circumstances.

Higher standards are expected in particular situations where the professional has in fact been trained and provided with resources to use in an emergency. For example, occupational health nurses working in a factory must attend an injured worker and, while interventions may be limited by the circumstances, that assistance would be expected to utilise training and equipment that should be up to date and ready for just such an emergency. A higher standard could be expected in this situation.

In an emergency or at the scene of an accident if you attempt to volunteer assistance then all that is expected is that your interventions are reasonable. If you are responsible for the safety or care of others in an emergency or an accident, it is expected that you will take all reasonable steps to help those clients. Again the key is 'reasonable' in those particular circumstances.

- There is no imperative that you imperil yourself or others in trying to save someone.

In fact putting others at risk of injury or death in an 'unreasonable attempt' to save someone would be grounds for legal proceedings against you; however, courts are aware that in the chaos of the moment it is often impossible to attribute blame for such sad outcomes. However, you can bet that institutions, accident and emergency services and community organisations will implement policies, training and education to avoid a recurrence.

It is true that there may be investigations of accidents, especially if death has resulted. Whether health professionals volunteered assistance at the scene or were on duty when the injured were transported or admitted for care, it may be that all involved are required to give evidence in order to establish what occurred. This is the point of a coronial hearing, to gain information; it is not to attribute blame. Findings might give direction for further investigations, and any of us can be called as witnesses and must attend to give evidence if that happens.

Earlier in this chapter reference was made to the situations where the common law does expect a person to render assistance, that is, where the injured or at risk person is related or in the control of another.

- So, for example, parents are expected to take all reasonable steps to save their children.
- Health professionals are expected to take all reasonable steps to save their patients, to help those in their direct care.

Consider the situation of a fire in a nursing home, or where clients are physically or mentally at risk or injured during an emergency. Staff on duty and even those off duty are expected to do everything possible to help those in their care. This can extend to clients in the community who may be visited or who attend a clinic. Institutional policies may require staff using work vehicles to stop and attend at the scene of an accident.

- Should the professional suspect the client is at risk of injury, self-harm or accident there is an obligation for them to take all reasonable steps to prevent or reduce risks.

Writing your concerns in client notes is insufficient. Telling someone who lacks the standing or skills to intervene is equally insufficient. It is expected that a health professional will refer the matter appropriately *and* follow up to ensure that appropriate steps are taken. Only if there was evidence that the professional was inadequate in their assessment of the risk, that they failed to carry out reasonable steps or from a professional point of view fell below the basic standard expected would there be a possibility of a finding of negligence.

Again, policies and protocols are often in place to avoid 'individual problem solving'. Rather than hope all staff will know what to do, there are rules governing clients deemed to be at risk. The law specifically addresses through legislation the rights and issues relating to children and those with a mental illness. We will explore these later.

Witnessing documents

Another area of confusion is whether you can sign as a witness to a consent form, a will or a contract. When you sign as a witness you are saying you actually saw the person sign the statement, will or contract at that time. You cannot witness a signature if you were not there, nor could you witness a signature if you were blind; you are signing that you saw that person actually sign the document.

There is no obligation for you to know what the document is about or what the document actually says. A witness is not the signatory, a witness is not claiming they agree, approve or know anything other than they saw that person sign this paper.

Where a person signs that they observed or were part of an activity such as being present when a patient was informed of the risks of removing themselves from care, or they were present when the patient or patient's family were informed about treatment or the patient was warned about consequences of refusing treatment, then signing the document carries a much higher obligation.

'What am I signing?' is a good question to ask. On wills or some agreements it is only that you saw the person put their mark or signature to a document that matters. If it is a contract, however, you may be a party to it, that is, even if you are not the person buying something, you might be signing that you guarantee to take on a debt, or that this person who is signing is known to you and not an impostor. This is common with passport applications.

To be a witness it is preferable for you to be over 18 years of age but except for wills this is rarely an issue. However, government papers such as passport applications are very specific about who can witness a signature.

- The witness should be independent of the matter being agreed, contracted or willed. So if you were going to benefit from a will, if the contract directly affected you, then your being a witness could lead to argument about the validity of the document.

Anyone of sound mind and independent of the matter addressed by the document can be a witness to a signature. The reason behind most institutions having policies strongly advising staff not to be a witness to such documents is the potential for later legal proceedings. It doesn't take much imagination to work out that clients in hospital may organise with a lawyer, friends or family to make a new will, to contract to give away valuable possessions or money or may promise in writing something that others disagree with. The likelihood of the aggrieved person claiming the author was confused, affected by medication, tricked or taken advantage of is high. Therefore to protect staff from proceedings or investigations where not only the question of the signature is at issue but also all the circumstances and interpretations of the client's state of mind are being questioned, a policy directing staff to notify someone nominated by the institution is often in place.

It is not illegal to witness a document unless you did not see the signature made. It is not an issue from a witness's point of view that the author was not who they claimed to be.

In Chapter 4, dealing with consent, the matter of witnessing a client's consent to treatment was dealt with at that point; however, many of the considerations discussed here are behind policies specifying just who should witness these documents. To reiterate, the information given to gain consent and the signature to witness that consent for a medical procedure should be by the practitioner performing that specific procedure.

Certifying and signing legal documents

Although a will and contract have legal standing there are documents that are required by law to meet certain requirements and as such the person signing and witnessing these must be recognised by law. Affidavits are legal documents used in court proceedings, there is a requirement for an oath or affirmation attesting to the truth of the document is taken before signing. Statutory Declarations need to be witnessed by authorised (by legislation) people. The person making the statement (the declarant) must sign the declaration in the presence of an authorised witness and make a solemn declaration that it is true and correct.

Some documents such as an application for National registration with AHPRA must be certified as true copies of the original documents. Only specific people are authorised to sign these.

The same rule exists for passport applications.

For these types of documents the application will specify who can sign.

Gifts and payments

There are stories about how people have been tricked into giving away valuables or while in care given gifts to those they admired or perhaps feared. Some of these are true stories. Perhaps the giver genuinely wished to repay service or kindness or ensure disposition of their possessions to people of their choice.

Where an argument arises about the right of a beneficiary or recipient over the rights of family it is assumed that the giver's wishes are valid and the court will uphold these. If the family can show that pressure, such as fear or threats, was brought to bear on the giver, or the gift giver was confused or mentally unstable or misled, then the courts may identify that a crime has been committed or may simply cancel the gift.

When providing care, the balance between a client showing appreciation and feeling obliged to give 'bribes' to ensure attention is sometimes an issue. In many countries unless the family pays the staff directly with cash or gifts their relative will not get care. The offer of money 'to make sure mum is cared for' can be quite a shock to an Australian health worker. If employed to provide care, and the health professional is contracted to do this as an employee, taking money independently to give that care is unacceptable. It could be argued that the employee had entered into two contracts to provide the same thing. If the double payment is discovered the employee might even be required to show that there was no fraud or coercion involved. Certainly no accredited health facility would be satisfied with the behaviour and it could be grounds for termination of employment.

Tipping, that is, giving a gratuity over and above an agreed price or in return for a service, is a normal practice in many countries. Australians have adopted (usually reluctantly) the practice of adding 10% or so to the cost of meals, taxi rides and other activities. Tipping is not an accepted practice in health service provision; accepting cash as a thanks for service the client feels was above and beyond that expected would be considered unethical, thus putting your professional standing at risk, even if not unlawful.

To avoid any confusion or risk of embarrassment, most facilities have a written or unwritten policy specifying that cash is never accepted by staff. A lavish gift is equally risky. Gold watches or jewellery have been given and here again the recipient is vulnerable. What is always at the back of people's minds are the concepts of theft, fraud or deception whereby a health professional takes advantage of the client. There have been criminal charges laid and successful prosecutions against nurses who have benefited from clients, whether the client was willing or not in handing over something of value.

Not only might other staff members suspect the motives of the health professional, but it may be considered professionally unethical.

The Nursing and Midwifery Board's *A nurse's guide to professional boundaries* (2010 p.3) states: Nurses recognise that involvement in financial transactions (other than in a contract for the provision of services) and the receipt of anything other than 'token gifts' within professional relationships with persons in their care is likely to compromise the professional relationship.

The odd box of chocolates or small gifts of toiletries, books or such like are not going to draw attention or questions about ethical standards but, remembering that Australia is a multicultural country, clients may have quite different interpretations about their obligations and attitudes to gift giving, and it requires some delicacy in refusing gifts. Even where there is no policy it is not unusual to hear staff members claim 'they can't accept due to the policy'. These professionals are treading a line between risking giving offence and adhering to good ethical standards.

Yet another myth

Surely I can answer questions and give information. That is my job; why should I be scared of the law if I am doing my job?

Here again it is necessary to refer to the concept of negligence. If a person suffers damage as a result of your information then you can be found liable. No matter how well intentioned, you must ensure that what you are saying, recommending or giving advice about is accurate.

What would be easily discounted or ignored if it came from a family member or neighbour is likely to be taken as gospel and acted upon if suggested by a professional. There is a category of negligence known as negligent misstatement; this covers giving wrong advice. The elements of negligent misstatement considered for a legal action are:

- Whether there is a special relationship between the person giving the information and the person receiving it.
- The level of competence of the person who gave the advice.
- How reasonable was it for the person getting this advice to act upon it and how much damage resulted from acting upon it.

While there are few cases specific to health professionals or health agencies the risk of such an action is predictable. Should you give advice thoughtlessly or lack knowledge about an issue, even if you think you have qualified your statement and alerted a client about the limits of your information, you should assume that the level of trust in you as a professional may be so high that anything you say has great credibility.

This does not mean you are gagged and silent. It does mean that you need to recognise that there is always a special relationship between health carers and clients, thus trust in your information. Therefore consider your words carefully and avoid throwaway lines or guesses; if you don't know and no one else does either then let the client know this. You must accept that, rather than be personally embarrassed, here in this situation you do not know that answer, and you must be competent and professional enough to recognise the fact. Refer the client to the right person or seek that information on their behalf.

Questioning orders; deciding to notify

We explored professional standards and professional governance in Chapter 7. These have relevance here to the myth of 'a nurse must obey the doctor's orders without question'.

A nurse has an obligation to check anything they do not understand. Following a written or verbal instruction that directs activities that are beyond their skill or experience or failing to provide sufficient information are obviously issues to be dealt with. Further, there is a professional and legal obligation to question an order if the nurse believes the treatment ordered is medically inappropriate or incorrect. As the client advocate, the nurse has a responsibility to question an order if they believe the client has been misled or inadequately informed about the risks or consequences of that treatment.

In assessing and reviewing a client, where a nurse identifies that the client status has altered, especially if there is a suspicion they are deteriorating or experiencing problems, the nurse must notify the doctor to inform them and, if necessary, request their attendance. The option of 'wait until the routine visit' is not acceptable. Of course your first steps may be to discuss concerns and seek advice from more experienced nursing staff but the decision of whether or not to call the doctor must be made with the client's best interests in mind.

There have been a few common law cases to do with whether the damage caused to the patient was a result of the nurse(s) failing to notify the doctor. In Australia an investigation into the death of a small boy identified that (trained) nurses did have the expertise and obligation to contact the doctor and express their opinions and concerns (*Coronial Inquest Adelaide Coroner's Court* 1989).

The manner and place where the discussion is held may influence the situation. It needs to be said that in a busy and stressful situation the style of communication between the nurse and doctor could affect the outcome. Professional discretion and courtesy are the ideal. Recall the case study in Chapter 1 where the nurse, after questioning the doctor's orders, proceeded to administer the excessive dose of medication. The standard of care expected of a nurse is now clearly articulated in both codes of practice and the Australian nurse and midwife competencies.

- Should the nurse hold any doubts these must be expressed to the doctor; if the nurse continues to believe the order puts the client at risk the nurse is entitled to refuse to administer or implement that treatment.

Institutional protocols may not exist for this type of situation or there may be identified staff members who should be involved before refusing to carry out an order. Expert staff may understand the rationale and be able to direct you to evidence that supports the treatment. At the least seek advice before refusing to do something. It is quite reasonable for you to ask the doctor to carry out the order.

Grounds for dismissal and discrimination

In 2005, changes occurred to legislation governing the rules of dismissal in some workplaces. Health professionals contracts will be discussed in Chapter 9 but here we will deal with the pervasive myth that it is possible to be 'sacked on the spot'. In reality the employer risks a great deal should they do this. Grounds to dismiss an employee are clear and legislation offers protection as do the courts for unfair dismissal. Changes to Australia's Industrial Relation law in 2005 appear to limit court and tribunal arbitration processes for employees who claim they have been unfairly dismissed. These changes are reflected in new legislation:

- Fair Work Act 2009
- Fair Work Regulations 2009
- Fair Work Commission Rules 2013

Unfair dismissal proceedings covered under the *Fair Work Act* is handled by Fair Work Australia, who may be able to handle a claim up until its conclusion. However, if the issue cannot be resolved by the process of conciliation, the claim may be pursued in the Federal Court or the Federal Magistrates Court.

There are some categories of employees who are excluded from bringing an action of unfair dismissal that also apply at a state and federal level. Those who may be excluded are:

- an employee who is still on probation
- an employee on contract for a specific task

- a casual employee who is engaged for only a short period
- some apprentices and trainees
- In NSW under the national workplace relations system administered by the federal government employees of private sector employers if dismissed after 1 January 2010

Employers of less than 100 workers can dismiss employees without following previous award procedures. This does not lessen the risk of industrial unrest and media attention on a business although the same legislation does impose penalties for industrial actions where none existed previously.

However while the extent and future of this legislation remains to be tested, health services continue to employ staff within the constraints of enterprise agreements and awards. Avoiding a claim against unfair dismissal will continue to remain a priority for most employers.

What is more likely is that an employee can be 'suspended from duties' pending investigation into the situation or behaviour that has caused a problem, which removes a potentially unsafe or problem employee. Employers need to be able to point to pre-dismissal procedures that evidence fairness in their dealings and show that opportunities were given for the employee to acknowledge and correct problems. These are often referred to as 'warnings' and most employers keep careful records to show that the employee had every opportunity to correct the problem.

A case that shows how problematic dismissal can be is worth a read. The reasons for the result for the case will give you some insight into the way a situation is assessed.

Go to: www.vmia.vic.gov.au/~/...?201105-Case1-EmployeeDismissal.pdf (accessed 7 August 2014)

The concept of fair and reasonable will be the key to any questions about dismissal. It is entrenched in legislation that it is unfair to dismiss a worker on the basis of their race or ethnicity. Other grounds that are held to be discriminatory are sex, religion, skin colour, pregnancy or family responsibilities, political or social affiliations, age or disability. Australian residents are covered by the provisions of federal legislation (*Racial Discrimination Act*, *Sex Discrimination Act*, *Disability Discrimination Act*). There is in addition state legislation prohibiting discrimination on a variety of grounds (there are some minor differences between states). However, while there is very broad protection against discrimination, all legislation identifies exemptions. Particular work needs may require workers of one sex only to be available for clients; hospitals that are operated by religious orders may have the right to employ staff who adhere to the same beliefs and practices.

Recall from Chapter 7 the discussion about Gross Misconduct; grounds for dismissal were:

dishonesty, theft or fraud;
malicious damage;
fighting or assault on another person;
serious incapability through alcohol or illegal drugs;
actions which endanger employees' safety;
falsification or unauthorised removal of company records

or property;
a serious act of insubordination".

As long as the employer could prove the allegation and demonstrate fair procedures were followed and has documentation to support the matter, any appeal by the dismissed employee would probably fail.

Activity

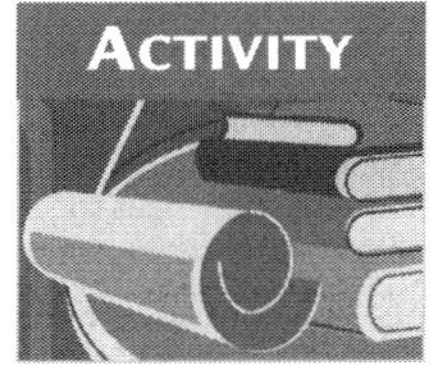

Scenario. In a small surgical facility, following the 11 September terrorist attack in New York staff refused to provide a client of Middle Eastern origin with care. Meals were not delivered or were supplied late, treatments were delayed and the client was told by more than one staff member he should go and get treatment from 'one of your own kind'.

- Is this an example of discrimination? What might be the legal or professional consequences to a health professional who does not provide care for a client because of issues of discrimination?
- Was there a failure of duty of care?

Clinical realities: frequently asked questions

With little effort most experienced clinicians can think up any number of 'what if . . .' 'what about when . . .?' situations. By now the principles that govern professional standards, negligence and ethical reasoning should provide some insight into what circumstances could have legal consequences.

Frightening ourselves to the point of putting clients at risk because of our own fear of legal liabilities is to be avoided at all cost. No matter how often principles are explained most nurses still seek clear direction and concrete answers. Some real-world situations that are often raised by qualified staff are given below.

What happens if I go off duty and have forgotten to document something?

If you realise the oversight but cannot 'reasonably' return to correct it, one option is to notify a colleague on duty and let them know. It is not illegal to document at a later time. What would be negligent is failure to notify staff about essential facts that could affect the client. The colleague can note: 'written on behalf of X – they can provide essential details and sign the note'. Leaving a blank space is not recommended. A simple written statement that X will complete notes on return to work is fine if there is no essential data to be included. On return to work you add to the notes beside the current date and state that this entry is for a previous date and time.

What happens if I forgot something and others have since written their notes?

Again, put in the current date and time and state this information is an 'addit' or additional to the relevant date and time entry.

Why is there a policy that I cannot wear my uniform outside of work? All I want to do is pick up some groceries on the way home?

In earlier times the argument was about infection control more than anything else. Today many institutions don't actually have such a policy. However, it may be in your own best interest to remove your uniform before going home as, should you be a passer-by at an accident or incident, the expectation created by your uniform that you can deal with the situation may be far higher than your capability and experience to deal with the situation.

Can I lengthen the time between observations when I have established that the patient is stable and no longer needs close monitoring?

If you as a registered nurse have the skill and expertise and clinical standing to assess the client accurately, know all the relevant details and there is no written order to the contrary you can change the times. It is likely that the standing order for intensive monitoring has not been updated and now in the nurses' opinion is no longer valid. Check first with the author of the order or their representative if possible. Should there be some health risk you are unaware of, for example cardiac irregularities, that provided the rationale to maintain frequent observations, you will at least understand the need to continue close monitoring.

Who can mobilise a client? Is it the physiotherapist only or can nurses do this?

Unless there are specific orders requiring a physiotherapist only, as long as the client is approved for this and the nurse has the skill and experience and has carried out a risk assessment then it is a duty within the nurse's role.

What is the rule about nurse-initiated medications?

Policies exist in most facilities about what (if any) medicines can be given without a prescription or a written order. Generally Schedule 2 medicines (available over the counter) can be given by a registered nurse who has full knowledge of the patient's current medication regime and allergies as well as the ability to assess the client appropriately. Some Schedule 3 medications are recognised as essential and permitted without an order in some situations. Asthma-relieving drugs such as puffers and inhalations, pain-relieving gases in midwifery practice and drugs to reverse the effects of narcotics are examples. If there is no policy, professional discretion in light of assessment and circumstances will support the nurse, but getting a policy in place is far preferable.

As a student or enrolled nurse can I get into trouble if I do something I was told to do but the act was specifically prohibited by policy?

Yes. If you are aware that the action is outside of your scope of practice you are personally responsible for undertaking it. However, the rules of delegation mean that the person directing another to act must establish the competence and confidence of that individual, although some circumstances such as an emergency can override policy. If the student or enrolled nurse fails to admit they lack the skill or experience then the senior staff members who reasonably 'relies' upon them to do the job correctly is not at fault. Delegation by a registered nurse to a student, enrolled nurse or less experienced graduate can be seen as them simply becoming 'an extension of the hands of the registered nurse'. The registered nurse, using their professional judgment and having considered all the circumstances, can delegate duties such as 'take these Panadol to Mr Jones', but is obliged to follow up delegated activities.

- The registered nurse remains responsible for making that judgment and for directing actions outside of policy.

If 'it was reasonable in the circumstances' and if the registered nurse can show good professional rationale for directing a competent junior there is little risk. However, when it becomes a habit rather than a considered decision then such delegation would be seen as flouting policy and all staff involved would risk censure.

How do I deal with situations where someone consistently refuses to carry out directions because they say 'that's not my job, I'm not paid to do that, that's 'illegal'?

First, establish if the delegation is within policy. The more high risk an activity the more certain you can be that it is a qualified staff responsibility; delegating to less qualified staff puts the onus to justify back on to the senior person. Second, is the action within the skill and expertise of the person being directed? Supervisors and managers are expected to know the levels of competence of their staff. Look at the Australian Nurse and Midwife competencies and check the qualifications and course content of certificated and enrolled staff. This situation is usually a personnel problem that requires communication, reference to job descriptions and a dialogue between staff to establish what constitutes 'authorised direction', 'reasonable circumstances', 'professional obligations and responsibility'. The matter will be revisited in Chapter 9, on contracts.

Occasionally the refusal of duties situation arises in an industrial dispute. For example in 2014 in WA in response to Government cost cutting, nurses initiated bans. "When there are no orderlies around because jobs have been cut, nurses have to do it - under the work bans they will refuse to do any jobs they are not being paid for" (*Bunbury Mail* August 8). This is a different context from those arising from an individual being asked to step in and undertake housekeeping duties that are outside the role of a nurse. The question there becomes is the duty essential for patient safety and patient need? Providing food, cleaning hazardous spills, infection control measures through cleaning may all justifiably fall back on the nurse IF there is no other staff immediately available. These jobs cannot be routinely added to their duty list.

Who signs?

When someone signs medication records, charts or files they are signing that they actually performed the tasks or care described in that record. If a registered nurse countersigns a notation it signifies that they supervised the action. Supervision can be direct or indirect. For some duties indirect supervision is reasonable if the delegation is within the scope of practice of the other person. For medications, complex or high-risk procedures direct supervision and countersignature protects the registered nurse. Teaching institutions have clear policies and restrictions on delegation of tasks. Other facilities may not. Schedule 2 medications and 'routine' but complex procedures are frequently delegated to other staff. If the registered nurse signs then it is 'evidence' that they take full responsibility for the action.

Can an enrolled nurse without medication endorsement actually administer medications?

Administration of medications in most states requires proof of knowledge and competence. This is what endorsement provides. Dispensing and administering medication by any route unless directly supervised should not be done by anyone other than a qualified or endorsed practitioner. Legislation protecting staff in remote and rural situations is discussed in Chapter 6.

What about leaving the medications on the client's locker for someone else to administer?

Dispensing, signing for but not giving medications is actually an example of withholding care. Signing the medication record indicates that the drug was given by the person who signs. Leaving the medications unattended has risks. This is not the same as putting the medication into the hands of a competent delegate who then immediately gives the medication following all the medication administration rules. Here the chain is broken. Most facilities have strict policies prohibiting leaving medications unattended.

Delivering and observing a client taking medications on behalf of the dispensing registered nurse can, *depending on the circumstances*, be a simple situation of having someone be 'an extension of the registered nurse's hands'. This often happens in clinics, aged-care facilities and remote situations. Again, the registered nurse is the one risking consequences but if they are confident of the skill and competence and it is 'reasonable in the circumstances' such delegation can be justified.

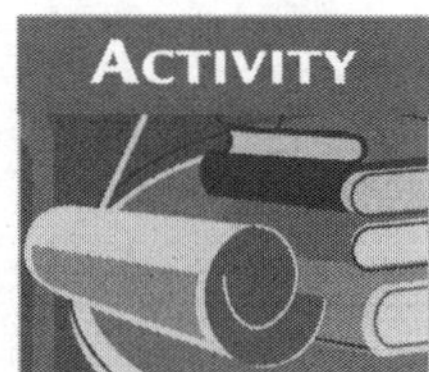

Activity

Read these two true stories and answer the questions.

A registered nurse needed a small quantity of Betadine (Povodine Iodine) so poured a little into a medicine cup. When the registered nurse went to the bedside the patient was not there. The registered nurse left the cup and went on to other tasks. On return she found the client had drunk the solution.

- What might be the legal consequences of this true story?

In an aged-care facility the registered nurse had left medications to be given with lunch by the assistant nurse. The registered nurse had clearly delegated and confirmed that the assistant was aware the medicines were there and were to be given immediately before she commenced feeding the patient. A confused and wandering client entered the room and took the medicines.

- Who is responsible?

The issue of 'whistle blowing'

We have explored various areas that health staff identify as confusing or worrisome in their practice. Here we extend upon that general information by looking at a particular situation: the issue of reporting a problem. Generally known as 'whistle blowing' it is a contentious and difficult area.

You have already been introduced to the legal concepts of defamation, slander and libel. Making unfounded claims that injure the reputation or character of another person or result in serious business losses can lead to court actions. However, the responsibility to protect the public from unethical or dangerous practices is one that most professionals take seriously. The health professional does not have the same protection that lawyers do of keeping confidences secret. If required by the courts to give information nurses are obliged, in spite of their codes of practice demanding respect for privacy and confidentiality, to respond to the court. This applies to providing all records and documentation as well.

It is generally accepted that there is a duty to report or warn the public. Should there be no appropriate response from the service or management internally, then most people tend to 'go public' with their complaint. Some states have legislation to protect whistle blowers; in fact under the *Equal Opportunity Act 1984* (SA) a whistle blower in South Australia can take civil action if they have been exposed to retribution or discrimination as a result of their complaint.

Below is information from the Australian Nursing Federation policy document on whistle blowing 2011 <http://www.anf.org.au/pdf/policies/P_Whistleblowing.pdf> (accessed 29 July 2014).

> It is the policy of the Australian Nursing Federation that:
>
> 1. Nurses and other health care employees should be able to speak out without fear of reprisal when misconduct or corrupt conduct is found to be taking place or has occurred.
> 2. Responding appropriately and in a timely manner to employee concerns and complaints will improve the health, safety and general wellbeing of employees and of people accessing health services.
> 3. Health care employers and employees should maintain the privacy and the anonymity of the person making the complaint or report, and be warned against any type of retaliation against them.
> 4. Nurses and other health care employees should not be victimised or discriminated against in any way, by either their employer or other employees, or have their employment terminated, as a result of making a complaint or reporting misconduct or corrupt conduct.
> 5. Health care organisations should have policies and procedures in place to assist employees, including managers, to deal with making, receiving and responding to complaints or reports of misconduct or corrupt conduct.
> 6. These policies and procedures should include the steps to be taken when immediate supervisors are implicated in the misconduct or corrupt conduct or where the outcome of the investigation does not satisfy the employee's concerns eg identifying a senior person within the organisation responsible for responding to complaints or reports or nominating an independent external person or body to receive complaints or reports.

7. Employees should utilise internal procedures wherever possible to notify employers when misconduct or corrupt conduct is found to have taken place. All complaints or reports of misconduct or corrupt conduct should initially be investigated internally and with procedural fairness as soon as practicable.
8. Health care managers who receive complaints or reports of misconduct or corrupt conduct should comply with the organisation's policies and procedures, including investigating the complaint or report and protecting the employee making the complaint or report. (ANF *Whistleblowing and Nursing*, 2004, p. 1)

Since 5 January 2014 the Australian Public Service whistleblowing scheme has been replaced by the *Public Interest Disclosure Act 2013* (PID Act). The PID Act aims to:

- encourage and facilitate disclosure of information by public officials about suspected wrongdoing in the public sector
- ensure that public officials who make public interest disclosures are supported and protected from adverse consequences
- ensure that disclosures by public officials are properly investigated and dealt with.

While not directly relevant to health professionals this does give insight into the legal standing of whistleblowers. Although there is no specific reference to whistleblowers, the *Fair Work Act and the OH&S (CE) Act* also provide some protection.

Sub-section 772(1)(e) of the *Fair Work Act* states that employment cannot be terminated for: 'the filing of a complaint, or the participation in proceedings, against an employer involving alleged violation of laws or regulations or recourse to competent administrative authorities.'

The *OH&S Act* includes a similar provision where an employee who complains about a work-related health, safety or welfare matter cannot be dismissed (s. 76).

Further information can be obtained from Whistleblowers Australia at <www.whistleblowers.com.au> (accessed 29 July 2014).

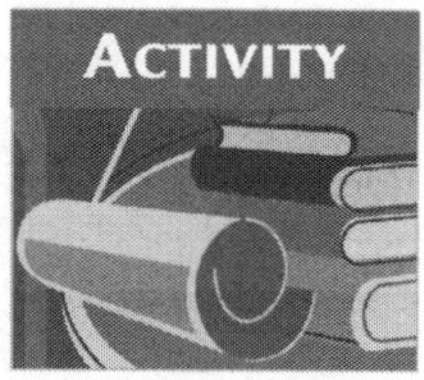

Activity

Go to Google and key in 'whistle blowing and nursing' to read more articles.

It is important before taking any steps or making any claims for the health worker to be familiar with the institutional policy for managing information and lodging complaints. Failure to follow those procedures can be a serious oversight. If there are no procedures or policies to address such an issue, written requests for them to be developed should be initiated.

The source of claims must be well understood before acting on a claim.

Summary

This chapter has explored various areas that health professionals identify as 'worrisome or confusing'. Often when hearing such tea room chatter one has to wonder whether some people just like to scare themselves and others with myths and exaggerations. The sense of insecurity and anxiety some of these types of discussions raise is a source of unnecessary stress. We know we are not lawyers, we know the law is complex and we know there are circumstances that create risks to us and our colleagues. Failing to go to a credible source and get factual information about issues is unprofessional. It is true that there are many areas of confusion hidden among the complexities of law that we do not have the time or skill to explore efficiently. However, it is equally true that professional bodies, unions and senior staff have dealt with these issues and probably know where to find answers. At the least a quick web search for information to confirm or reject these worries can save a great deal of anxiety.

A possible assignment question

Length 500 words

Refer to the NMBA code of ethics to discuss the issues below.

As an RN you are working with Kelly who you consider a friend since you both went through university together to graduation. After a few shifts you notice when you are together at tea or meet in the treatment room she looks a bit dazed, seems a little forgetful or distracted. On one occasion you actually wonder if she has been drinking as you detect a faint alcohol smell. You hear other RNs discussing Kelly very negatively, they seem to think she is slow and unreliable. You talk with Kelly and she admits she is using recreational drugs and alcohol regularly; she begs you not to tell anyone and insists it is not affecting her work.

Sources

Australian Nursing Federation (2004) *Whistleblowing and nursing*, Policy Document <www.anf.org.au/anf_pdf/P_Whistleblowing.pdf>, (accessed 14 April 2011).

Bailey, P. & Deveraux, A. (1998) 'The operation of anti-discrimination laws in Australia', in D. Kinley (ed.), *Human Rights in Australia*, Federation Press, Sydney, pp. 292–318.

Commonwealth Treasury (Ipp Report) (2002) *The Review of the Law of Negligence*, < http://revofneg.treasury.gov.au> (accessed 14 April 2011).

Fleming, J. G. (1987) *The Law of Torts*, 7th edn, The Law Book Company Ltd, NSW.

Forrester, K. & Griffiths, D. (2005) *Essentials of Law*, 2nd edn, Harcourt, Sydney.

Forrester, K. & Griffiths, D. (2010) *Essentials of Law for Health Professionals*. Elsevier, Australia.

Kennedy, R. & Richards, J. (2004) *Integrating Human Service Law and Practice*, Oxford University Press, Melbourne.

Kennedy, R., Richards, J. & Leiman, T. (2013) *Integrating human service law, ethics and practice*, Oxford University Press, South Melbourne, Victoria.

MacFarlane, P. J. & Reid, S. J. (2003) *Queensland Health Law Handbook*, Queensland Dept of Health, Brisbane.

McIlwraith, J. & Madden, B. (2014) *Health Care & the Law*, 6th edn, Lawbook Co., Australia.

Morris, G., Cook, C., Creyke, R. & Geddes, R. (2001) *Laying Down the Law*, `5th edn, Butterworths, Sydney.

Morris, J. (2000) 'Insuring against negligence: medical indemnity in Australia', *Policy*, Spring, <www.cis.org.au/policy/Spring02/polspring02-2.htm> (accessed 9 June 2005).

Staunton, P. & Chiarella, M. (2003) *Nursing and the Law*, 5th edn, Elsevier, Sydney.

Staunton, P. & Whyburn, B. (1997) *Nursing and the Law*, 4th edn, Harcourt Australia Pty Ltd, Sydney.

White, B., Wilmott, L & McDonald, F. (2014) *Health Law in Australia*, 2nd edn, Thomson Reuters, Australia.

Cases

Inquest touching the death of TJB (1989) Adelaide Coroners Court.

Medical Board Of Australia v Dekker [2013] WASAT 182

Lowry v Mayo Newhall Hospital 64 ALR 4th 1191 (Cal 1986), 1196;

Vaughan v Webb (1902) 2 SR(NSW) 293

Mid Density Developments Pty Ltd v Rockdale Municipal Council (1993) 44 FCR 290

Employment contracts and obligations

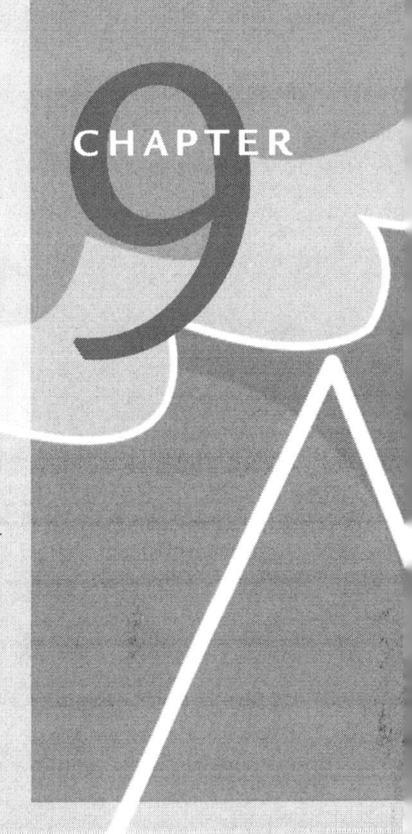

Learning outcomes

After studying this chapter you should be able to:

- Demonstrate an understanding of the Australian legal system and relevant statutory bodies that create or interpret law and policies for health professionals and health agencies.
- Identify the sources of legislation and common law affecting employment.
- Relate the obligations in law of the employee to practice.

Overview

A contract is an agreement between parties and a contract creates rights and obligations between those parties. A contract will be enforced by the law. While all of us enter into contracts almost daily (an example is retail purchases such as going to a shop and buying your lunch), most people tend to think of a contract as a written document setting out relevant details of a deal, purchases or agreements to do something.

Contract law is a particular area of law. In the past every contract was enforceable, whether it was fair to all parties or not. You may have heard or used the term 'let the buyer beware'. This was the principle of contracts in the old days. With the complexity of modern financial dealings there was an obvious imbalance between the consumer and large corporations and businesses. During the twentieth century through legislation there have been many limitations and rules imposed on parties entering into a contract in order to protect the consumer. There is now extensive consumer protection and legislation imposes limits on the types of contracts that are valid and requires companies to ensure consumer advice is given about the risks that some contracts might hold.

An overarching Commonwealth statute is the *Trade Practices Act 1974*. This provides consumers with protection although it is an Act that primarily deals with trade and commerce. At the state and territory level additional consumer protection is given through fair trading legislation, which provides for mechanisms for dispute resolution through tribunals as well as setting rules and expectations about dealings.

As a separate and historical area of the common law, contract law has its own jargon and concepts. Any reading in this area will introduce you to terms such as:

- Unconscionable or deceptive practices
- Misleading and deceptive conduct
- Misrepresentation
- Terms and conditions
- Warranties

As a citizen and a consumer you need to have some knowledge about the area of contract law but as a citizen you, like anyone else, can find advice and seek legal counsel for your own business dealings.

- A basic premise for a contract is that the parties involved intend the agreement to be *binding*. The existence of a contract creates an agreement such that, should one or other party to that contract fail to fulfil their promises or obligations, the law can enforce those obligations or demand a compensation.
- Domestic and social agreements do not create a binding contract.

The most relevant issues to health practice and health professionals are the contracts that a client enters into for care and services when they are admitted or seek treatment, which create obligations that must be met, and health professionals' own employment contracts. Of course, institutions enter into many contracts and finance officers, purchasing officers and others will have to know the rules involved in establishing a contract and what actions are available to ensure these are fulfilled. Were you to find your career moving in this direction, further study in this area would be essential. At this stage we will focus upon the legal issues arising from contacts for employment.

Employment contracts

Fundamentally a contract of employment is based on the employee being engaged to perform work under the employers' direction and control in return for payment. As you well know, there are constraints on such a contract. Industrial law is another specialty area, and embedded within industrial law is *industrial relations*. The focus of industrial relations extends to every part of the working situation. Wages and conditions and recognition of the need to balance productivity with human rights are all captured within this concept. Dispute resolution procedures and the grounds for dismissal or termination of employment fall within this area. Most places of work are covered by an industrial agreement and this might be an award or an enterprise agreement.

Industrial agreements and the common law have the same underlying principles. While some contracts spell out these, other employers may simply follow the 'implied' or known rules of employment in their contracts. If the contract or the award does not specify a matter that becomes grounds for dispute the courts will rely on 'usual practice in that industry' to determine what is expected or implied. For example, one of these implied obligations is the employee's obligation to obey all lawful and reasonable directions of the employer.

Obligations of the employer

There are obligations imposed on both employees and employers. The employer's obligations and issues arising from them include the following.

- The employer's obligation to provide a safe working environment means that the employee can sue for compensation should an injury occur. The injury or disease must have arisen in the course of employment. Workers' compensation claims tend to be based on the elements of a negligence case; however, legislation provides the worker with a number of benefits, not the least of which is speed of resolution of the case. If the claim is made under workers' compensation then it is not possible to initiate later a civil action in negligence against the employer.
- The employer is held to be vicariously liable for the acts of the employee (recall Chapter 6). Unless the employer can show the employee caused damage while working outside of the role, functions and policies of the job, it is the employer who must meet the costs of a successful negligence action.
- The employer can only require the employee to function within the law. An employee cannot be directed to carry out work that is prohibited by legislation or the common law.
- The employer cannot discriminate against people in employment on the basis of age, race, sex or disability (recall Chapter 8).
- The employer is obliged to remunerate the employee for the work done. In the health industry the amount paid to a worker is most often governed by industrial laws that are translated into awards. Various categories of staff are entitled to a fixed wage. That wage may vary due to special allowances such as shift penalties or between grades of staff within categories.

Private health sector awards may differ from public sector awards. There is flexibility in many awards permitting an employer to pay more than the recommended salary but never less. Annual leave, superannuation contributions, study and family leave allowances are usually prescribed by the award, which is lodged by a union with the Industrial Court after formalities of agreement with employer and employee representatives have been met, or through enterprise agreements where terms and conditions have the force of law for the life of that agreement.

As well as the obligations on the employer to uphold the contract and satisfy both common law and industrial requirements there is legislation aimed at ensuring employee safety. This has been referred to in previous chapters. New work health and safety (WHS) laws commenced on 1 January 2012 in many states and territories to harmonise occupational health and safety (OH&S) laws across Australia.

Occupational health and safety legislation is yet another source of direction and standards for employment. While occupational health and safety is primarily regulated by legislation, common law principles continue to have some application in certain jurisdictions. For example, employers may have a duty arising from implied terms in the common law employment contract to take reasonable care for the safety of their employees, breach of which may give rise to a cause of action.

Employees may also be able to bring a common law action for damages for negligence where an employer is in breach of its duty to take reasonable care for the health and safety of employees (Macken, 2002 p. 118).

Who is an employee?

An employee is not the same as an independent contractor. Recall your readings on vicarious liability. There the damage caused by an employee might be compensated by the employer if the damage was caused in the course of employment. A private contractor has a contract to provide work for someone but is liable for their own actions and must be indemnified (have insurance) to ensure protection of the public or service they provide work for.

There are many common law cases that have explored this issue. If someone works under the direction and control of the institution or the institution's representative this is taken to be an indication of employment status. Often the issue in the courts has been whether a visiting medical officer or specialist doctor is liable for damage to a client or whether under the doctrine of vicarious liability the responsibility rests with the facility.

It can be difficult to determine whether a specialist is an 'employee' in the real sense. Establishing if there is a relationship with the client that is independent of the facility is necessary. In the case *Ellis v. Wallsend District Hospital* (1989) the court determined that the doctor was personally liable as that doctor was engaged by the patient privately and the treatment carried out at the hospital was simply a use of the facility's resources for that private patient. If the client had been admitted and the medical officer was allocated by roster or other facility rules then that doctor would be deemed an employee.

Employers may elect to take on independent contractors rather than engage their own staff. While the independent contractor has benefits such as freedom to choose when to work and some taxation allowances, the employer gains advantages as well, saving on payroll taxes, allowances and annual leave, for example. The law will look very hard at contracts to establish if the worker is genuinely self-employed.

Casual employees are often disadvantaged as they do not receive the benefits of permanent full- or part-time staff that are enforced by the award or industrial agreements. In many environments, to protect workers employers are obliged to offer permanent employment after a worker has taken on a specified number of short-term contracts.

Hours of work may be controlled by legislation if there is a public safety risk, for example for airline pilots and long-distance drivers. Most positions pay wages against an hourly rate and the normal working week varies between industries between 35 and 40 hours per week in Australia.

Overtime is work done beyond those normal hours. Some industries' awards include overtime and the employee is obliged to work 'reasonable' extra hours.

Rates of pay, allowances for breaks, compensation as 'time in lieu' is usually detailed in the awards. In the health system shift penalties and overtime are expressly covered by industrial agreements.

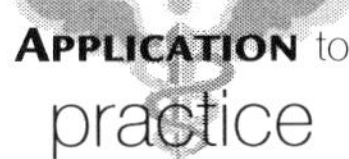

Application to practice

Health practitioners are able to establish themselves as independent contractors. They can have their own business and take on clients in a private capacity. While they may have links with other service providers and utilise the resources of a hospital or clinic in return for seeing other patients or paying for the right to use the service, the health professional would remain liable unless the facility or facility staff could be shown to be directly negligent or have failed the agreement.

Working for an agency is not the same as being an independent contractor. The agency finds the position and in return receives a commission for doing so. The individual undertakes to work for a client or facility directly as an employee, so the individual is bound by the rules and obligations of employee–employer relationships.

Overtime is usually a matter of requesting an employee to work longer hours or extra days. If there is a genuine emergency, under the obligations to the client which demand appropriate and adequate care the facility must ensure the staff coverage to meet these needs.

There is a constant tension between the institution's obligations and the employee's right to choose whether to work overtime or not. Professional ethical obligations are another consideration in times of short staffing. Satisfying the ethical obligation to ensure that client safety and needs are met has to be balanced against 'what is reasonable' to expect an employee to do.

Obligations of an employee

Industrial awards and enterprise agreements do not specifically address the obligations of employees. However, the common law obligations, while they can be expressly spelt out in a contract for work, are understood to be part of every employment contract. These are, in the language of the common law, *duties* of the employee.

- The employee has a duty to obey all lawful and reasonable commands of the employer. This is not a matter of opinion. 'Reasonable in the circumstances' may require some investigation but if direction for an activity is for an activity that falls within the professional role, within scope of practice or under supervision to meet the needs created by an unusual or emergency situation, then obeying the direction is expected.
- There is a duty to be faithful and loyal to the employer's interests.
- An employee has a duty to display due care and be competent in their work.
- There is a duty to account for all money and property received in the course of employment.

- There is a duty to make available to the employer any products or process that the employee has invented during their employment.
- An employee has a duty to give the employer any information that is relevant to the business.
- Unless prohibited by legislation the employee may have a duty to reimburse (indemnify) the employer who has been made vicariously liable to pay for damage caused by that employee.

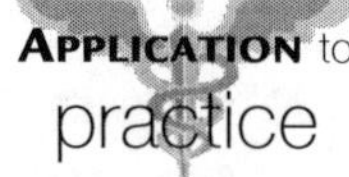

Application to practice

Most of these common law duties are obvious; however, two are worth relating to practice as they have been grounds for disputes.

It is not unusual to hear someone complaining bitterly about being required to work in another area, 'backfilling' a vacancy created by an absent employee. 'I wasn't hired to work in X ward.' Unless a contract of employment specifies a work area and duties specific to that role, the facility can require a (suitably qualified) staff member to work anywhere. Most contracts imply this with a clause along the lines of 'and any other duties as required' in the job description.

If you were asked to work outside of your skill and qualification, then it might not be 'reasonable in the circumstances'; however, holding a qualification indicates a proven competence. Identifying to the manager that you have reservations about your knowledge and skill and identifying that certain duties are outside of your knowledge and experience are reasonable and recommended. This imposes on the manager an obligation to supervise, teach or delegate duties outside of your abilities. If the work is carried out by another of the same education and credentials then it falls within your duties as an employee.

Many positions involve development or creation of new material or methods. Designing a procedure manual, research, a lecture series or education materials are examples. If these have been created as part of your job the product belongs to the employer. While you can claim authorship or the invention, you cannot withhold or take the product as your own.

Creating a contract

It might seem obvious to state this but there must be an intention to enter into a contract by both parties. There have been cases where inquiries about a property, test driving a vehicle or trying on an outfit were deemed by one party to be a commitment and the other as simply an expression of interest.

Going for a job interview, even after the time and expense involved in providing all the necessary pre-interview paperwork, is not a commitment to take the job. One of the difficulties for employers is the time and expense involved in advertising, preparing for and interviewing candidates who are not actually interested in taking up the position. Equally, applicants have the right to find out about potential employers by using the interview process and the right to apply for as many positions as they wish. Applying for and attending an interview does not establish a contract unless promises are made.

Contracts may be verbal or written. Most employment contracts are standard written documents. After (usually) an interview, confirmation of credentials and checking references an employer makes an *offer* of a job and the individual *accepts* this offer. There is generally no formal contract until the employee signs an agreement.

- This may not be the case where special services or a reliance on the employee's promise to start work is involved. The verbal commitment may be upheld if the employer has suffered loss because they relied on the agreement.

Typically a written offer would include the date of commencement of the employment, the position, information regarding wages and any other important aspects of the employment relationship that differ to or are not set out in Australia's employment legislation, the *Fair Work Act 2009 (Cth)*.

Most health staff commit to a contract which has been discussed and often the contract may contain a duty statement. This duty statement or job description will specify the role and functions of the position and any special obligations such as attendance at orientation, participation in annual review of CPR and manual handling skills. The existence of an industrial award or enterprise agreement means that the contract does not have to list all the various matters of salary, leave entitlements and superannuation.

Application to practice

APPLICATION to practice

Most facilities have clear policies and procedures in place for the process of determining which applicants proceed to interview and the interview process. Inexperienced interviewers may be so friendly that they mislead hopeful job seekers. Some candidates have interpreted extremely positive interview experiences as a promise of the job; however, until a formal offer has been made and accepted there is no contract.

The employer can select any applicant as long as there is no discrimination or deviation from the published 'essential criteria' that the job required. A number of government agencies have systems for appeal available to unsuccessful candidates. An employer can choose to offer the position to an applicant who was at interview a poorer candidate after the first, second or other choices of applicant have not taken the position. Equally an employer can elect not to offer the position to any applicant and choose to re-advertise or leave the position vacant.

Interviewers may well have reservations about a candidate but are prohibited from asking questions that may verge on personal grounds or provide grounds for claims of discrimination. As the whole business is stressful and relies on quality communication, the reality is that parties need to be aware of exactly when the legal obligations for contract arise rather than assuming rights that do not exist.

Discipline and termination of employment

The common law recognises termination as the only sanction available to an employer. It is through awards, enterprise agreements or individual contracts that matters of probation, sanctions or discipline are detailed. For example, being absent from work without reason can be grounds for an employer to withhold the wages for those hours. This is called 'docking' the pay. The employer is not obliged to pay for work not done.

Chapter 7 explored the various professional disciplinary grounds available through legislation. Misconduct of an employee can be defined, depending on all the circumstances, as failing the duties/obligations of an employee. Employers must have good grounds for taking action against an employee. Before dismissing an individual and risking a claim of unfair dismissal a number of considerations and investigations should have been in place.

- Employment history – if the individual has given long and faithful service and/or if there is no previous disciplinary record then dismissal or sanctions should be balanced against this record.
- Refusal to carry out duties – the employer must be able to show that in fact the required activity was lawful and within the role and function of an employee of that education and training. Referring to the duty statement, professional registering authority and even the relevant union will establish this.
- Was it habit or just this one occasion that the employee failed to meet standards? If the facility has tolerated or turned a blind eye to some activity or failure then opportunity to correct and change behaviour must be given before it is grounds for dismissal.
- Has everything/anything been done to assist the employee to overcome the problem? Some behaviours may be evidence of a need for counselling, treatment or short-term support and assistance. Domestic matters, bereavement or illness may affect an employee and with support or referral to appropriate professionals the problem could be resolved.
- Is there written evidence clearly stating what the employee must do and that termination will be the result of failing to rectify matters? This is often referred to as a 'written warning' and is frequently the final step in a series of oral warnings, interviews and monitoring as well as documenting in employee assessment records prior to dismissal.

An employer must give the employee notice of dismissal. Summary dismissal is 'on the spot' dismissal and grounds for this usually involve matters of safety, competence or outrageous behaviour. Most employers even with good grounds for dismissal will choose to pay out notice of one pay period rather than get into a protracted argument with the employee. Dismissal with notice, as long as reasonable steps have been taken to inform, warn, educate or train the employee, will be upheld.

Recognised grounds for dismissal can be categorised as:

Breach of the law If the employee has lost their right to practise in a professional capacity as a result of professional disciplinary actions or has breached legislation, has a criminal history or proven to be involved in criminal activity they can be dismissed. Employers cannot 'assume' the employee is guilty, it must be a fact. Health services tend to await the outcome of a tribunal investigation of a professional before dismissing that person.

Incapacity If age, infirmity or disability interferes with the safe or required job performance an employee can be dismissed. Medical rather than managerial opinion should provide the evidence.
Redundancy If the position (not the person) is no longer required then the organisation can dismiss the person filling that position. This must be genuine: the organisation must show the position itself is superfluous to the organisation's needs. Opportunity to retrain an employee to fill new or different functions if refused by the employee will deny the employee the right to a financial payout to compensate for redundancy.

An employment contract can be terminated by agreement between the employer and employee.

In reality an employment contract is usually terminated by the employee who submits their resignation. Again industrial agreements direct the length of notice that must be given to the employer. Generally 14 days or one pay period is the normal practice.

Fixed-term contracts are common in many industries. Being seconded or 'backfilling' a position and working on a project are common examples. The duration of the contract is clearly spelt out and when either the date or completion of the project arrives that contract is terminated.

Application to practice

As a professional it is often assumed that you will know and adhere to the written and unwritten rules of employment. Recognising that the employer is limited by the awards means that in most facilities all staff of the same grade or level of employment receive the same level of pay. The varied benefits and rights of employees for leave, time in lieu and sick leave are again governed by the award.

A national Nurses Award was introduced on 1 January 2010. The Nurses Award 2010 covers nurses in primary health care and general practice, including registered nurses, enrolled nurses, nursing assistants and midwives. It determines the minimum pay and conditions for a nurse working in Australia. Regularly updated this document includes all aspects of employment. <http://www.apna.asn.au/lib/pdf/Careers/NursesAward_Dec2013.pdf>

There are state awards, for example: Public Health System Nurses' and Midwives' (State) Award 2011 in NSW. Updates can occur during the life of an award, for example: Nursing wage rates as at 1 April 2014, Qld Health.

Note, however, that legislation in 2006 has opened the way for employers to develop individual contracts for individual employees. Consistency between classes of professionals may not continue.

The hours of work and break times may be assumed to be 'understood and adhered to' and an employee who has been casual about punctuality could find themselves in difficulties on the basis that they failed to adhere to the agreement. Staying late to finish up your work may not be recognised as grounds for coming in later the next day. Employment contracts in service industries tend to be fairly inflexible.

Failure to notify the employer that you will not be at work could be construed as abandonment of the job if it extends beyond a 'reasonable' period. What is considered reasonable will depend on the circumstances. Policies may govern aspects of employment and usually include administrative requirements like provision of a doctor's certificate, notice when leaving the ward and formal application for time in lieu.

Workplace realities and discipline

- When knowledge, skill or behaviour deficits are identified, the workplace will often interview and work out with the employee, a solution.
- Often it is further education opportunities and assessment, guided, supervised practice or referral to a counsellor that are put in place.
- Records are kept.
- If the situation requires management to "issue a warning" then a contract/agreement may be put in place, reporting and surveillance may be considered.

Under Equal Opportunity Legislation, employers must ensure that employees are not treated unfairly or harassed because of personal characteristics or attributes. Harassment is defined as any form of behaviour that the other person does not want in return. It is behaviour which offends, humiliates or intimidates them, or targets them because of race or sex.

It is not uncommon for a nurse who has been corrected/disciplined to claim they were the victim of bullying. This claim in its own right, must then be investigated as workplace bullying is a serious issue.

WorkSafe Victoria defines workplace bullying as: persistent and repeated negative behaviour directed at an employee that creates a risk to health and safety (WorkSafe Victoria, 2012). Negative behaviour includes actions such as: yelling, ostracising, belittling, blaming, invading personal space, verbal abuse, excluding or isolating someone, or assigning meaningless tasks unrelated to the job. In other words, negative behaviour is behaviour that a reasonable person would anticipate would victimise, humiliate, undermine or threaten the other person. Bullying occurs when negative behaviour is persistent and repeated, not a one-off incident, although such incidents must be addressed (Shaw & Blewett, 2013). Legislation addresses bullying in the workplace. From 1 January 2014, the Fair Work Commission has jurisdiction to deal with bullying complaints raised by workers and powers to make an order for the bullying to stop. Whilst the incoming workplace bullying provisions under the *Fair Work Act 2009 (Cth)* will not create powers to make orders on reinstatement or compensation, there will nevertheless be increased pressure and onus on businesses to be proactive about preventing workplace bullying and promptly dealing with any related complaints, in order to avoid an intervention by the Commission.

Making a claim that bullying rather than justified discipline processes were experienced must be supported. It might be a "heat of the moment" statement or an attempt to defend self-esteem but it is an accusation that the employer must take seriously. If there were lack of processes and clarity in the interview it could lead to someone misinterpreting what was in fact acceptable performance management actions so they have responded to these as if they were bullying. Before making such a claim it would be worth seeking advice. If, on investigation the claim is unfounded it might be interpreted as malicious.

Activity

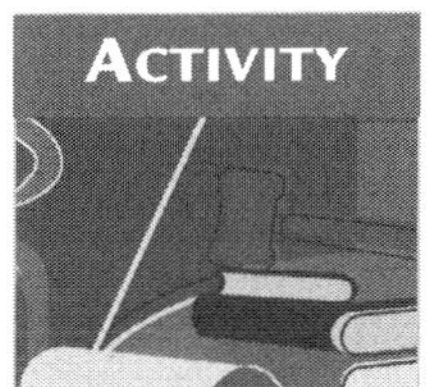

Below is a summary from one of many Practice Nurse Employment kits that were developed in consultation with peak nursing and industrial bodies. Around Australia these kits were disseminated by Divisions of General Practice. While focused upon practice nurses, the document contains many relevant points for every nurse by clarifying terms and expectations of the employer and employee.

EMPLOYMENT CONTRACTS GUIDE FOR NURSES IN GENERAL PRACTICE

The preamble identifies that these are minimum conditions so the nurse and employer might negotiate to increase salary and benefits. However the contract cannot offer less than the minimum. Section 1 recognises the various position titles of nurses employed in a general practice environment.

Section 2 describes the Terms of Employment. Where a contract does not specify a set period of time, it means the nurse is employed on a week-to-week basis. This means for employees who have worked for less than a year, either the employee or the employer can terminate the contract on one week's notice. If the nurse has been employed for 5 years or longer, notice is up to 4 weeks.

Every contract should specify whether the employment is full-time, part-time or casual. Full time is 38 hours per week. Part-time is varied hours, usually up to 20 hours per week. A casual employee is hired for short periods; the minimum is usually 2 hours for each period of work. Casual employees do not receive annual leave or other benefits so their wage includes a casual loading, between 10% to 15% additional salary. The contract should specify remuneration, the salary, shift loadings, allowances and relevant matters.

In Australia it is a legal requirement for full and part-time employees to have superannuation payments made on their behalf by the employer. The amount varies but the minimum is 9% of the basic salary.

Every contract should identify the hours that the employee should work, the shifts, the days of work and, if there is a roster, what that means. Where there is a system of time in lieu, the number of days to be worked to accrue a leave day is specified. If the employer requires the nurse to work official public holidays, the contract will be clear as to what the compensation or pay scale is for working on these holidays. Penalty rates vary between time and a half, double or triple time. This means that the hours worked on a public holiday are paid at that rate. Time in lieu is another form of compensation.

For nurses the award directs that a minimum of 4 weeks annual leave is entitled after a full 12 months of employment are completed. Employers are required to pay a leave loading for full time employees of 17.5%. Part-time annual leave loading is calculated against hours per week. Casual employees do not (usually) get paid leave or loading.

Sick leave is a right for employees, but there are differences as to the number of days allowed in every state. A contract may specify between 15 to 20 days and the requirement to produce a doctor's certificate for the allowance to be paid. State and Territory awards allow for long service leave, carers leave, compassionate leave, parents and maternity leave. These details vary and the contract may specify these leave entitlements or assume adherence to the State legal requirements.

Most contracts identify the procedures for dispute resolution and staff complaints. If disputes are unresolved at local level, matters may be referred to the *Fair Work Commission. The main of disputes and dismissals that can be referred to the Commission are:*

- *disputes under the terms of an award or a collective or enterprise agreement*
- *bargaining disputes*
- *disputes arising under the general protections provisions of the Fair Work Act 2009, and*
- *unfair dismissals.* (Italics signify changes to legislation since the original document was published).

While most contracts do not specify detail of workers compensation, there are laws that govern the procedures for reporting and seeking compensation for a work place injury.

Most contracts do identify that the employee is expected to adhere to Occupational Health and Safety legislation and undertake to maintain safe working practices. The law requires employers to provide a safe working environment.

Contracts may be very specific about the laws of confidentiality, but the need to maintain confidentiality and the procedures and policies of the workplace are often included, as are the expectation for nurses to adhere to their professional codes.

Legislation to protect employees and ensure the rights of employers and employees are maintained exists in Australia. A contract may not specify matters that could arise in the future such as redundancy or the focus of the business but the contract will usually identify the length of notice required to terminate employment.

There are professional requirements for nurses to demonstrate ongoing education and maintain their professional development. There are various awards that provide for either hours per week or days per year. The contract may not specify this training requirement time but the contract of employment will be assumed to satisfy the award (Wentwest, 2008, p.17).

As you can see there are many areas covered by contracts of employment. Awards protect both employees and employers. In state health services the awards are often assumed to be inherent in the contract of employment, in private practice the contract may be very specific and every entitlement spelt out.

Service contracts and obligations

The common law recognises that a contract exists when a client attends a health facility or seeks treatment and, as Lord Justice Denning states, 'The hospital has a duty to employ competent staff' (*Cassidy v. Ministry of Health* (1951)). The facility or independent practitioner owes the client a duty on the basis of a contract. As you have seen in Chapters 5 and 6, a failure to fulfil a duty of care that results in damage is grounds for an action in negligence. A service owes a client a duty of care.

The duty in contract is not as obvious as negligent failure of duty. With contracts the duty may be 'implied' and, while the elements of negligence are relevant, should there be damage suffered by an individual contractual obligations also exist and these duties are enforceable at law; remedies exist should there be a contractual failure.

Patients have a contract with their doctors, dentists and other professional staff. If they enter or are admitted to a health facility then they have a contract with the administrators of that facility. This may be a public or private facility. Employees or volunteers who deal with the client in the facility are considered to be servants/agents acting for the hospital.

Health care agencies also have a duty of care to visitors and tradespeople who are lawfully on the premises. Occupational health and safety legislation spells out the standards for ensuring the safety of those entering and using resources on the premises.

In determining if a contract exists between a service provider and client the same principles for any contract must underpin the relationship. These include the following:

- There is an intention to create a legal relationship. An agreement to provide a service in return for some benefit is inherent in providing access to treatment. Here benefit may be the client paying a fee or nominating an insurer to cover costs.
- The contract may be oral or written, formal or informal.
- The parties understand what the bargain involves and what the costs will be. This area is often where contentious issues arise. 'I came to be cured, I paid my bill, however I still suffer the symptoms of my disease'! Courts look at what is customary service, reasonable and possible in the circumstances. While a contract may exist, the courts will not impute onerous or impossible obligations on either party.
- Parties to a contract must have the capacity to understand and enter into a contract. Mental disability, influence or duress is grounds to put aside a contract.
- A contract to illegal acts will not be enforced.

Discharge of a contract

The contract is discharged when the conditions of the agreement are fulfilled. Creating a new contract renders the old contract void. However, a new contract cannot be substituted if one party has fulfilled their obligations but the other party has not.

There may be specified or legally recognised time limits to a contract, for example a sunset clause may be built into the contract. This will be a termination date.

Legislation or law may override the intentions or plans for a contract. If one party becomes bankrupt (legal bankruptcy, not just a statement of being broke but bankruptcy being officially filed) means that standing contracts are void.

Death of a party to a contract can be grounds for termination of that contract. This is not always the case as debts may be satisfied by the estate.

Breach of contract by one party can provide grounds for a legal action allowing the party who has been 'injured' to be discharged from their obligations. If the breach is not severe but only a partial failure to meet obligations, the court may not set aside the contract but instead award damages to the injured party.

Circumstances may 'frustrate' the contract. Natural disasters or war may interfere with the ability to fulfil a contract so it is said to 'lapse'.

Considerations for the future

Health professionals may embark on many career paths, from partnerships in private business, consultancies and project workers to being casual, temporary and permanent employees. The risks and rules governing partnerships, business and consultancies in private practice are important aspects of such career choices. It is vital to seek professional guidance before entering such agreements as the varied taxation and insurance obligations need close attention. It is also important to be aware that individuals can be liable for the debts of partners. As the majority of us start our careers within an institutional framework, the priorities are to know our rights as an employee and recognise that we have obligations to our employer. With so many changes to industrial laws there are now various options available to employees. These range from individual contracts to work within an Enterprise Bargaining Agreement or an Award formalized by the Fair Work Commission. All these arrangements require an attention to detail that was once irrelevant to people working under an Award. Part of your own pre employment research might be spent in determining your own contractual requirements and exploring what other practices entail whether this be opportunity for paid study leave, further education or competitive salary levels. Currently, the majority of health staff do not have to contemplate these issues, their Awards and benefits have been gained through Union activities and representation. In the future, taking personal responsibility for your own contract of employment inclusions could be likely.

Summary

This large and complex area of law and legislation has been presented in a very limited form to provide information in relation to employment and service contracts. The principles of contract law in relation to employment are upheld in common law. The intricacy of modern financial and trade agreements as well as the new industrial laws introduced in 2006 means legislation provides for a variety of employer/employee agreements. These new agreements are still contracts and the duties and obligations of the employer and employee remain.

Sources

Creighton, B. & Stewart, A. (2000) *Labour Law: An Introduction*, 3rd edn, The Federation Press, Sydney.

Forrester, K. & Griffiths, D. (2005) *Essentials of Law*, 2nd edn, Harcourt, Sydney.

Kennedy, R. & Richards, J. (2004) *Integrating Human Service Law and Practice*, Oxford University Press, Melbourne.

MacFarlane, P. J. & Reid, S. J. (2003) *Queensland Health Law Handbook*, Queensland Dept of Health, Brisbane.

MacFarlane P. J. & Reid, S. J. (2006) *Queensland Health Law Handbook*, GoPrint, Brisbane.

Macken, J. (2002) *The Law of Employment*, 5th edn, Lawbook Company, Sydney.

Price, R.B.E. & Nielsen. J. (2012) *Principles of Employment Law*, 4th Edn. Thomson Reuters, Australia.

Shaw, A. & Blewett, V. (2013) *Good Practice Guide to Performance Management for Nurses and Midwives in Victorian Public Health Services.* http://www.health.vic.gov.au/__data/assets/pdf_file/0005/764321/Final-guide_April-2013.pdf

Staunton, P. & Chiarella, M. (2003) *Nursing and the Law*, 5th edn, Elsevier, Sydney.

Staunton, P. & Whyburn, B. (1997) *Nursing and the Law*, 4th edn, Harcourt Australia Pty Ltd, Sydney.

Stewart, A. (2013) *Stewart's guide to employment law*. The Federation Press, Annandale, N.S.W.

Wentwest Ltd (2008) *Practice Nurse Employment Kit* (version 5). Wentwest General Practice Support, Parramatta, Sydney.

White, B., Wilmott, L & McDonald, F. (2014) *Health Law in Australia*, 2nd edn, Thomson Reuters, Australia.

Cases

Cassidy v. Ministry of Health (1951) 1 ALL ER 514.

Ellis v. Wallsend District Hospital (1989) Aust Torts Reports 80-289.

New South Wales Nurses Assoc. v. Elizabeth Drive Nursing Home (1979) AILR 46(9).

New South Wales Nurses Assoc. v. St George Hospital (1980) AILR 133(1).

Industrial hearings

M I Gregory v. Jimboomba Community Care Association – re Termination of employment – jurisdiction – probation/award employee – 22 November 2001 – Hoffman C.

Guevarra v. Seton Medical Center, No. C 13-2267 CW, 2013 WL 6235532 (N.D. Cal. Dec. 2, 2013)

Bendigo Health Care Group and others v. Health Services Union of Australia (Victoria No. 2 Branch) – re Imposition of bans in relation to staffing levels and workloads – 22 November 2001 – Blair C.

Australian Nursing Federation re Health and Community Services Industry Sector – Minimum Wage Order – Victoria 1997; and others re Minimum Wage Orders – re Applications for minimum wage orders for certain Victorian employees – 16 August 2001 – Ross VP, Watson SDP, Lewin C.

Coronial inquests

Learning outcomes

After studying this chapter you should be able to:

- Demonstrate an understanding of the Australian legal system and relevant statutory bodies that create or interpret law and policies for health professionals and health agencies.
- Describe the role of the coroner in providing direction for health care practice.
- Demonstrate a knowledge of procedures and policies for investigation of health matters, professional and legal hearings and sanctions for failure to meet standards.
- Demonstrate an understanding of the legal ramifications for incident reporting, report writing and documentation.

Overview

The office of Crown Coroner is one of the oldest legal institutions. While a number of functions have altered over the centuries a common thread remains. This is the investigation of an unusual, unexpected, suspicious or violent death or death through unnatural circumstances, with the particular aim of detecting unlawful homicide. In reality the number of inquests that lead to criminal proceedings are very few; generally the focus of an inquest is upon identifying causes and giving direction to prevent recurrences.

A coronial investigation aims to identify whether there is a case to answer and, if so, the coroner can refer (commit) the matter to go before a judge and jury. Investigations relating to health care matters may not expose fault or causes that justify criminal charges but can give the coroner grounds to criticise or make recommendations about the behaviour of health staff or health systems.

The report of the coroner's findings, recommendations or criticisms of health staff are made available to the registering body, administrative authorities or other relevant authorities. When such findings are brought to the registering authorities' attention this can lead to allegations of professional misconduct on the part of the health professional and the registration board will require that these allegations be addressed. (Recall your readings on professional governance, tribunals and sanctions in Chapter 7.) If the coroner's findings identify that negligence has been a factor in the death then this can lead to the family initiating a civil action. Findings can also be used by the employer to decide whether a civil action against the health professional is justified.

Recall your learning in relation to the system of law in Australia. You have already explored the structure of the legal system and have learnt about the various courts and the hierarchy of the courts. In large cities the Coroner's Court is often a separate court; in smaller centres the magistrate, in the role of coroner, holds inquests in the Local Court. The procedures are similar to other court cases.

Legal representation is sometimes sought by witnesses who are called to give evidence. Cross-examination of witnesses occurs. Thus, procedurally, the inquest is inquisitorial in nature. Any documents, records or witnesses sought by the coroner must be provided, and failure by a witness to present at the inquest is against the law. One difference between a coronial inquest and other types of court cases is that many of the rules of evidence do not apply. This means that the coroner is able to draw upon any type of evidence that in other courts might be kept out on the basis of hearsay or other common law rules.

In summary, then, the State Coroner is a judicial officer (usually a magistrate) whose role is to:

- determine the identity of the deceased person; inquire into the place of death, medical cause and circumstances of death;
- bring to the notice of any relevant authorities practices or laws which could be changed to prevent any similar deaths in the future;
- explore other matters of public interest;
- investigate fires, accidents and the disappearance of missing persons as well as deaths;
- inquire into every death that is reported in accordance with the Coroner's Act.

The inquest/inquiry is to establish the cause and circumstances of death, and is required when a person dies violently or from an unusual, suspicious or unknown cause. Death in certain other circumstances, such as deaths in custody and some deaths in institutions, must also be investigated.

Legislation

Every state and territory has its own Coroner's Act and in recent years many of these Acts have been reviewed and revised. The decision by the coroner as to whether to investigate a death by holding an inquest has in some states been curtailed and in others closely regulated. Generally all states' legislation is similar in identifying the role and responsibilities of the coroner. For example, in Queensland the legislation that governs the role and office of the coroner has been recently updated. The *Coroners Act 2003* commenced on 1 December 2003 and allows coroners to examine the circumstances surrounding a person's death more extensively. In NSW, the *Coroners Act 2009* has been confirmed as current in 2014. Coroners can comment on matters relating to public health and safety or the administration of justice and make recommendations designed to reduce the risk of future fatalities.

While generally the categories of reportable deaths remain the same as in all other jurisdictions, the new Act in Queensland is location specific, as well as identifying relevant categories of reportable deaths. A reportable death in Queensland is defined as one in which the following circumstances apply:

- it occurred in Queensland; or
- the person ordinarily lived in Queensland; or
- the person was on a journey to or from somewhere in Queensland; or
- the death was caused by an event in Queensland. (Department of Justice and Attorney-General, 2005, Office of the State Coroner, Coroners Act 2003 Information for Health Professionals pp. 1–3.)

Go to <http://www.courts.qld.gov.au/courts/coroners-court/reportable-deaths> (accessed 30 July 2014), and at the moment just read the sections `Health care related deaths' and `Deaths in care'. Bookmark the site as below you will be asked to return to it.

Registration of a death

Nationally all deaths must be registered with the Registrar of Births, Deaths and Marriages in the jurisdiction. Before a death can be registered there must be a medical certificate specifying the cause of death. If a doctor is unable to specify the cause of death or has not attended the deceased recently a certificate cannot be issued (unless legislation allows).

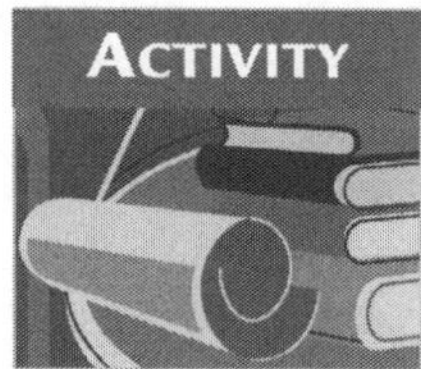

Activity

Go to the home page of the Queensland Government Department of Justice and Attorney-General web site at <http://www.justice.qld.gov.au/>
Click on Births, Deaths and Marriages menu option. Scroll down to Deaths. This section explains the standard procedures required by the law. These procedures are essentially identical in every state and territory.
For example, in NSW, the Department of Justice NSW administers the *Births, Deaths and Marriages Registration Act, 1995 and the Commonwealth Marriage Act, 1961.*

A doctor is legally bound to report a death to the coroner in every state and territory if:

- it is not known who the person is; or
- the death is violent or unnatural death; or
- the death was not reasonably expected to be the outcome of a health procedure; or
- a cause of death certificate has not been issued and is not likely to be issued; or
- the death was a death in care; or
- the death was a death in custody. (Coroners Act, Information for Health

Professionals, 2003, p. 1; available online at <http://www.courts.qld.gov.au/courts/coroners-court/information-for-health-practitioners> (accessed 30 July 2014)

Go back to Queensland Courts, Reportable Deaths at <http://www.courts.qld.gov.au/courts/coroners-court/reportable-deaths> (accessed 30 July 2014), and read the definitions of each reportable death.

Traditionally a death certificate could not be issued if the deceased had not seen a doctor within the previous three months. Now, the Queensland Act specifically deals with this by referring to another updated piece of Queensland legislation, the *Births, Deaths and Marriages Registration Act 2003*, commenced on 1 February 2004. This Act allows a doctor to issue a cause of death certificate without having seen the deceased in the three months prior to the date of death.

A death certificate can only be issued if there is a body. At common law, where a person has disappeared after seven years the state Supreme Court can provide an order to the effect that the person is presumed dead. Where there is no doubt about death but no remains can be identified/found the family can apply to the court for an order immediately.

Activity

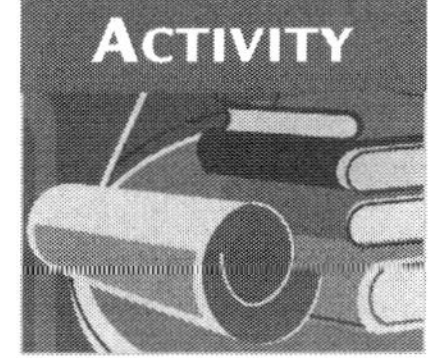

The site below is one hosted by the Australian Museum. Created for the general public it is an easy and informative site about death and practices in Australia. Nurses often feel bewildered when families turn to them for advice about 'what do we do now?'. This exercise is aimed to give you some insight into the processes and procedures. The relevant page for the purposes of this chapter is 'Who ends up in a morgue?'.

This page provides statistics and a summary of reportable deaths.

Go to the homepage of the Australian Museum, Deaths: the last taboo; click 'What happens after death?' and scroll down to 'morgues and mortuaries'→Who ends up in a morgue? and read the article 'What happens after death?' <http://australianmuseum. net.au/Death-The-Last-Taboo> (accessed 30 July 2014).

<www.deathonline.net/what_happens/morgue/who.cfm>

Application to practice

APPLICATION to practice

As stated earlier, legislation in most states specifies the grounds for an inquest. The medical officer who certifies death has occurred may elect to sign the death certificate if all the facts are known and the death is a natural death. However, in most states legislation still prohibits signing the death certificate if the medical practitioner had not attended the client during the last three months. Other situations that require an inquest be held are:

- If the person died while under or within 24 hours of receiving an anaesthetic that was administered for medical, surgical or dental treatment.
- Where the person dies within a year and a day of an accident that may be attributable as the cause of death.

- If the person was 'in care', as an in-patient or out-patient at a mental, welfare, disabled or residential facility.
- If the person died in detention, police custody or 'in the care' of police or responsible officials.

The facility will usually notify staff where a death is subject to an inquest, and the list above makes it clear that there are potentially many deaths that could be investigated in a large health facility. Once death has been pronounced (certified) the police are notified. The police are required to take statements whether or not there have been suspicious circumstances.

These inquiries are usually routine and staff simply make available all relevant documents and provide their report. The coroner will use these statements to decide whether a formal inquest should proceed. Should there be issues, if the circumstances of the death are considered a problem or if you can see that the matter is not just a case of giving a routine statement you may delay giving the statement until after you get legal advice.

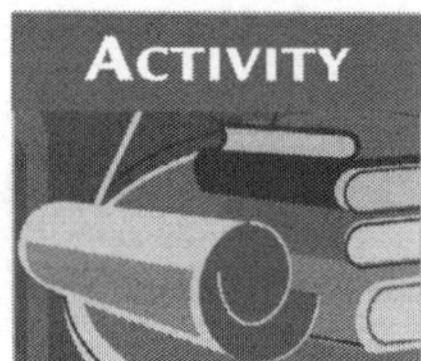

Activity

Legislation in each jurisdiction is specific about reportable deaths, one area in the Queensland Act that does need to be well understood by health professionals as their work is frequently related to general or particular care of the groups listed.

Go to the homepage of the Queensland government Department of Justice and Attorney-General website at:

<www.justice.qld.gov.au> (accessed 5 August 2014). Click on Births, Deaths and Marriages menu option. Scroll down to Deaths. This section explains the standard procedures required by the law. These procedures are essentially identical in every state and territory.

The law is concerned with protecting the public, particularly those who are vulnerable or unable to defend themselves. This extends to the death of someone who was the responsibility of another person or service. While there may be no inquest, it is the law that a person in direct care of a government service or who was the responsibility of such a service when they die, the death must be reported.

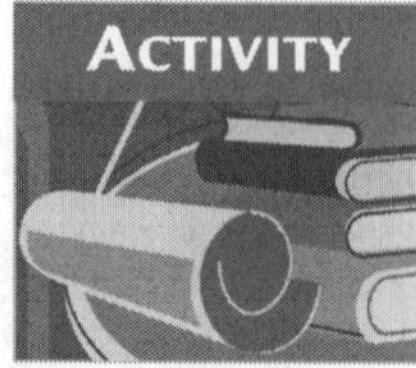

Activity

Go to the homepage of the Queensland Government Department of Justice and Attorney-General web site at:
<http://www.courts.qld.gov.au/__data/assets/pdf_file/0006/84561/m-osc-deaths-in-care.pdf> (accessed 5 August 2014)

A very informative fact sheet explaining Deaths in Care is available at this website. The categories of disabilities and relevant legislation are linked. There are many services and facilities that are identified as 'care'. It will be obvious that many of us could find ourselves employed in these services.

APPLICATION to practice

Application to practice

Health professionals work with people who have a disability, whether physical, intellectual or mental. Clients may be placed in care, choose to reside in a care situation or be detained for their own health and safety under relevant State Mental Health Acts. Staff working in these environments must be aware of the obligation to report a death whether it occurred in their facility or somewhere else, for example after the individual transfers to a hospital.

Inquest procedure

The inquest procedure is inquisitorial; witnesses are questioned and cross-examined. Staff members required to attend an inquest have rights in law. While you cannot refuse to attend an inquest if summoned, all staff should be aware that they are not required to incriminate themselves; they are not required to deal with police or other figures during an investigation without a clear understanding of the issue. In practice it would be sensible if faced with questions about an incident, or a request for a statement about a problematic death, to seek legal advice. Sometimes giving the police a statement is merely a matter of policy; the death falls within one of the reportable death categories so statements need to be given but there are no issues or problems in relation to that death. What can cause anxiety or lead to more serious consequences are situations where staff are contacted by the police asking for a statement about the incident/circumstances *many months* after the situation occurred. Refusing to give a statement is not an option. Not all information gathered by the police will in fact be used, but taking time to get legal advice before providing the statement would be wise. Experience has taught some health workers the benefit of keeping their own records of an incident. At the time, when there were issues or conflicts these staff members noted their observations or experience, signed and dated their own record and kept it quietly in a bottom drawer for use should their fears of an investigation come to be realised. The diary is not a legal document but it may assist in recalling the incident. It should be understood that your 'private' records can be required by the court. What might be for you, a simple aid to memory should be written with care and considerations of confidentiality and professional obligations.

The coronial hearing

In legal terms the whole inquest is considered 'a verdict'. The final result, what the coroner decides, is, in general language usage, called 'the verdict'. The distinction is not of great importance but should you be exploring the area or find yourself working with court staff involved in the process their use of the term may be confusing.

The magistrate acting as coroner at the inquest usually sits alone although a jury is required in cases of death occurring in prison or police custody or where death has resulted from an accident, poisoning or disease, or as directed by legislation. Like other court proceedings the inquest is often tape recorded and evidence and any discussions are written down.

The coroner is not bound by the rules of evidence that control what may be examined by the court and the coroner has the right to direct what questions can be asked, what information can be sought and who will be called as a witness.

Who can be a witness?

To establish the identity of the deceased and to provide a factual, sequential report of the events that preceded the death the coroner will call as witnesses those who knew the deceased and those involved in the events. Where there is a person identified as being 'responsible for the death', that person is usually the last to be called as a witness.

Each witness is required to swear an oath or affirm that they will tell the truth and each witness must identify themselves. The statements provided to the police will already have been given to the coroner prior to the inquest and these statements are explored with each witness.

Depending on the circumstances and the relationship of the witness to the events and the deceased, they are asked questions to clarify their relationship and provide insight into their knowledge and actions. The coroner can invite anyone present at the hearing to voice any questions once the witness has covered the matters described in their statements. Finally, cross-examination of the witness to get a better understanding and insight into events is undertaken.

Medical experts and professional evidence may be called for. The standards, custom and practice of those involved in the event may be elicited before the coroner investigates the specific facts of this case.

The process is not adversarial; while there may be a finding of fault the process is focused upon discovering facts.

After hearing all the evidence, if a jury is present matters of law, review of key issues and evidence are summed up prior to the jury being asked to come to a finding. As it is quite rare for a jury to be present, the coroner usually thanks those present and sets a date for presenting findings to the court.

The verdict

If there is no clear cause or there is no evidence to support a finding the coroner can return an 'open verdict'. If the cause of death is identified but the evidence shows that the deceased contributed to their own death through neglect or lack of care, that finding is appended to standard verdicts such as:

- Natural causes
- Industrial disease
- Dependence on drugs; non-dependent abuse of drugs

Other verdicts that are standard causes of death might be:

- Want of attention at birth
- Killed himself or herself while the balance of the mind was disturbed
- Attempted/self-induced abortion
- Accident/misadventure
- Killed lawfully
- Killed unlawfully
- Still birth

As there is no longer capital punishment in Australia there is no longer call for an inquest to establish:

- Execution of sentence of death

Results of an inquest

All states and territories have procedures to deal with recommendations arising from a coroner's report in relation to health care and health service provision. Evidence of wrongdoing during a coronial inquiry documented in the court transcript can be forwarded by the coroner's office to the Attorney-General if there is a crime involved or statutory authorities for safety, environmental or disciplinary actions.

For example: A state coroner may refer a finding of an inquest to AHPRA or the Board to bring to the attention of the profession. AHPRA will publish a case summary of each referral from the Coroner on its website, naming the deceased person, with the coroner's recommendations in full (AHPRA, 2012).

The Coroner is not a judge: The coroner is prohibited under the Coroners Act 2003 (Qld) from making any finding that a person is guilty of an offence or civilly liable. The coroner's findings and recommendations cannot be used as evidence in any other court or tribunal. This is because the focus of the Act is to help to prevent further deaths from occurring in similar circumstances. However, the coroner is able to refer a matter to the Director of Public Prosecutions or to a disciplinary body for consideration and possible action by that body.

It should be obvious that a coronial inquest can be a very worrying matter for health staff. The coroner can refer matters to the police and the Attorney-General for criminal matters or to professional statutory bodies for disciplinary or deregistration procedures and provide the family of the deceased with grounds to initiate a civil action against negligent staff.

An example of a case (in the UK) of the coroner referring a matter to the police was: A locum anaesthetist was sent for trial for manslaughter on a coroner's warrant after an inquest into the death of a 9 year old boy during an appendectomy. The locum had used a thin walled nasotracheal tube, but had passed it through the mouth into the trachea and then secured a loose connection with sticking plaster. The thin walled tube had kinked under the sticking plaster. After about 10 minutes the boy was noticed to be blue, and he subsequently died. Charged with a crime the doctor was convicted.

Another example: A Brisbane Professor at the Mater Hospital allegedly sliced open a woman's vein in a botched hysterectomy operation and then prescribed blood-thinning drugs that hastened her death.

The Coroner has charged him with manslaughter. (30.10.07)

Yet another example: Mother dies giving birth- coroner, rules her death was preventable.

Piyanat Siriwan began hemorrhaging uncontrollably after labour at the South Eastern Private Hospital, but her transfer to another hospital for life-saving surgery was delayed. The coroner found obstetrician and gynaecologist Maurice Lichter and anaesthetist Emlyn Williams contributed to Ms Siriwan's death.

She recommended the Medical Practitioners Board take whatever action it deemed appropriate against the doctors. (26.01.08 VIC).

Practice issues at time of death

There are numerous staff involved in communication with relatives and the protocols that are implemented at time of death. Some staff believe that the responsibility to inform the family and assist them to deal with these protocols lies with the medical officer or social workers. The reality is that the family can turn to anyone in time of need, and any staff members may be called on to provide accurate information, with care and consideration.

When a person dies in hospital the likelihood that an autopsy will be carried out is very high. In some circumstances this is policy – by law the coroner may require a medico-legal autopsy – in other situations it is a desire to research causes. Permission is sought from the family as it is not 'law' that an autopsy for such research should be carried out but rather a matter of science. If autopsy findings establish that the death 'was a result of natural causes' then the coroner may dispense with an inquest.

- Legislation allows for relatives or guardians of the deceased or the Commissioner of Police or Minister of Justice to request an inquest.

Some families do not want an internal autopsy performed. The coroner is required to consider these views, if known, when deciding whether an internal autopsy is necessary. Any information about the family's view on the autopsy should be provided to the coroner as soon as possible. Cultural and religious prohibitions to autopsy are considered very carefully but the law takes precedence. Not every autopsy is an extensive and intrusive examination of the deceased. In some circumstances the examination may be complete with minimal tissue samples or external examination.

While an autopsy is an investigation of the body, a post mortem is an examination of all the events and circumstances relating to the death. The public tend to use the term post mortem examination rather than autopsy so it is common to hear the terms used interchangeably among staff.

Tissue can be removed for testing during the autopsy. However, if the tissue to be removed and retained is a whole organ or foetus, then the doctor must inform the coroner.

At the end of the autopsy the doctor must complete particular legal forms to give notice to the coroner. On this form the doctor must advise the coroner that they want to retain a whole organ or foetus and why this is considered necessary. The doctor must also inform the coroner that they have advised the person's family of the need to retain tissue and whether the family has any objection. If the coroner approves the release of the body for burial the institution/researcher holding the whole organ or foetus will be advised of the coroner's decision. The decision to retain the whole organ or foetus is required to be reviewed by the coroner every six months.

An organ or foetus kept for testing can only be disposed of when it is no longer required and with the consent of the coroner. This can be sought at any time by writing to the coroner or when the coroner reviews the decision to retain the tissue after six months.

While the consent of the coroner is not required to retain samples of tissue other than a whole organ or foetus, consent by the coroner is required for tissue disposal. The doctor/researcher retaining these samples must request the authority of the coroner in writing prior to disposal. Once consent for the release of samples has been granted by the coroner the institution that is in possession must arrange for their disposal. If the family of the deceased have advised the coroner that they wish the organ or foetus to be returned to them, the institution must release it to the family or the family's nominated funeral director.

Application to practice

APPLICATION to practice

Nurses tend to clients who have died. Some facilities may require only that the client is transferred to a room or mortuary to await collection by the nominated funeral director. This is common in aged-care facilities and private care. In acute hospitals there are considerably more steps to be followed.

When the client has been pronounced dead by a medical officer the usual practice is to remove appliances such as monitors, ventilators and other machinery. Where there is to be an autopsy, policies are often in place dictating that any central or peripheral lines be disconnected, *but* the cannulae are left taped *in situ*, which is also usual for wound drains and the like. Open wounds are covered appropriately.

Many patients die while engaged in some activity other than bed rest. Some staff fear to move a client found on the floor or in the bathroom until the doctor has seen the patient and certified that they are dead. However, circumstances may dictate that moving the body is essential. In a private home or residential facilities there may be considerable delays before a medical officer can attend. Leaving someone sitting on the toilet after suffering an embolism, or in the dining room or on the floor is neither respectful nor necessary. The relatives often see their family member even before the doctor attends. If there is any question of criminal or other interference, then of course, for a police investigation to be effective, leaving everything, including the deceased, untouched is required.

The practice of washing the body, changing the clothes and allowing relatives to view the client is still common in a number of areas. Requests for the deceased to be dressed in personal attire rather than the hospital gown or 'shroud' are usually easily satisfied, unless circumstances may dictate otherwise. Jewellery is often given to the family with an explanation that it can be returned to the deceased at the funeral home. Wedding rings are usually taped in place if left with the deceased.

Transfer to the hospital mortuary with accompanying documentation and ID is usually managed in a timely manner. The body, whether or not it is to be subject to autopsy, *belongs* to the executor of the deceased's estate. In practice the body is released to the next of kin by the coroner or, if there are no formalities involved, the institution. It often happens that there is no next of kin or there has been no will nominating the executor of the deceased's estate. In this situation, before the body can be disposed of by either cremation or burial, a legally nominated or legally recognised person who has sought standing from the court to 'administer' matters is required.

Your nursing texts will provide further information on basic clincial procedures and the facility will have written policies and procedures providing guidelines. As it is a stressful situation for everyone involved, including other patients who are usually well aware of a death on the ward, the professional needs to be aware of the heightened sensibilities and anxieties of all; inappropriate comments and 'black humour' may reduce the tension of some staff but could be construed as unprofessional behaviour and be grounds for disciplinary action.

Recommended reading

This short article available on ProQuest describes a coronial inquest (Case No. 1887/97, 21 May 1999 (Vic) State Coroner Graeme Johnstone) and also highlights the nursing issues of safe lifting and incident reporting and documentation that arose at the inquest.

Amelda Langslow, 'Nursing and the law', *Australian Nursing Journal* October 1999, 7(4):36.

Activity

Answer true or false to the questions below.

- The coroner is required to investigate the circumstances of deaths in many health care facilities where nurses may work, including psychiatric facilities, homes for mentally disabled people, mental institutions and children's residences. When a person dies in a nursing home or home for the aged, the coroner must be notified, but an investigation is discretionary.

  True False

- The coroner has broad powers to conduct their investigation, including the power to enter and inspect premises and to seize evidence where necessary to the investigation.

  True False

- The coroner may delegate to the local police who typically assist the coroner's investigation.

  True False

- Nurses may be questioned when an investigation is held into a death at their place of work. It is against the law to obstruct or interfere with a coroner's investigation.

  True False

- A coronial investigation can lead to criminal charges, civil litigation or professional discipline. If you fear that your involvement may lead to this, what are your rights?

  Refuse to cooperate?

  True False

  Refuse to provide full and complete statements that could incriminate you?

  True False

  Right to seek legal advice prior to making a statement?

  True False

Right to legal representation during any proceedings?

True False

- It would be highly recommended that you have your own legal representative even if your employer has offered representation.

True False

Activity

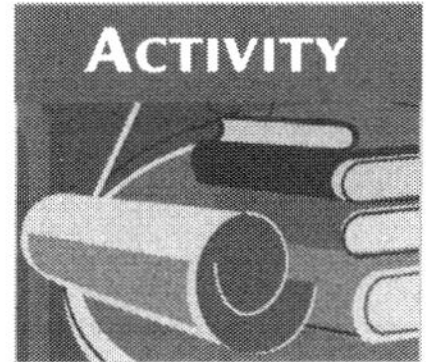

- What is the difference between an autopsy and a post mortem examination?
- What is the difference between a 'hospital autopsy' and a 'medico-legal autopsy'?
- If a person dies without leaving a will and appointing an executor, who has claim to the body of the deceased?

Practice considerations

Your communication skills, emotional intelligence, empathy and the professional attribute of recognising boundaries of practice will all contribute to meeting the obligations and responsibilities which arise surrounding the death of a client. Legal aspects are often outside of the clinical sphere but some awareness of these key issues can help health professionals deal with the physical and emotional requirements of the situation. The perceptions of family members and their response to staff at this time need to be considered. Poorly supported family members may interpret behaviours of staff very negatively and the circumstances can easily generate complaints or demands for investigations. The legal requirements of a shocking, unforeseen death impose added burdens on relatives and staff. Policies and procedures may give staff some comfort and sense of security but it is often empathy without intrusion, guidance and explanations by a professional that provides comfort and security to the family who have to deal with their grief and formalities.

Summary

This chapter explained the law relating to formalities of death and the rules governing particular deaths that must be investigated by the coroner. Understanding these rules means the nurse can assist the family to understand procedures. Recognising there are a number of circumstances where the health professional could be involved in an inquest adds still more weight to the professional requirement for accurate and timely documentation. As you have seen there have been many inquests where findings led to changes in policies and procedures. One way of looking at these inquiries into client deaths is to appreciate that the law has helped to change and improve practice.

Sources

Abernethy, J., Baker, B., Dillon, H. & Roberts, H. (2010) *Waller's Coronial Law and Practice in New South Wales*, 4th edn (eBook) Lexis Nexis.

AHPRA (2012) Findings from the Coroner. http://www.ahpra.gov.au/News/Recommendations-from-the-Coroner.aspx

Forrester, K. & Griffiths, D. (2005) *Essentials of Law*, 2nd edn, Harcourt, Sydney.

Health Law Update (2001) *Retention of Body Parts Following Post Mortem in New South Wales*, June.

Kennedy, R. & Richards, J. (2004) *Integrating Human Service Law and Practice*, Oxford University Press, Melbourne.

MacFarlane, P. (1995), *Health Law*, 2nd edn, The Federation Press, Sydney.

MacFarlane, P. J. & Reid, S. J. (2003) *Queensland Health Law Handbook*, Queensland Dept of Health, Brisbane.

Middleton, S. Buist, M. (2014) *The coronial reporting of medical-setting deaths: a legal analysis of the variation in Australian jurisdictions*. Melbourne University Law Review, Vol 37:699.

Morris, G., Cook, C., Creyke, R. & Geddes, R. (2001) *Laying Down the Law*, 5th edn, Butterworths, Sydney.

Office of the State Coroner Queensland, Information for Health Professionals' <http://www.courts.qld.gov.au/__data/assets/pdf_file/0006/92868/m-osc-fs-information-for-health-professionals.pdf> (accessed 9 August 2014)

Queensland Courts, Office of the State Coroner Deaths in Care <http://www.courts.qld.gov.au/__data/assets/pdf_file/0006/84561/m-osc-deaths-in-care.pdf> (accessed 9 August 2014).

Staunton, P. & Chiarella, M. (2003) *Nursing and the Law*, 5th edn, Elsevier, Sydney.

Staunton, P. & Whyburn, B. (1997) *Nursing and the Law*, 4th edn, Harcourt Australia Pty Ltd, Sydney.

White, B., Wilmott, L & McDonald, F. (2014) *Health Law in Australia*, 2nd edn, Thomson Reuters, Australia.

Cases

Coroner's inquiry into the death of Mark McCabe (1981) Glebe Coroners Court.

Coroner's inquiry into the death of Clinton Norwood (1984) Westmead Coroner's Court.

Coroner's inquiry into the death of Sara Slapp (1993) Westmead Coroner's Court.

Criminal law and health professionals

CHAPTER 11

Learning outcomes

After studying this chapter you should be able to:

- Explain criminal law in context of the Australian legal system.
- Describe the relationships between professional governance an criminal offences by a health worker.
- Recognise the value of professional behaviours in avoiding legal risks.
- Identify the legislation relevant to criminal investigations and procedures.

Overview

Criminal law differs in many key concepts from civil law while remaining at its core a part of the common law. Many criminal offences have been created by legislation rather than being part of the inherited common law. Some jurisdictions have all crimes and rules for criminal procedure incorporated into a code, the Criminal Code. This is the situation in the Australian Capital Territory, Northern Territory, Queensland, Tasmania, and Western Australia. In New South Wales, South Australia and Victoria the common law, modified by state legislation (Crimes Act), is the chief source of criminal law. In Queensland in 1899 a Criminal Code was enacted and this came into force in 1901. This code was adopted in Western Australia and later, in a modified form, introduced in Tasmania. Decisions in states using the common law as the chief source of criminal law may have no relevance to similar cases in those states governed by the code.

To understand this area from a health professional's perspective it is necessary to delve a bit into the complexities of the law itself. Then it may be easier to see the points where a health professional's work or actions may cross paths with the legal concepts.

Crime and punishment are what this area of law is all about. We have explored in civil law the idea of damage and compensation and, in relation to professional governance, standards and sanctions. As you have seen, penalties exist for failure to adhere to legislative and professional standards but in a legal sense these are not 'punishments' as defined in a criminal law action.

The legislature and the courts determine in any given legal system what acts should be classified as criminal. Normally it is the combination of two factors which are to be found in the decision to treat a certain class of conduct as criminal. The first is *publicness* of the conduct. This means that it will only be labelled a crime if it is thought to be an offence against one or more individuals. It must be injurious to the public in general. The second element is *moral wrongdoing*. Recall from Chapter 1 that the issue of ethics in relation to law was discussed. That blurred line between morality as a philosophical concept and morality in relation to a crime against society comes to light in this area. Recall also that not every instance of conduct that might be considered morally wrong or against the public interest is treated as a crime.

Here, however, in criminal law we are discussing behaviour where the risks or harm to society are so great that there must be deterrents in the form of punishment both to encourage conformity and thus social harmony, as well as visit upon the wrongdoer a punishment that society feels is equal in severity to the harm done.

A moment's reflection will no doubt enable you to list the various matters that are considered crimes:

- Invasions of a person's right to life
- Invasions of a person's right to liberty
- Invasions of a person's property

These are the crimes most commonly dealt with by courts. Invasions may be direct, such as theft and assault on a particular person, or indirect, such as driving offences which break laws aimed at protecting all road users.

A variety of terms used commonly in American police and court room dramas can lead to confusion. From a purely administrative point of view crimes are divided between major and minor crimes. In the past major crimes were called felonies and minor crimes were called misdemeanors, and these terms are still used in US jurisdictions. In Australia today major crimes are termed *indictable offences*; these are serious offences against persons and/or property. Minor crimes are termed *summary offences*. The Magistrate's Court tends to deal with summary offences from the stage of charges being laid, the accused's claim of guilty or not guilty, through the hearing (if a not guilty plea was entered), to a verdict and penalty being finalised. Magistrates do not hear trials for indictable offences, only the first stage of the charge and plea of the accused. For indictable crimes where the accused pleads not guilty, the magistrate will commit the accused for trial to be heard by the District Court or Supreme Court.

Victimless crimes

An area of criminal law that has undergone much debate is that of 'victimless crimes'. Usually these are activities where there has been consent by adults to conduct but the society at large has a strong belief that the conduct is morally wrong. Conduct that is considered criminal carries a real stigma. An investigation by the police can damage the reputation and standing of a person whether or not a criminal charge is finally laid. The process of arguing a case where criminal charges have been laid and are presented to the court by the prosecution further puts the individual at risk in relation to the wider society. Even if found innocent, there is usually great damage to reputation and employment and family relationships for the individual. This stigma means law makers have a great responsibility to balance the concept of what is 'moral' at any given time and place against a desire to protect society at large.

For example, homosexuality is no longer a crime in most jurisdictions of Australia but incest remains a crime. This is not the place to argue the social or moral justice issues but as health workers dealing with both victims and perpetrators of crimes it is important to remember that what is a crime in one place and time may not be in another. Professional standards of care must take priority in spite of opinions about the individual and labels. Finding yourself identified as a criminal due to your own attitudes, communication or behaviours towards a client who you have been told is a 'criminal' would be a disaster.

Criminal acts

A fundamental concept in criminal law is the belief that individuals have free will and this gives them a choice to act or not to act. Blame attaches to acts that are considered intentional. The Latin term *mens rea* is used to explain this idea of free will. It captures the ideas of intention and awareness of what one does. So if a person does something reprehensible a defence could be 'lack of awareness, unintentional, didn't understand'. This is the basis of a defence of insanity.

This concept of *mens rea*, or the mental element of a crime, is not a simple matter. Over time the meaning has changed somewhat; the belief that a person's state of mind makes something a crime is tricky to prove. In reality it is the behaviour of the accused that is closely examined. The actions (*actus rea*) give insight into the mental state. For example, pointing a loaded gun, bashing someone over the head or participating in 'violent' activity is evidence of a 'will' or desire to harm.

This doesn't quite cover situations described by statements such as 'I didn't mean the person to get hurt', 'I never thought it would cause harm', 'we were just fooling around'. Here the law considers in modern terms the idea of recklessness. When someone is reckless about the consequences they still actually had some desire to produce some consequence; in current legal jargon this is still 'intention', therefore a criminal act can be attributed to a thoughtless or reckless behaviour. In spite of changing times and psychology this mental state concept still flows through the criminal law.

Criminal negligence

Negligence in criminal law results from a higher degree of failure to meet standards and directly cause damage than is recognised by civil law. Even if a person simply did not consider the risks of their action or omission, if they had a responsibility to do something and their work or that activity has risks, then whether or not they had no intention to harm or there was no mental component to hurt it will not negate the fact that the action was criminally negligent.

Mistakes do happen and we have explored these in a number of chapters, particularly those relating to civil law. For the matter to be criminal, even if there was no intention to harm, the level of negligence is far more than 'could have happened to anyone'. A case which demonstrates the level of negligence that amounts to criminal negligence is *R v. Bateman* (1925, p. 51), in which it was stated that 'the accused showed such disregard for the life and safety of others as to amount to a crime against the State and conduct deserving punishment'.

Murder and manslaughter

- Murder is homicide. There was an intention to kill.
- Manslaughter is where a death has occurred but there was (usually) no intention to cause that death. The death may have been caused through recklessness, an unlawful act or behaviour that amounts to criminal negligence.

Manslaughter is classified as voluntary or involuntary. It may be that the accused actually *did mean* to kill the person, they did have intention, but the circumstances were such that the court can't find for murder based on the facts in evidence. Circumstances that give rise to the finding of voluntary manslaughter would be killing in self-defence or killing to protect your child or another person who was under threat. Another is provocation: the behaviour of the victim was such that the reaction of the accused is mitigated or less reprehensible.

Involuntary manslaughter is when the death was caused by reckless or thoughtless actions, or where there was intent to hurt someone – inflict bodily harm – but that harm resulted in an unintended death. This may be the finding when someone who has diminished responsibility caused the death of another. Each jurisdiction has legislation covering diminished responsibility. The causes and levels of impairment of mind that will permit a finding of murder to be reduced to involuntary manslaughter are described by relevant legislation.

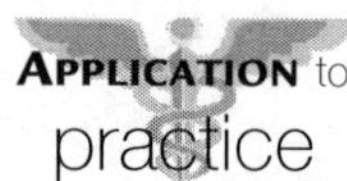

Application to practice

An incorrect drug has been administered by the wrong route, in the wrong dosage. The patient dies.

- Is this murder?

Was there an intention to kill the person? No: therefore it is not murder.

- Is this manslaughter or criminal negligence?

There was an intention to give the drug. The issue is, however, wrong drug, wrong dose, wrong route. This was so *reckless*, a mistake of such a degree that the death of a person occurred. It could only be seen as manslaughter due to criminal negligence.

Whether or not a death occurs, criminal negligence arises where the level of recklessness, incompetence or choice to deviate from practice norms is beyond any acceptable meaning of the word 'mistake'.

Strict liability

Legislation imposes the concept of strict liability for many actions considered crimes. For this type of legislation, rather than exploring issues of mental state or intention, simply proving that someone did something is enough to guarantee punishment. Usually these types of crimes and their punishments are not as severe as those investigated by courts where a sentence has severe effects on life or liberty. For these less serious situations the individual can still defend themselves and suggest mitigating circumstances but, generally speaking, these types of actions are *summary* crimes and brought before a magistrate who awards a penalty as specified by the legislation. This is usually a fine but may be community service or imprisonment.

Evidence and the standard of proof

Strict rules of evidence and procedure exist for criminal trials. Factual evidence, not hearsay, is required. The judge or legal representatives cannot bring to the trial matters that fall outside the protocols.

When a person is charged they are brought before the appropriate court as the 'accused'. There they may plead guilty or not guilty to the charge. It falls to the police to provide evidence to uphold the charges in a court hearing and in criminal cases this is referred to as the *burden of proof*. Any evidence tendered to satisfy the court must meet the *standard of proof*, which is to a higher requirement than other legal matters.

At common law there is the presumption of innocence. The evidence presented must satisfy not only the standard of proof but must provide the court with sufficient certainty to be able to conclude that the accused is guilty *beyond reasonable doubt*.

The judge or jury decides on the issue of guilt or innocence only after all evidence and witness statements and the legal representatives' arguments have been heard.

Legal identity

Above, reference was made to defences based on the individual's mental state. Insanity and diminished responsibility are defences. Inability to perceive or understand actions is a defence. Taking this idea a step further, there are individuals who, in law, are not considered liable for their actions.

Infants and children are unable to judge the rightness or wrongness of their actions. While the common law generally considered a child under the age of seven years to be incapable of 'committing a crime', whether or not their actions caused harm, this age is now eight years in some jurisdictions and ten in others as a result of legislation such as the *Children's Protection and Young Offenders Act 1979* (SA).

Under the age of 14 for a child to be charged it is usually a case of having evidence that the child not only did the act but admitted they knew it was wrong. Then the matter can be treated as a criminal action by a young offender. Children's Courts provide another safety net and have been set up in every state. These are the usual courts dealing with offenders under the age of 17 years.

To round off this concept of who is a legal 'person' note that the entity of a corporation is considered a legal person. A corporation can be liable for the criminal acts specific to that corporation of its officers or employees. While a corporation can't be sent to gaol, the revocations of licences or fines are options to penalise a corporation.

There is a concept of sovereign or diplomatic immunity that extends to adults. Should a crime be committed by someone of this status they are immune from prosecution. However, accomplices who are not diplomats (or the sovereign of a nation) are just as liable as anyone else. Diplomatic immunity does not provide umbrella coverage to non-diplomats involved in the criminal activity.

Crimes and professional practice

You have learnt that coronial findings can be referred to the police if there is evidence of an unlawful death arising from the inquiry. You have seen that a criminal record can affect registration in relation to professional governance. In your readings of torts in civil law you learnt that failure to obtain consent can be construed as assault (the old-fashioned term battery, that is, laying hands on someone to cause harm, is rarely used today). Generally, however, rarely does the work of a health professional lead to a criminal investigation or charges that must be defended in court.

Murder, manslaughter and criminal negligence or, a less used action, professional malpractice, are concepts most of us have heard of. We will explore these now.

Homicide

Homicide is the term that includes murder, manslaughter and infanticide. Recall from the overview above that crimes have a mental element.

- Murder is where a person at the age of discretion, having a sound mind, unlawfully kills another and does so with intention or malice and the death occurs (within a year and a day) as a result of causing that harm.

This definition is a reconstruction of a very old definition by an English judge but in essence the concept has remained unchanged since 1797. Note the following:

- The definition considers the issue of legal capacity (age of discretion); children under the age of 14 years must be proven to have known that what they did was wrong.

- 'Unlawfully kills' covers the idea of withholding treatment or actively assisting someone to die. In the Northern Territory in 1995 there was a legislative attempt to provide immunity from prosecution to doctors for activities which assisted patients to die in order to meet patients' requests as terminally ill clients. This Act has been overturned and there are no jurisdictions in Australia that provide immunity for actively assisting a terminally ill client to die.
- The year and a day rule in the definition was in common law the limitation set for proving the death related to a specific action. This is irrelevant in this day and age with advances in technology allowing identification of unlawful killing and discovery of evidence at times far removed from the original murder. Legislation has overridden the common law rule in most jurisdictions.

Here is a summary of the various types of homicide.

- *Manslaughter* is the same as murder except that there was no *mens rea*, there was no intention. It is in common law an unintended, wholly unexpected and unlikely killing as a result of an act which is unlawful, dangerous or of reckless negligence.
- *Voluntary manslaughter* is where there was an intention to harm or kill but the accused did this act in self-defence or was provoked to such a degree that the court will accept that the provocation is a defence.
- *Involuntary manslaughter* is the result of dangerous, unlawful, reckless or grossly negligent acts. This has been the finding in cases where health professionals have acted in ways that are deemed outside of an objective expectation of safe and reasonable practice. Drug administration is a good example. Miss any of the six checks and the action is not only negligent but should a death result this could be the verdict. A defence of impaired understanding, where there was no comprehension of the risks of the activity that causes a death, can result in involuntary manslaughter.
- *Negligent manslaughter* arises where there is a duty of care and the acts or omissions on the part of the professional/responsible person fall well outside what is considered to be a reasonable standard of care.
- *Reckless manslaughter* is where the accused knew the activity/treatment carried real risks but proceeded to do this anyway. High-risk treatments and operations would not fall into this category if there was evidence of informed consent and that the professional standards were adhered to.
- *Infanticide* is the killing of a newborn by its mother. This is closely linked to another criminal offence, concealment of birth. The courts recognise that the mother may be affected by pregnancy and birth and this may affect her mental state.
- *Child destruction* is the deliberate destruction of the foetus after a certain time of pregnancy. In common law this is considered to be mid or late pregnancy. The difference between abortion in the sense of public usage and this crime lies with the concept of viability. In some common law jurisdictions the courts currently accept that at 28 weeks a child is capable of being born alive so any deliberate or unlawful act to prevent that is potentially a crime. Interventions to save the mother 'done in good faith' would of course fall outside the criminal jurisdiction.

> The *Queensland Criminal Code* (s. 224) makes it an offence to procure the miscarriage of a woman. Section 282 does provide for a surgical operation carried out for the benefit of the mother or to preserve the mother's life. Interventions are taken with regard to the woman's state and circumstances. There is no criminal liability because the code does not recognise an unborn child as a legal entity. It cannot be murder unless the child is delivered: once delivered the child is a 'person'.

The decision to terminate a pregnancy made by the woman herself is generally referred to as abortion. There have been changes to the laws in various states to remove abortion from the Crimes Acts or Criminal Codes.

In both Queensland & New South Wales: Abortion remains a crime for women and doctors. However abortion is legal when doctor believes a woman's physical and/or mental health is in serious danger. In NSW social, economic and medical factors may be taken into account.

Australian Capital Territory: Abortion is legal, the procedure must be provided by medical doctor.

Victoria: Abortion is legal up until 24 weeks. If induced after 24 weeks it is only legal when signed off by two doctors.

South Australia: Abortion is legal if two doctors agree that a woman's physical and/or mental health endangered by pregnancy, or for serious foetal abnormality. If this is not evident the abortion is unlawful and counted as a crime.

Tasmania: Abortion is legal up until 16 weeks on request, and after 16 weeks with the approval of two doctors.

Western Australia: Abortion is legal up to 20 weeks, after that it requires two doctors approval, these doctors are selected from a Ministerial panel. For girls under 16 years of age the Act includes a parental notification clause. This requires one parent to be informed, and given the opportunity to participate in counselling before an abortion can be performed. However, young women may apply to the Children's Court for an order to proceed with an abortion if it is not considered suitable to involve her parent(s).

Northern Territory: Abortion is legal to 14 weeks if 2 doctors agree that woman's physical and/or mental health endangered by pregnancy, or for serious foetal abnormality. Abortion is considered legal up to 23 weeks in an emergency.

Case Study 1

The extract below is one of the few cases for murder against a nurse.

In the early hours of 18 November 2011, a fire was deliberately lit at the Quaker's Hill Nursing Home. As a result of the fire, three people died at the scene and a further eight died in hospital after suffering the effects of burns and/or smoke inhalation. Eight people were seriously injured from burns and/or smoke inhalation who survived the fire. The offender, Roger Dean, pleaded guilty on 27 May 2013 to eleven counts of murder under s18 of the *Crimes Act 1900 (NSW)* "by way of reckless indifference to human life, and eight counts of recklessly cause grievous bodily harm" s 35(2) of the

Crimes Act 1900 (NSW). He was sentenced to life imprisonment. Judge applied section 61 (1) *Crimes (Sentencing Procedure) Act 1999 (NSW)* in sentencing Dean to life imprisonment.

R v Dean [2013] NSWSC 1027, NSW Supreme Court, Latham J, 1 August 2013

Case Study 2

An 18-day-old baby died after treatment with herbal drops by a naturopath. The baby was born with a heart defect, aortic stenosis. The parents failed to attend appointments for planned surgery in the belief the child had been cured by the naturopath.

It was not the herbal remedy that killed the child, it was the belief that this treatment had in fact cured the child and the naturopath's recommendation that the parents cancel the hospital appointments as surgery was no longer necessary.

The naturopath was found guilty of manslaughter. The problem was curable and any professional would know that the treatment was surgery. Even if the naturopath lacked that knowledge, as a professional it would be expected that investigation of the diagnosis and treatments would be carried out.

During his nine-day trial, the New South Wales Supreme Court in Newcastle was told Fenn (the naturopath) had treated baby Mitchell in September 1999 with herbal drops and a 'Mora machine' before declaring him cured.

Justice Newman said that the sentence should act as a deterrent to other alternative practitioners, saying that the full weight of the law would fall on them if tragedy followed their treatment of people.

Assault

The term assault and battery is commonly used but is rarely found in case law although it exists in some legislation. Assault covers a threat as well as actual harm in criminal law. Recall that in civil cases relating to refusal or lack of consent to touching we talked about the possibility of that being construed as damage (physical or mental), thus being captured by the tort of negligence. In criminal law the victim needs only to *believe* they will be harmed for it to be criminal assult. Making someone fear imminent violence or harm as a result of a threat or abusive language amounts to criminal assault.

There are categories of assault in criminal law. The degree of harm is referred to as common assault, bodily harm and grievous bodily harm or wounding.

Verbal aggression and obscene language

The law deals differently with written and spoken language, and charges relating to offensive language have frequently been brought under laws relating to obscenity.

Legislation about offensive language is intended to protect people from the detrimental effects of speech (Jay 1999) and to control behaviour in public places (Brown et al 2006).

To warrant criminalisation, offensive epithets must:

- constitute personally abusive insults;
- be addressed in a face-to-face manner;
- target a specific individual and be descriptive of that individual; and
- be addressed to an individual unable to avoid the assaultive message

Use of offensive language may result in exclusion from schooling, healthcare and other services, in fines or even imprisonment.

Rape and sexual assault

In earlier times common law rules about rape were very narrow. Rules of procedure and evidence led to a perception that victims did not fare well if they proceeded to report rape. Legislation has intervened not only with many changes to what constitutes rape but also to recognise that men as well as women can be victims. Rape within marriage, anal penetration and other sexual offences have been identified as crimes and are generally now referred to as sexual offences. Most states have updated legislation and broadened concepts of consent in the 21st Century.

Rape and sexual assault cases usually hinged on the concept of consent. Consent can be withdrawn at any time and if this consent is disputed then the behaviour and conduct of the victim can be used as evidence. An example of legislation that gives direction to courts in relation to consent issues are the legal changes to the definition of rape in South Australian legislation Criminal Law Consolidation (Rape and Sexual Offences) Amendment Act 2008- The laws have been strengthened to provide a clearer definition of offences and what constitutes consent. This legislation reflects every other jurisdiction in identifying who cannot give consent, thus if the person was "not legally capable" the action will be held to be sexual assault.

The law also states that some people cannot give consent to sexual intercourse. This includes:

- A person who has sexual intercourse with any person under the age of 14 years shall be guilty of an offence and liable to be imprisoned for life.
- A person who has sexual intercourse with a person under the age of seventeen years is guilty of an offence. Maximum penalty: Imprisonment for 10 years.
- A person who, being in a position of authority in relation to a person under the age of 18 years, has sexual intercourse with that person is guilty of an offence. Maximum penalty: Imprisonment for 10 years. The person in a position of authority could be a teacher, foster parent, step-parent, guardian, religious official or spiritual leader, medical practitioner, psychologist, social worker, person employed in correctional institution or training centre, or employer.
- Sexual intercourse with a person with intellectual disability, unable to understand the consequences of sexual intercourse.

The legal age for consensual sex varies across Australian state and territory jurisdictions. The age of consent is 16 years of age in the Australian Capital Territory, New South Wales, Northern Territory, Victoria and Western Australia. In Tasmania and South Australia the age of consent is 17 years of age. Queensland is the only state that makes a distinction between different forms of sexual activity and the age of consent. In Queensland, the age of consent for anal sex (referred to as sodomy in legislation) is 18 years of age, while the age of consent for all other sexual behaviour (described as carnal knowledge) is 16 years of age.

In situations where consent is given for what might be 'intrusive or inappropriate medical examinations' that the victim believed were necessary as a result of professional advice, the consent is invalid.

From a professional point of view, fraudulent or misleading advice to obtain consent to an intimate procedure is a category of rape. Current ethically sound practice is to ensure that explanations and consent are witnessed as well as having another professional present during the procedure.

Victims of rape often present to hospitals or clinics after some delay. There are protocols and policies for providing support to these victims. Police protocols for evidence gathering have led many institutions to have specialist staff work with clients to ensure their needs are met concurrently with the gathering of evidence such as swabs, photographs and statements. It is important that evidence is not lost through showering or wound cleansing and that the victim is treated with dignity and respect. Issues of privacy, confidentiality and protection of identity have sometimes been overlooked in clinical environments.

Female genital mutilation

As a result of Australia being a signatory to international treaties, conventions and declarations female genital mutilation is now a crime in Australia. In all jurisdictions it is an offence for a person to perform any type of female genital mutilation. Although in some cases different language is used to define female genital mutilation, all definitions essentially cover the same conduct and are consistent with the definition of female genital mutilation accepted by the World Health Organization.

Importantly, in all jurisdictions the consent of the victim, or their parent or guardian, is not a defence to female genital mutilation and specific exceptions have been granted for legitimate medical purposes (including those related to child birth and sex reassignment procedures).

All State and Territory offences also operate extraterritorially to protect Australian residents from being subjected to female genital mutilation outside their jurisdiction of residence, including overseas. For example, it is illegal in New South Wales and the Northern Territory to perform female genital mutilation on another person irrespective of where the female genital mutilation occurs, so long as the victim is normally resident in New South Wales or the Northern Territory respectively. Further, in all jurisdictions except New South Wales it is an offence to remove an individual from that jurisdiction with the intention of having female genital mutilation performed on that person other jurisdictions this practice would be caught under child abuse legislation and health workers are required by law to report suspected, intended or performed genital mutilation injuries (Review of Australia's Female Genital Mutilation legal framework, Final Report 2013).

Crimes against children

The criminal law creates a number of specific offences relating to child neglect and abuse. The creation of specific offences recognises that the criminal law has an important role to play in child abuse and neglect, on the basis that a function of the criminal justice system is to define acceptable standards of behaviour.

There is child protection legislation which to some extent duplicates the criminal law in specifying offences and those responsible for child protection work closely with police so a person may be charged under different legislative provisions. In four jurisdictions, Queensland, South Australia, the ACT and the Northern Territory offences relating to child abuse and neglect are contained in general criminal laws. In the other four jurisdictions, there are specific child abuse and neglect offences in child protection legislation. In Western Australia, a person with the care and control of a child must not do an act, or fail to do an act, knowing (or recklessly disregarding) that the conduct may cause significant harm to a child from abuse (physical, sexual, emotional or psychological) or neglect. In Victoria and Tasmania, it is an offence for a person who has a duty of care to a child to take, or fail to take, action that has either resulted in harm to the child, or has the potential to cause harm. The NSW child protection law makes it an offence for any person (not just one who has care of a child) to do an act intentionally that causes or appears likely to cause injury or harm to a child or young person. It is also an offence for a person who has care of a child or young person to fail to provide the child or young person with adequate and proper food, nursing, clothing, medical aid or accommodation (Australian Law Reform Commission, 2010).

Documentation

The issue of record keeping and documentation has been identified constantly as a key legal issue for health professionals. In criminal proceedings the patient records and all documents can and probably will be used to provide evidence for the charges and to give the court information. Client statements about the cause of their injuries such as happens when they present at the hospital after injury are critical documents. As well, documents such as evidence of consent, orders for restraint, records of observations, monitoring and status have all been at different times, in various cases, used by the courts.

There have been civil, criminal and coronial cases where medical and often nursing records have been found to be so poor, inadequate, subjective or adulterated that findings have specifically addressed the issue.

Objective findings rather than subjective statements are necessary. Clarity, legibility and accuracy are expected in all documentation.

Patient statements and patient complaints should be reported exactly and either quote marks or a note to the effect that these are the client's own words is needed.

As you already know, reports and documentation should occur at the time of an incident. Trying to recall progressive stages of an incident after the event can lead to mistakes. Real-world pressures do cause delay and client status may be altering hour by hour. Writing up at 4 pm, after the client has died, that it was noted he was pale, sweating and complaining of chest pain at 1000 hours then steadily adding in the incidents and actions that occurred before the death from memory is going to be very difficult to justify should that entry be used in court proceedings.

Courts use documents in a very literal manner. If the observation chart says that it was at 11 am that the blood pressure was 90/40 the court will be unimpressed when the nurse who took that blood pressure later says it was actually 11.15, just moments before the client died. Nurses work to time periods for many activities. Some areas still have standard times for 'pill rounds', 'dressing rounds', 'routine obs'. However, there can be long delays between the time the first client received their treatment or observation and the last client receiving treatment or observation. Charts should show the true times.

Future considerations: criminal law and health professionals

The United Kingdom is currently grappling questions about prosecuting health workers for reckless and negligent behaviours after systemic failures in care and treatment of patients at the Mid Staffordshire NHS Foundation Trust Hospital (MSNFTH) contributed to radically higher death rates than in comparable hospitals elsewhere in the UK.

Australia's recent experience with the trials of former Bega gynaecologist Graeme Reeves and Bundaberg surgeon Jayant Patel are recent examples of criminal actions against medical staff.

In Wisconsin USA a nurse was prosecuted for a medication error that led to an obstetric patient's death. The case raised serious questions about staffing and overtime pressures being the underlying cause yet it was the nurse who was charged with murder.

Provisions criminalising wilful or reckless neglect or mistreatment of mentally ill and child patients already exist in the UK. In the UK there are strong arguments for these sanctions to be extended to cover all patients.

Unlike the UK in Australia practitioners can be charged with criminal offences for reckless or negligent acts. However it is usual that claims of negligence or misconduct are dealt with by professional disciplinary tribunals, or as civil claim in negligence or trespass.

'Australia is yet to experience a scandal on the scale of MSNFTH. To avoid it, a better strategy would be to ensure that our regime emphasises systemic improvement in health-service delivery rather than being driven by moral panics founded on perceptions that every incident has someone who should be punished – preferably with incarceration' (Bonython & Baer Arnold 2014).

Principles of criminal law

While this is a major area of the law and of interest to every citizen, from a health professional point of view, criminal law is somewhat removed from our day to day work.

Previous chapters have introduced many of the issues discussed here. Anything in civil law that can lead to an action could, if there were evidence of deliberate and considered intent to harm, be found to be a crime. You have now seen how assault and negligence can be grounds for a civil or a criminal action. Similarly, misleading statements aimed to deliberately defraud rather than confuse would be a crime.

Other specialist areas of law such as Industrial, Taxation, Insurance and Corporations law have developed from common law and legislation. Powers to investigate using the police and prosecute using the office of the Attorney General may be the same as those we have considered in criminal law. There are many activities identified as crimes that carry severe sentences for punishment that we have not covered here.

Health institutions and their staff may well find themselves 'under investigation' for failure to adhere to financial or statutory expectations. Legal responsibilities increase with management responsibilities of health staff as there are rules of partnership governing medical practices as well as those governing health institutions. There are taxation and accounting rules that govern large and small health providers and depending upon your future career choices some or all of these areas may need to be understood.

Rather than be anxious about whether something could be a criminal offence, refer to the eight principles of criminal law provided by Wallace (1995) as an outline . It provides the concepts that underpin criminal offences in an easily understood manner.

1. A criminal offence must be established at law
   (Imposing new legislation to make an earlier activity a crime has been attempted at different times in various jurisdictions. This has been allowed in taxation and financial fraud cases, but usually the act must have been a crime at the time of the activity for a court to accept the charge as valid.)
2. There must be an act or an omission
   (The accused must have done some positive thing which the law prohibits, or omitted to do some act which the law required).
3. There must be an intention to do an act (or to refrain from acting)
   (An accident is a defence in criminal law).
4. The intended act (or omission) must be voluntary
   (If it can be shown that coercion, duress or the influence of drugs was an issue this is a defence. However drink driving is not a permitted defence should an accident have occurred.)
5. The liability is personal
   (The accused can not point to another to take responsibility, there is no vicarious liability in criminal law).
6. A person must be guilty as charged
   (The act committed must be the act specified in any charge brought against the person).

7. If an act is specified by law to be a crime, ignorance of the law will not be an excuse.
8. A person is innocent until proved guilty (Wallace 1995: pp. 250-57)

Summary

This chapter explored the rationale for labeling a behaviour a 'crime' and the various crimes that are relevant to health practice. Whether a particular State or Territory has the criminal law entrenched in a legislated code or crimes fall within the common law there is consistency in Australia as to what constitutes a crime and how criminal matters are dealt with. The links between a number of grounds for civil and professional actions such as consent, negligence or reckless behaviour and a crime have been discussed. From a practice point of view, the health professionals intent will often make the difference between something being a mistake or seen as a crime. The importance of documentation was again highlighted in this chapter.

Sources

Andrewartha, D., Bagaric, M., Harvey, I. & Harvey, Y. (2013) *Investigating Crime - The Laws of Australia*. Thomson Reuters, Australia.

Australian Government, Attorney-General Office (2013) Review of Australia's Female Genital Mutilation legal framework. Final Report. Barton: ACT.

Australian Institute of Criminology (2002) *Australian Crime: Facts and Figures*, Australian Institute of Criminology, Canberra.

Bonython, W. & Baer Arnold, B. (2014) *Health-care providers - a different class of criminal?* <http://theconversation.com/profiles/bruce-baer-arnold-1408> (accessed 2 August 2014)

Forrester, K. & Griffiths, D. (2005) *Essentials of Law*, 2nd edn, Harcourt, Sydney.

Johns, P. (2003) 'Crimes compensation: three approaches to a common purpose', *Plaintiff*, 58, (August): 20–24.

Kennedy, R. & Richards, J. (2004) *Integrating Human Service Law and Practice*, Oxford University Press, Melbourne.

Legislative Council Standing Committee on Social Issues (1993) Sexual Violence, The Hidden Crime: Inquiry into the Incidence of Sexual Offences in New South Wales, Part 1. Parliament of NSW.

MacFarlane, P. (1995) *Health Law*, 2nd edn, The Federation Press, Sydney.

MacFarlane, P. J. & Reid, S. J. (2003) *Queensland Health Law Handbook*, Queensland Dept of Health, Brisbane.

Mathews, B. (2011) Female genital mutilation: Australian law, policy and practical challenges for doctors, *Med J Aust*, 194 (3): 139-141.

Morris, G., Cook, C., Creyke, R. & Geddes, R. (2001) *Laying Down the Law*, 5th edn, Butterworths, Sydney.

Richards, K. (2009) Juveniles' contact with the criminal justice system in Australia, Monitoring Report No. 7, Australian Institute of Criminology, Canberra.

Staunton, P. & Chiarella, M. (2003) *Nursing and the Law*, 5th edn, Elsevier, Sydney.

Staunton, P. & Whyburn, B. (1997) *Nursing and the Law*, 4th edn, Harcourt Australia Pty Ltd, Sydney.

U.S. Department of Justice Office on Violence Against Women (2013) *A National Protocol for Sexual Assault Medical Forensic Examinations Adults/Adolescents*. 2nd edn, Washington.

Victorian Law Reform Commission (2004) *Defences to Homicide*, Final Report, Victorian Government Printer.

Wallace, M. (1995) *Health Care and the Law*, 2nd edn, The Law Book Company, Sydney.

Waller, L. & Williams, C. R. (1989) *Criminal Law Text and Cases*, 6th edn, Butterworths, Sydney.

Cases

R v. Bateman (1925) All ER 45 p. 51.

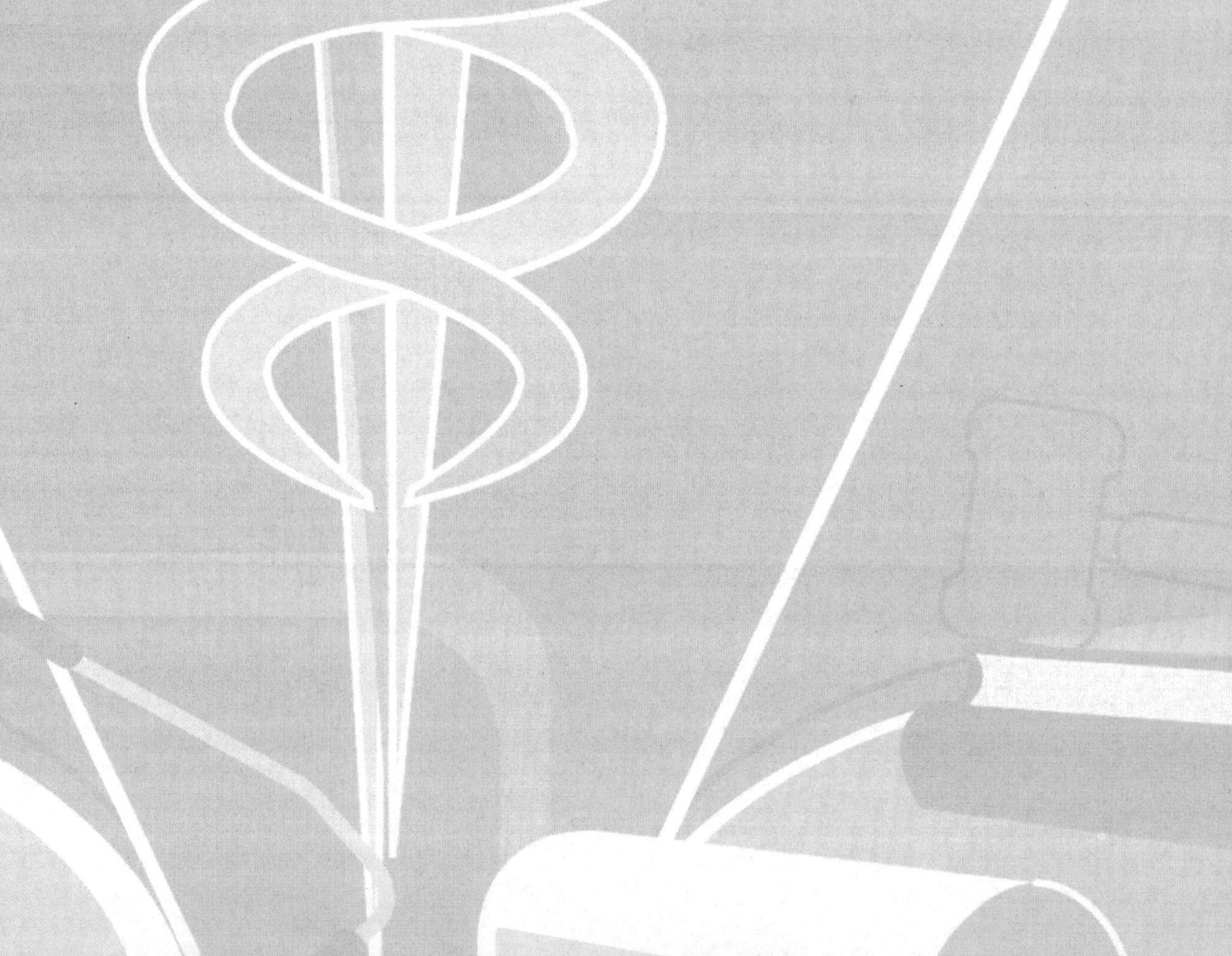

Legal issues for special areas

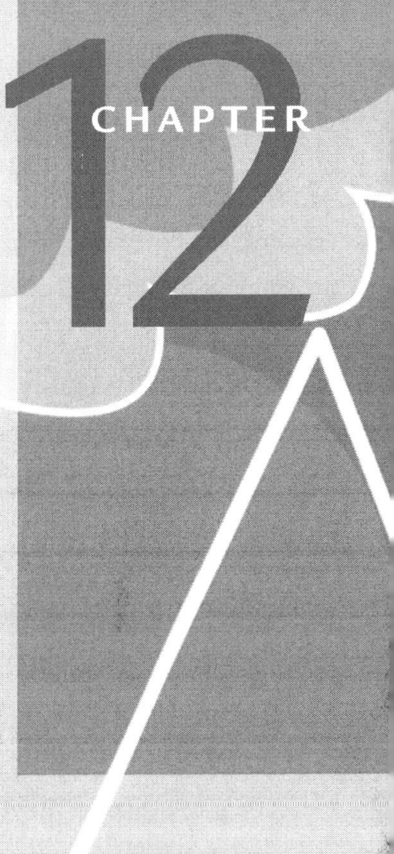

Learning outcomes

After studying this chapter you should be able to:

- Relate Commonwealth and state legislation to policies governing drugs and their administration.
- Demonstrate an understanding of the legal ramifications for incident reporting, report writing and documentation for drug management and clients with special needs.
- Display an understanding of key legislation affecting health policies and procedures.
- Describe the role of the law in providing direction for health care practice.
- Apply legal and professional standards when assessing and responding to client needs, practice and policy situations, professional reporting and communication.
- Discuss guidelines for effective recording that meets legal requirements.

Overview

No matter which text is selected for an undergraduate nursing law course, a quick look at the list of contents will alert you to the breadth of relevant law and by now you will have realised that each subject area is potentially huge. Identifying key areas for learning that have relevance to the workplace can depend on whether the health worker is in private practice, working in the community environment, contracted as a private worker or an employee in the public sector.

All health professionals, however, need to be alert to special risks or special needs of particular client groups. The law in relation to administration of medication is an area of special risk, and the legal obligations and protections for mentally ill or mentally disabled clients and those for children should be understood by all health professionals. While it is true that mental health is a specialist area of practice, often many of the legal requirements and standards expected in this area are relevant to clients attending any health practice.

Drug administration

As the policies and procedures related to drug administration are incorporated into various areas of your program of study only specific legal issues will be covered here.

Legislation tends to refer to drugs as poisons. The idea here is that drugs are dangerous and there must be strict rules governing all aspects of their use. You are familiar with this legislation already from earlier chapters. The Commonwealth and every state and territory has enacted legislation in regard to poisons and therapeutic substances. In Queensland the Health (Drug and Poisons) Regulation (1996) is complemented by sections of the *Health Act 1937* and the *Drugs Standard Adopting Act 1976*. In other states the legislation may be simply the Poisons Act.

The Commonwealth has considerable control over drug research, drug approval, drug availability and marketing through the *Therapeutic Goods Act 1989*, and the Pharmaceutical Benefits Scheme and Adverse Drug Reporting Scheme contribute to monitoring and availability of medicines in Australia.

State legislation is concerned with scheduling and regulations governing the use and supply of poisonous substances. Scheduling is the term used to explain the various categories into which drugs have been placed. In some states, which drug falls within which schedule is found in a separate list, as in New South Wales and Tasmania; in other states this information is incorporated within the primary Act. Schedules mean that drugs are categorised into classes such as controlled substances, restricted substances and regulated substances.

There are regulations governing each classification or schedule. For example, knowing a drug is classed as a Schedule 8 drug means that the health professional should follow the rules governing its prescription, dispensing, labelling, accounting and use. Regulations also direct storage and security arrangements for drugs.

Schedule 8 drugs are often called dangerous drugs, narcotic substances, drugs of addiction or restricted or controlled substances. These are kept in a separate area from other medications in a cupboard that is kept locked and whose key must be kept on the person authorised to carry the drugs. Drug registers are kept and accounting for these drugs is required.

In remote or emergency rescue facilities special approval can be given to permit these drugs to be kept in approved first-aid kits. In an emergency these drugs can be administered on a verbal order from a medical officer following the same strict requirements for all verbal medication orders, that is, double checking the order, documenting the time and facts of the order, if possible having another person witness the order and the medical officer being responsible for writing it up within (usually) 24 hours.

The majority of medications administered by nurses fall within Schedule 4. These are restricted substances and can only be obtained by prescription. In a health facility a medication order correctly and legibly filled in by a doctor is a prescription. Legislation allows for situations in health facilities where there is no pharmacist to fill a prescription for a restricted substance. Senior nursing or medical staff may be authorised to dispense the drug in these circumstances.

Like those in Schedule 8, some Schedule 4 substances must be stored in a secure cupboard, and must also be documented in a drug register. When drugs requiring recording in the register are delivered they must be counted in by two authorised staff and signed for. Every time a drug is used, wholly or in part, this must be accounted for. Damaged, destroyed or unused portions of a medication must be documented. A common policy is for daily counts of secured drugs by two staff members who sign that they have checked and accounted for these drugs. When the senior staff member carrying the keys leaves the ward they must be handed over to an authorised person (usually another registered nurse). The keys cannot be left unattended for any reason.

Legislation does not specify how to administer medication, rather it focuses on who can administer drugs and by what methods can drugs be ordered. For nurses there have been areas of uncertainty about drug orders.

- Generally a verbal order is recognised as being spoken, telephoned or faxed. The order must be issued by an approved person (medical officer), however, and in most states that verbal order must be documented in writing (usually within 24 hours).

Most facilities have strict policies about who can administer medications. All registered nurses under the *Health Practitioner Regulation National Law Act (2009)* are deemed legally qualified to administer medications. Enrolled nurses, unless their registration states they do not hold medication endorsement (that is, on the register it states "does not hold board approved qualification in administration of medicines") can, under the supervision of a registered nurse. In spite of proven competence in the area, some nurses are prohibited from some or all types of medication administration. The facility may initiate special training and credentialling of staff to carry out routine or specialised drug administration. Should a nurse disregard these policies or prohibitions this perhaps in the narrow sense would not be illegal, but it could be professional malpractice and a serious breach of employment contract.

Policies about nurse-initiated medication are another institutional variable. Legislation does not require Schedule 2 medications (over the counter drugs) to be prescribed so registered nurses can administer these unless there is a policy to the contrary. It is obvious that the nurse must know what drugs are covered by Schedule 2. Some areas are approved to have Schedule 3 (prescription needed) drugs on hand for use in emergencies. An example might be asthma medication kept in the first-aid room of a factory.

It is usually recommended that drug checking is done by the registered nurse administering the drug, with another registered nurse being present. This is not always possible. *There is no legal requirement as to who can check*, only as to who can order or administer medications. Policy may dictate that it must be medical officers or registered nurses in every circumstance, while some institutions have taken the uncertainty out of the matter by documenting that an enrolled nurse may check. In the community, usually the registered nurse must do the checking alone and there circumstances dictate the need for a high level of awareness and care.

The reason that so many facilities have drawn up policies restricting staff from carrying out duties involving medications, in spite of their education and having satisfied assessments proving competence, might be better understood through reference to the prevalence of drug-related errors found in a major Australian study:

> Twenty-six per cent of 27 000 hospital-related incidents were medication-related, as were 36% of 2000 anaesthesia-related incidents, and 50% of 2500 general practice incidents.
>
> Results (errors): Errors occur in 15–20% of drug administrations when ward stock systems are used and 5–8% when individual patient systems are used. Previous allergic reactions to drugs may not be recorded more than 75% of the time (Runciman, Roughead, Semple & Adams, 2003).

Illegal or misused drugs

Drugs classed as illegal or misused may well be drugs from Schedule 8 or Schedule 4 and as such quite familiar to health staff from their therapeutic use. In some states there is legislation covering drug misuse, in others the Criminal Code specifies what constitutes unlawful possession, trafficking, producing and handling of illegal drugs. When restricted/regulated therapeutic medicines from Schedule 8 such as pethidine and morphine or Schedule 4 drugs such as sedatives and analgesics are prescribed, in the possession of or dispensed by other than authorised practitioners within their authorised role it is a crime. There are drugs that are illegal substances in every situation, for example cannabis, cocaine, designer drugs. The police have powers to investigate, search and seize evidence in relation to possession and trafficking of drugs.

Should drugs go missing or the drug counts fail to satisfy audit, the facility is obliged to notify the police. Should there be evidence of theft or misuse of a drug, indicating a crime has been committed, charges can be laid. Convictions for illegal drug possession, dealing or drug use vary depending on the amount of the drug and circumstances.

From a professional governance aspect, lending oneself to aid in the theft or misuse of drugs or carrying out any activity construed as illegal, negligent or reckless that promotes such activity will be investigated and result in deregistration or at the least strong penalties and professional sanctions.

While not directly a health controlled medication, staff do care for clients who have used or may continue to use illegal substances. This can be a dilemma for staff focused on treatment not legal aspects of drug misuse.

There are usually protocols in health facilities giving staff direction. An example is: Queensland Health, Management of patients with psychostimulant toxicity: Protocols for emergency departments (2008).

What does cause confusion is the sheer number of drugs that are available and questions about "legal/illegal?" arise. One group of drugs is particularly problematic. These are the new psychoactive substances (NPS) (synthetics), including synthetic cannabis. The laws surrounding NPS are complex, constantly changing and differ between states/territories, but in general they are increasingly becoming stronger. In Queensland, New South Wales, and South Australia there is now a 'blanket ban' on possessing or selling any substance that has a psychoactive effect other than alcohol, tobacco and food. In other states and territories in Australia specific NPS substances are banned and new ones are regularly added to the list.

There are various names for these drugs in the literature and street names; new and emerging drugs (NEDs), synthetics, legal highs, herbal highs, party pills, herbal ecstasy, bath salts, drug analogues and synthetic cannabis (Australian Drug Foundation, 2014).

The use of inhalants, usually a volatile substance, is not a criminal offence in any Australian state or territory. In recent years, some Australian states and territories have revised police powers to intervene in inhalant use in two main ways. Police are authorised to:

- Take away inhalants and related equipment
- Pick up young people who are misusing inhalants, and release them into the care of a responsible person, or a place of safety.

The use of amphetamines is restricted. They can only be prescribed by a medical practitioner for medical reasons. The same rules apply to benzodiazepines. In 2014, in response to concerns about the use and harms associated with the benzodiazepine, alprazolam (Xanax®), it was rescheduled under the Pharmaceutical Benefits Scheme (PBS) as a Schedule 8 drug.

Activity

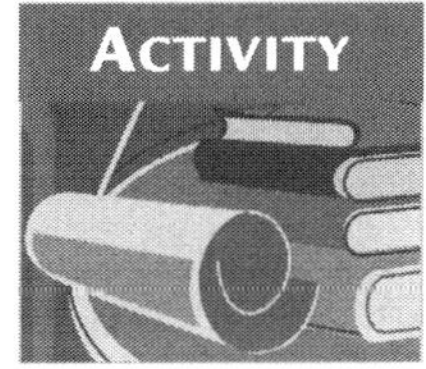

The Australian Commonwealth Department of Health has published, Alcohol and other drugs: a handbook for health professionals.

http://www.health.gov.au/internet/main/publishing.nsf/Content/phd-aodgp (accessed 2 August 2014)

Just scan the Overview and Chapter 1 which identifies the role of nurses as well as giving some good insight into the extent of drug (legal and illegal) related problems.

Nursing and Midwifery Board Hearing related to medication errors:
HCCC v Santos [2012] NSWNMT 8

- **Findings against Nurse S of unsatisfactory professional conduct and professional misconduct (under National Law) on the basis of competence issues and medication errors.**
- **Between** 2009 and 2010, Nurse S was assessed 5 times by her employer. During those assessments various failings were identified in relation to her administration of medication, communication skills, making and recording adequate observations and response to emergency situations. The Tribunal was also satisfied that there had been repeated near miss medication errors by Nurse S throughout her employment as well as actual medication errors on some occasions.

Registration cancelled and Nurse S **disqualified from seeking review of the cancellation** for one year. **Costs** awarded against S.

Take a moment to reflect on the possible consequences to every client who had been involved in these medication errors. There are any number of media reports and research papers about negligent medication administration. Few court cases have been published, mostly in the UK and USA but the trend is obvious, nurses may be charged with a criminal offence particularly if there is death of a patient attributed to a drug administration error. Patients or their families will seek legal advice for harm caused by health staff and medication errors are by numerically far more common than any other health mishap.

Mental health issues

There have been major changes in the way society and thus the law have dealt with matters of mental illness. History tells us that management strategies have not always been kind but the changes that have occurred have also meant that the courts and society, through legislation, have had to adjust to keep up with these changes. Diagnostic and therapeutic advances have added complexity to the situation; disorders can be classified in many ways and clients may be involved in dealing with many facets of the health and social welfare systems.

Different states have defined mental illness in different ways in their legislation and what are 'certifiable' situations (involuntary admission) differs between jurisdictions. This has relevance for health professionals involved in referral or taking steps to provide care. As every health worker will at some time or other find themselves working with clients who have mental disorders (given that one in five adults are likely to have or experience a mental disorder), awareness of client rights and legislation is necessary.

Clinical Resource: Major reviews of current mental health legislation and practice have been ongoing since the new state's Mental Health Acts have been introduced. Constant research and monitoring have produced numerous guides. One that may be of help in practice is: National practice standards for the mental health workforce (2013). This document is available as a PDF on the internet at <www.health.gov.au>. (accessed 3 August 2014).

Staff working with mentally ill clients deal with complex situations, the demands on them to balance the needs of the client, the professional and legal standards for assessment and care are high. There is a need to be cognisant of these sometimes competing pressures. A concept that has become a current term is risk assessment. Risk assessment may be legally relevant to mental health professionals in two ways. First, in the forensic context, psychiatrists and psychologists may be called upon to assess the risk that their patient or client may be violent in the future. Risk assessment may be relevant in civil and criminal law as well as in professional conduct contexts. In the civil law field, risk assessment is necessary in relation to the involuntary commitment of those diagnosed with a mental illness or intellectual disability, detention to prevent the spread of infectious diseases, assessing the risk of child abuse in family law matters, child protection proceedings and workplace occupational health and safety. In the criminal law field, mental health professionals may also be asked to write reports in relation to the risk of an accused person reoffending, for the purposes of bail applications, sentencing and preventive detention, the disposition of offenders with mental disorders, and parole. Second, one of the most difficult questions for health staff concerns knowing when they should disclose a patient's confidential communication on the basis that the patient may be at risk of harming others. If they breach confidentiality, they may leave themselves open to a legal claim for negligence, breach of contract or breach of confidence by the patient, as well as professional disciplinary action. If the mental health professional does not breach confidentiality, there may be a risk of the patient committing a serious offence, engaging in self harm, or putting other people's lives and well-being at risk (McSherry, 2004).

The law also does not consider confidentiality to be absolute. In Australia, statutory provisions exist that require a health professional to breach confidentiality in circumstances such as reporting child abuse or notifying the authorities of certain infectious diseases. However, a common law public interest exception to confidentiality has yet to fully develop.

Over 20 years ago, the Supreme Court of California held in *Tarasoff v Regents of the University of California* (1976) that a duty to protect potential victims may override the confidentiality of the relationship between psychologist and patient. Tarasoff's case dealt with a situation where the patient had disclosed to a clinical psychologist working at a University student health centre that he was going to kill a woman who could be readily identified.

In England, New Zealand and Canada, the courts have recognised a common law public interest exception to confidentiality (McSherry 2000, 2001). For example, Bingham of the English Court of Appeal stated in *W v Egdell* [1990] that 'the law treats [confidentiality] not as absolute but as liable to be overridden where there is held to be a stronger public interest in disclosure'. It remains unclear what this 'public interest' means in a legal context.

The Supreme Court of Canada case, *Smith v Jones* (1999) has significantly broadened the public interest exception to enable disclosure where there is a potential risk to a class of victims. Judge Cory in *Smith v Jones* set out three factors to be considered in weighing up breaching confidentiality in the interest of public safety:

- First, is there a clear risk to an identifiable person or group of persons?
- Second, is there a risk of serious bodily harm or death?
- Third, is the danger imminent?

If a client has admitted to past criminal conduct, then a mental health professional may still be compelled by the courts to disclose this information: *R v Lowe* (1997).

However, there is no legal duty to report to police a client who discloses past criminal offences except in Queensland. In that state, a medical practitioner is guilty of professional misconduct if he or she does not disclose to police any information received concerning an attempted or completed crime, or if he or she attends an injured victim or perpetrator of a criminal act and does not report the incident: *Medical Act* 1939 (Qld) s 35.

A case that discussed if there had been knowledge of a risk and a failure to inform was: *Coronial Hearings: 127902 Mr X*

This inquest concerned the death of Mr X (name suppressed) (aged 53 years), who died from multiple large incised defects to the head and a single stab wound to the chest. Mr X's son, Mr A, was charged with his murder.

At the time of the stabbing, Mr A was on a Community Treatment Order supervised by Peninsula Health Mental Health Services. On 19 April 2004, when

Mr A appeared at the Supreme Court of Victoria before Justice Teague, the jury returned a verdict of not guilty on the grounds of mental impairment. ...

The Coroner (Audrey Jamieson) found that Mr A's management on a CTO by Peninsula Health Mental Health Service was reasonable and appropriate and that it did not contribute to Mr X's death.

In 1991 the United Nations General Assembly resolution, *Principles for the Protection of Persons with Mental Illness and for the Improvement of Mental Health Care*, was adopted. The Australian Human Rights and Equal Opportunity Commission and the Australian government played a major role in drafting these principles. The principles were endorsed at the Australian Health Ministers' Conference in March 1991. In their statement they assert that consumers have the right to:

- respect for individual human worth, dignity and privacy;
- appropriate and comprehensive information, education and training about their mental health disorder, treatment and services available to meet their needs;
- interact with health care providers, particularly in decision making regarding treatment, care and rehabilitation;
- mechanisms of complaint and redress;
- refuse treatment (unless subject to mental health legislation);
- advocacy;
- have their cultural background and gender taken into consideration in the provision of mental health services; and
- contribute and participate as far as possible in the development of mental health policy, provision of mental health care and representation of mental health consumer interests.

All states have undertaken major reviews of legislation, administration and coordination of all aspects of mental illness. This preceded the enactment of new Acts early 2000 by most states. These statutes in some states have been revised, in Tasmania the *Mental Health Act 2013* April 2013, came into force, in Victoria the *Mental Health Act 2014* has been passed. In every state and territory the framework for the provision and regulation of mental health services is within legislation. This has been controlled to some extent by Commonwealth planning but within every state where a review has occurred the incorporation of the United Nations Principles has been deliberate. For example, in the *Mental Health Act 1990* (NSW) Section 4(2) (a) and (b) requires that persons with a mental illness be treated in the least restrictive environment for that treatment to be effectively given, and that any restriction or interference with their rights, dignity and self-respect are kept to the minimum necessary in the circumstances. In Section 6(2) it is required that persons with a mental illness be informed of their legal rights and other entitlements under the Act, and that reasonable steps be taken to ensure that all relevant parts of the Act are explained in the language, mode of communication or terms that they are most likely to understand.

Generally each state's Mental Health Act includes provisions for:

- Initiating involuntary assessment, authorising involuntary treatment and independent review of involuntary treatment and patient rights.

- Processes for admission of mentally ill offenders from court or custody and decisions about criminal responsibility where the person has a mental illness or intellectual disability.
- Notification orders and non-contact provisions for persons such as family members and victims of crime, as well as other provisions addressing community safety.

Scheduling

This is a term often used when a health professional recommends that a client requires treatment but the client refuses or is incapable of recognising their own needs. In legislation this is usually referred to as involuntary admission. An individual can voluntarily admit themselves to a mental health unit, or a hospital or health facility if no unit is available. Most legislative regulations relate to involuntary admissions.

The people who can ask for an assessment or who can make an assessment and how to request such an assessment are strictly controlled. The criteria for making an order for an involuntary admission are specific. Under the New South Wales Mental Health Act there are five types of schedule:

1. S23 Health or care agency, for example crisis team, on request of a relative or friend
2. S21 General practitioner (valid for five days)
3. S25 Court order
4. S26 Welfare order
5. S27 Following order by magistrate

There are regulations governing the procedure and mandatory review of client status at periodic intervals. The police may be involved in a violent or escalating situation but before a client (or the consumer, the term used in the mental health field) is scheduled they must be examined within 12 to 24 hours of admission. Similar regulations exist in every jurisdiction.

Detaining a person for an assessment is usually limited to 24 hours; this can be extended for a further 24 hours by a medical practitioner. A treatment order follows the assessment, and the client may be in a facility or the community at this stage. Whenever an involuntary treatment order is created, it must be accompanied by a treatment plan, which gives specifics of duration, mode of treatment and the people who are responsible for providing care and monitoring the client. Mental Health Review Tribunals are responsible for reviewing a patient's status and their need to remain in hospital.

A key case in Australia reiterating the absolute requirement to satisfy legislative requirements and adhere to review timelines is *Kracke v Mental Health Review Board & Ors* 2009. Judge Bell found that the Mental Health Review Board breached Mr Kracke's human right to a fair hearing under s 24(1) of the Charter by failing to conduct the reviews of his involuntary and community treatment orders within a reasonable time.

Certifying a person as mentally ill involves ensuring that they are made as aware as possible of their legal rights. Where the client refuses to sign in as a voluntary client (or is unable to agree to voluntary treatment) a magistrate's hearing takes place, usually within a week to 10 days as a matter of law. Detaining a person requires health staff or the police to fulfil obligations to ensure early assessment, independent evaluation and appropriate placement and treatment of that individual. There is provision in all Australian jurisdictions for free legal representation for the client involved in such a review.

Common law and mental health

Legislation takes precedence over common law. Legislation in every state governs the management, assessment, care and safeguards for the mentally ill client. However there have been court cases that involve mental health issues.

In an action for negligence against the health care provider it was held there is a duty to take steps to protect a client who, on assessment, is identified as mentally unwell, even when there is no obvious threat. The case of *Crowley v Commonwealth of Australia, ACT and Pitkethly* [2011] is authority for the proposition that a mental health service provider can be held negligent in relation to, amongst other matters, failing to pursue a patient's admission to hospital, even if assessed at the time as no risk to themselves or others.

State of NSW v Coffey [2002] NSWCA 361, 7 November 2002 (Meagher, Heydon and Ipp JJA), the judge's decision was that under common law, an employee with a psychological injury may be able to sue an employer for negligence and be awarded damages.

Australia has now set legal precedents in support of Karoshi (a word that means death by overwork) and Karojisatsu (suicide as a result of overwork and stress). Mrs Matheson, as executrix of Mr Matheson's estate, brought a personal grievance and breach of contract action against the company. She claimed, amongst other things, that the company had unjustifiably dismissed Mr Matheson, and had failed to provide him with a safe working environment. He had committed suicide after being fired. (*Transmissions and Diesel Vs Mrs. Matheson* [2002] 1 ERNZ 22 (CA).)

A precedent was set in a 2000 Court of Appeal judgment which awarded a former child abuse officer, Beth Seedsman, $750,000 for NSW Police failure to provide a safe system of work or protection from mental injury (*Wood v State of NSW* [2004] NSWCA 122).

Guardianship Board

Reference to the Guardianship Board in relation to issues of consent has been made in Chapter 4. In relation to protection of mentally ill or mentally disabled people the board has statutory responsibilities. The Guardianship Board is a legal tribunal with the power to appoint guardians and financial managers for people 16 years and over who are unable to make decisions for themselves because of a disability, including a psychiatric disability.

- Any person, whether professional or otherwise, can make an application to the Guardianship Board if they are concerned about a person's welfare or capacity to manage their affairs. The guardian is a legally appointed person who has the responsibility to make decisions on behalf of an individual. These decisions relate to everything from living arrangements and finances to consent for medical or dental procedures.

The federal *Disability Discrimination Act 1992* is applicable to mentally ill patients as disability is defined within the Act so as to include a loss of mental functions. Should a client feel that their freedom to choose or their rights have not been considered, through legislation they can enforce their rights as well as having access to the protections afforded under state legislation. The client has the right to appeal decisions of the Guardianship Board and Mental Health Tribunals.

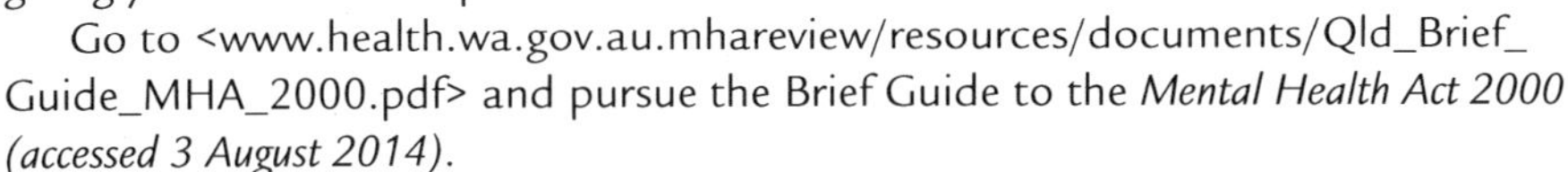

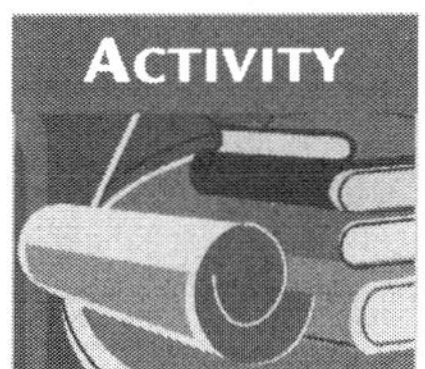

Activity

Review the document found at the site given below. This is a comprehensive summary of current Queensland mental health legislation. You are not expected to learn or come to grips with all the concepts in the document, but rather to see it as a current and future resource capable of extending your knowledge in the area and giving you direction for practice.

Go to <www.health.wa.gov.au.mhareview/resources/documents/Qld_Brief_Guide_MHA_2000.pdf> and pursue the Brief Guide to the *Mental Health Act 2000 (accessed 3 August 2014).*

Limiting interventions and force feeding

Mentally ill (and sometimes prisoners) clients may refuse sustenance. Forced feeding, or artificial hydration and nutrition, has been used to maintain life. Client rights and refusal to consent are obvious issues here. Involuntary clients are protected by state Mental Health and Guardianship Acts in Australia; however, below is an example (Keim & Williams, 2005) that required the courts to explore and determine the position of a client and the position of the health providers at law.

> The case of *Re: Langham & Ors (2005)* cited in Keim & Williams
> In Queensland a detainee under a forensic order was an inpatient in a secure unit. The client's psychotic behaviour led him to refuse food and drink. The Adult Guardian first provided health care consent on behalf of this man as Statutory Health Attorney of last resort, on 20 June 2003. The client had refused all meals since April 2004, surviving on a 'milky coffee' until July 2004. The Adult Guardian, under section 63(2) of the *Powers of Attorney Act 1998* (Qld), consented to the insertion of a nasogastric tube (NGT) for the purposes of giving artificial hydration and nutrition.
>
> In February 2005, after multiple hospital admissions, surgery for a PEG insertion and continued refusal to eat, two applications were made to the Guardianship and Administration Tribunal:
>
> - an application for the appointment of the Adult Guardian as guardian
> - and an application by the Adult Guardian for directions as to whether the artificial nutrition and hydration ('ANH') being given against the client's will should be consented to under the Guardian Act or the Mental Health Act.

This tribunal sought help from the Queensland Supreme Court on a number of legal questions. At the root of the problem was that one Act directed that the rights of the client were paramount while the other Act allowed the decision making to be put into the hands of another – the guardian. This was important because legislation allowed a guardian to consent to required therapy to treat the illness. Now the question was whether artificial feeding is actually a treatment for a mental illness, as under the Act only those types of treatments could be 'forced' without consent (Keim & Williams, 2005).

Justice Chesterman found that:

> The conduct in question, the fruit of the delusion, is the rejection of food and drink. To supply the first respondent with sustenance, even against his will, is to treat a symptom of his disease. It is therefore treatment as defined by the *MH Act*: it is done with the intention of alleviating his suffering, which is therapeutic. (Keim & Williams, 2005, p. 2)
>
> A case from the UK supports this approach, there the issue was an involuntary patient suffering from anorexia nervosa who refused food.
>
> Re A (A Child) (2014) EWCOP 920, (2014) MHLO 77 – 'A, the young person with whom I am concerned, will be 16 years old in June of this year. At the time I am hearing this application, brought by an NHS Foundation Trust, A weighs just 5 ½ stones and has been in hospital for 10 months. ... On the 9th January 20014 the Trust applied for declarations inter alia (i) that it is lawful and in the best interest of A to have a Nasojejunal tube inserted and reinserted on any occasion that it is removed; (ii) it is lawful and in the interest of A to receive fluids, nutrition and medications through a Nasojejunal tube; (iii) it is lawful and in A's best interest to receive treatment (to include psychiatric, psychological and medication as prescribed by her consultant treating psychiatrist) and assessment by the child and adolescent mental health team.

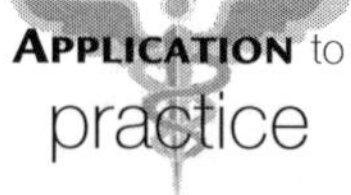

Application to practice

Force feeding a mentally ill client has been an issue ethically as well as legally in relation to consent. A person with legal standing such as a guardian can take responsibility to give consent for a therapy that, while not a mental health treatment in the traditional sense, is justified on the basis that refusal is a symptom of the illness.

This finding does not extend to clients who have no mental illness but have made the decision to refuse food and drink for other reasons.

Children and the law

Consent issues for children were raised in Chapter 4. A key case that addressed many of the clinical realities that occur with children was Marion's case. The case of *re Marion* (1991) originally came before the Full Court of the Family Court of Australia in June 1990. Marion (not her real name) was intellectually disabled, severely deaf, had epilepsy and an ataxic gait and behavioural problems. Her parents had applied to the Family Court of Australia for an order authorising the removal of her uterus (a hysterectomy) and ovaries (an ovariectomy). Both these operations involve major surgery, and either would result in Marion becoming permanently infertile.

The Full Court of the Family Court delivered its judgment in December 1990. At that time Marion was 13 years old and had reached puberty. She was considered to be incapable of caring for herself physically and did not understand the nature or implications of sexuality, pregnancy or motherhood. Her parents claimed that Marion was experiencing psychological and behavioural problems caused by hormonal changes and that it would be in the girl's best interests for her to undergo the operations they sought. A hysterectomy would prevent menstruation and pregnancy, and the removal of her ovaries would, they argued, eliminate her hormonal instability and associated stress and behavioural problems.

Marion's disabilities were so severe that she was unable to understand the nature or implications of the operation her parents were seeking on her behalf, and Marion presumably would never reach that level of comprehension.

The Full Court of the Family Court decided that the parents, as joint guardians of Marion, were able to authorise her sterilisation without a court order, although Strauss J considered that Family Court approval should still be obtained as a matter of prudence. McCall J found that the relevant provisions of the Family Law Act gave the parents responsibility for the long-term welfare of their child, and also independently granted them all the common law powers, rights and duties associated with guardianship. He concluded that these were sufficiently wide to enable parents to authorise sterilisation.

However, the joint majority judgment considered a number of aspects of assault, consent to medical treatment, parental responsibilities and duties and the particular nature of sterilisation. They held that the parents could not lawfully authorise a sterilisation procedure to be carried out on their daughter without a court order.

This case explored the legal relationship between parents and children. The rights of a child and obligation to protect them were important issues. Traditional attitudes about children and the belief that parents have unfettered rights to make decisions on the child's behalf have changed as society has changed, and this case explored such issues.

In all situations, regardless of any statutory provisions, parental consent is ineffective if given in relation to treatment which is not in the child's best interests. The amputation of a limb to enable a child to pursue a lucrative career as a beggar was mentioned in Marion's case as being an example of such treatment (Harrison, 1992).

Internationally Australia is a signatory to the United Nations Declaration on the Rights of the Child. The General Assembly of the United Nations unanimously adopted the declaration on 20 November 1959. The declaration sets out 10 principles including:

- The child shall enjoy special protection, and shall be given opportunities and facilities, by law and other means, to enable him to develop physically, mentally, morally, spiritually and socially in a normal and healthy manner ...

- He shall be entitled to grow and develop in health; to this end, special care and protection shall be provided both to him and to his mother, including adequate pre-natal and post-natal care ...
- The child who is physically, mentally or socially handicapped shall be given the special treatment, education and care required by his particular condition.
- The child shall be protected against all forms of neglect, cruelty and exploitation.

The changes in marital relationships, blended families, births outside of marriage and marriage breakdowns present the law with new issues to grapple with. At-risk and vulnerable children can become a state responsibility. Active protection from exploitation and abuse is accepted as a state responsibility.

Parental responsibility

Section 68F and Section 65 of the *Family Law Act 1975*, emphasise the responsibilities of parents. The Act recognises that both parents are responsible for the care and welfare of their children until they reach 18 years, and arrangements which involve joint responsibilities and cooperation between the parents are in the *best interests of the child*. The *Family Law Amendment (Shared Parental Responsibility) Act 2006* has replaced the definitions in the *Family Law Act 1975* concerned with dispute resolution, counselling and mediation, with the concepts of family counselling, family counsellor, family consultant, family dispute resolution and family dispute resolution practitioner. As well, the 2006 Act established two primary considerations: that children benefit from a meaningful relationship with both parents; and, the need to protect children from physical or psychological harm.

When making decisions involving children, a court exercising jurisdiction under the *Family Law Act* must make a decision based on the best interests of the child. When deciding what is in the child's best interests, the court must consider:

- the relationship with both parents;
- the wishes of the child and factors which might affect the weight they give to those wishes, for example how old the child is;
- the effect on the child of any separation from a parent or other child;
- the practical difficulty and cost of the child having contact with a parent;
- the ability of each parent to care for the child;
- the age, sex and cultural backgrounds of the child (including any need to maintain contact with Aboriginal or Torres Strait Islander culture);
- the need to protect the child from any physical or psychological harm caused by any abuse or violence;
- the attitude of the parents to the child and to their parenting responsibilities;
- any violence or violence order in the family;
- whether the court order will lead to further applications;
- any other factors the court thinks relevant.

Separated families: custodial issues

It requires a court order to alter the legal fact that both parents are considered to be guardians of the children of a marriage. If parents are separated and one parent has sole custody of the children, both parents have legal rights and responsibilities for their children's long-term welfare. In the short term, the custodial parent can consent to matters and medical treatments that are matters of 'the moment'.

Application to practice

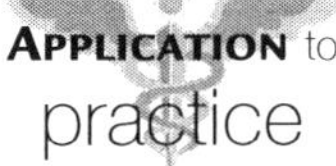

In a situation where one parent has sole custody they have the responsibility to make decisions and provide consent to treatment for acute and routine matters. If the treatment is to have lifelong consequences both parents have responsibility. Unless the court has specifically ordered that a non-custodial parent is restrained from contact with the child, they have the right to know and discuss issues. Even where there are no visitation or contact rights, that non-custodial guardian has the right to speak to health workers and be informed by them about a child's treatment and prognosis.

Should one parent inform staff that there are restraining orders against the other parent and no contact is permitted, this does not mean that there is a right to withhold information. Anxiety and a difficult history may underpin situations that may be exacerbated by staff failing to acknowledge the rights of a parent to be informed, even if they cannot visit their child.

Children at risk

Each state has legislation dealing with situations where a child has been charged with criminal offences, is uncontrollable or at risk of injury or harm. The Magistrate's Court or District Court will normally exercise the jurisdiction of a Children's Court under the relevant legislation. Applications for care and control or care and protection of a child are usually made by police or officers of the state Department of Children's Services.

Child abuse

Every state and territory has legislation aimed at protecting children from neglect, abandonment, ill-treatment or exposing a child to risk of injury or suffering. Mandatory reporting of any suspected or actual child abuse is required in every state. The professionals that are legally bound to report include medical practitioners, child welfare workers, registered nurses and school teachers. This mandatory duty to report requires notification to an authorised person such as the police, medical officer, state child care officer and, in Queensland, the State Director General of Health.

The Australian Government has published a fact sheet from the Australian Institute of Family Studies 2013 that compares each jurisdiction's rules as to who should report and on what grounds child abuse, neglect or child sexual abuse must be reported. Mandatory reporting of child abuse and neglect at: <http://www.aifs.gov.au/cfca/pubs/factsheets/a141787/> (accessed 3 August 2014)

Where a child is admitted to a hospital and it is reasonably suspected that the child has been maltreated or neglected, the child may be detained at the hospital for 96 hours (there are minor variations in each state) regardless of the wishes of the parents.

Summary

The aim of this chapter is to alert health professionals to the range of legislation and common law approaches to drugs administration, mental health and children. Community-based staff, social welfare and social service professionals as well as mental health professionals need to be aware of the legislation and procedures governing these areas. For those working in more general acute care areas these issues will rarely be part of their work. However, the principles of documentation, medication management and the rights of clients who are vulnerable are universally applicable.

Possible assignment questions

Question 1 Length 1000 words

Kelso is a 40 year old man with a 20 year history of bipolar affective disorder. His history shows that during depressive stages he frequently becomes suicidal and has in fact made several attempts to take his life over the last 6 years.

His wife discovered a large quantity of hidden medications, found a document "promising a number of valuable paintings" to people who were almost strangers and she reports he is neither eating nor communicating. The doctor confirms a diagnosis of depression and recommends hospitalization.

Kelso refuses to go to hospital, he claims he cannot be forced to consent to this.

Apply the bioethical principle of autonomy to the scenario

What actions under legislation are available to help Kelso?

Question 2 Length 1000 words

Consider in light of legal requirements and nursing professional requirements, the issue below.

Phillipa is 28 years old. She is married to Rob and they have 1 child Jason, who is five years old and who attends the local school. Phillipa has 10 year history of bipolar affective disorder. Her history shows that during depressive stages she frequently becomes suicidal and has in fact made several attempts to take her life over the last 9 years. Rob is familiar with her symptoms, he monitors her medication regime and tries to organize his work to ensure both Phillipa and Jason are supported and safe.

Today Rob called the community Mental Health intake nurse telling them Phillipa has been hiding her medications after spitting them out, she has been up all night threatening Jason's teachers as she claims they are making unreasonable demands. Phillipa is agitated and hostile towards Rob and Jason. Further, he reported Phillipa refuses to attend the doctor or mental health staff. The nurse recommends he call an ambulance and the nurse takes responsibility to inform the acute mental health admissions staff. When the ambulance arrives Phillipa is even more agitated and refuses to go voluntarily.

1. What procedures can be initiated that adhere to the Mental Health Act (in your State) in relation to her refusal and need for assessment?
2. Discuss Phillipa's rights should her assessment lead to admission.

Sources

Environmental Health Unit (1996) *The Health (Drugs and Poisons) Regulation: What Nurses Need to Know*, previously located at <www.health.qld.gov.au/phs/Documents/ehu /9101.pdf> (accessed 26 June 2006).

Forrester, K. & Griffiths, D. (2005) *Essentials of Law*, 2nd edn, Harcourt, Sydney.

Harrison, M. (1992) 'What's new in family law?', *Family Matters*, No. 33, December.

Jones, M. & Basser Marks, L.A. (2000) 'Valuing People Through Law – Whatever Happened to Marion?', *Explorations on Law and Disability in Australia*, The Federation Press, Sydney.

Keim, S. & Williams, K. (2005) A Case of Two Acts – the Rights of the Severely Mentally Ill and Forced Feeding, pp. 1–6, previously located at <www.qldalliance.org.au/resourcesitems/2005/12/64367-upload-00001.pdf> (accessed 14 September 2006).

Kennedy, R. & Richards, J. (2004) *Integrating Human Service Law and Practice* Oxford University Press, Melbourne.

MacFarlane, P. (1995) *Health Law*, 2nd edn, The Federation Press, Sydney.

MacFarlane, P. J. & Reid, S. J. (2003) *Queensland Health Law Handbook*, Queensland Dept of Health, Brisbane.

Mårtensson, G., Jacobsson, J.W. & Engström,M. (2014) Mental health nursing staff's attitudes towards mental illness: an analysis of related factors. *Journal of Psychiatric and Mental Health Nursing*. <http://onlinelibrary.wiley.com/doi/10.1111/jpm.12145/full> (accessed 9 August 2014)

McSherry, B. (2004) Risk assessment by mental health professionals and the prevention of future violent behavior. *Trends & issues in crime and criminal justice no. 281*. Australian Institute of Criminology Canberra.

Morris, J. (2000) 'Insuring against negligence: medical indemnity in Australia', *Policy*, Spring, previously located at <www.cis.org.au/policy/Spring02/polspring02-2.htm> (accessed 9 June 2005).

Office of the High Commissioner for Human Rights (1959) 'Declaration of the Rights of the Child', resolution 1386 (XIV) of 20 November 1959, Geneva Switzerland previously located at <www.unhcr.ch/html/menu3/b/25.htm> (accessed 20 November 2006).

Office of the United Nations High Commissioner for Human Rights (1991) 'Principles for the protection of persons with mental illness and the improvement of health care', Geneva Switzerland previously located at <www.ohchr.org/ english/law/principles> (accessed 20 November 2006).

Runciman, W. B., Roughead, E. E., Semple, S. J. & Adams, R. J. (2003) 'Adverse drug events and medication errors in Australia', *International Journal for Quality in Health Care*, **15**: 149–159.

Staunton, P. & Chiarella, M. (2003) *Nursing and the Law*, 5th edn, Elsevier, Sydney.

Staunton, P. & Whyburn, B. (1997) *Nursing and the Law*, 4th edn, Harcourt Australia Pty Ltd, Sydney.
'The Case of "Marion"', *Family Matters*, No. 32, August 1992: 10–12.
Williams, G. (1982) *Learning the Law*, 11th edn, Stevens and Sons, London.

Cases

Crowley v Commonwealth of Australia, ACT and Pitkethly [2011] ACTSC 89
Re: *Langham & Ors (2005)* QSC 127.
R v Lowe (1997) 2 VR 465
Smith v Jones (1999) 132 CCC (3d): 225
State of NSW v Coffey [2002] NSWCA 361, 7 November 2002
Re A (A Child) (2014) EWCOP 920, (2014) MHLO77
Re *Marion* (1991) FLC 92-193.
Tarasoff v Regents of the University of California 17 Cal d 425; 131 Cal Rptr 14, 551 P 2d 334 (1976)
Transmissions and Diesel Vs Mrs. Matheson [2002] 1 ERNZ 22 (CA)
W v Egdell [1990] 1 All ER 835: 848
Wood v State of NSW [2004] NSWCA 122

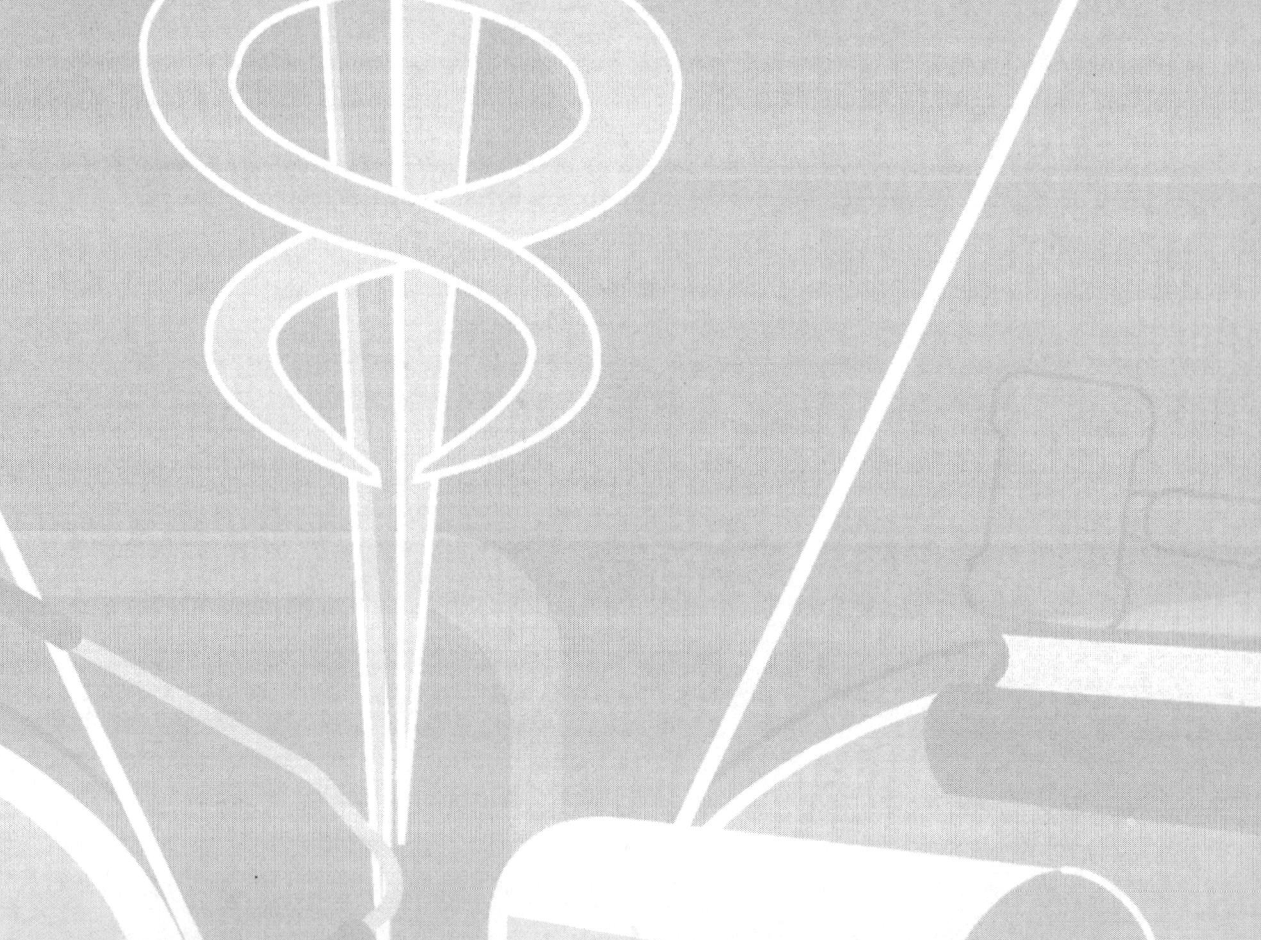

Current health issues and the law

CHAPTER 13

Learning outcomes

After studying this chapter you should be able to:

- Describe the role of the law in providing direction for health care practice.
- Demonstrate a knowledge of procedures and policies for investigation of health matters, professional and legal hearings and sanctions for failure to meet standards.
- Demonstrate an understanding of the legal ramifications for incident reporting, report writing and documentation.

Overview

With some reflection you can see that no matter what the 'legal issue' is, the fact is that the involvement of people in various situations will give rise to the expression of many human emotions. There are conflicting needs and pressures in our professional lives; our clients experience anger, grief and fear, and inevitably so do we. Often it is an unresolved or unrecognised emotional state that can lead to legal consequences. As health professionals, our advantage is that education, experience and our particular skills of assessment and insight into human reactions and needs can help us to assist and negotiate problematic interactions to lessen tensions and identify risks. Attention to protocols and our documentation methods further lessen risks. Acknowledging that developments and technology may move faster than institutional policies and procedure manuals, the advantage of our being 'legally literate' means that we can identify gaps in knowledge or work practices and take appropriate steps to move ourselves and our colleagues toward best practice.

Instead of looking for situations and asking 'can I do that? Is it legal?' you should now be able to analyse situations and identify: What are the risks? What is the policy? What is best practice? What steps and documentation should be implemented to ensure the client and staff are not at risk?

During your clinical experience you may well have noted incidents, behaviours and activities that go against your own professional and ethical values. You should now be able to judge if something is a professional governance issue or potentially has legal consequences or both. Nothing is static in our work or our lives and remaining up to date and informed is a professional obligation.

As society changes so too does the response of the law. Protection of the vulnerable and recognition that populations are made up of individuals who may have different cultural, religious and social beliefs is seen in the creation of laws aimed at ensuring that the less able are not exploited, the different are not discriminated against. However, this in turn raises tensions between the ideals of human rights and self-determination while still ensuring the community at large is protected.

Abortion, withholding of treatment, forced treatment, euthanasia, in-vitro fertilisation (IVF or 'test tube babies') and treatment for severely handicapped babies are all issues which attract a great deal of emotional response from health care professionals, patients and their families. Emotional responses occur when an individual *chooses* to do something society does not agree with and, equally, when laws limit an individual's freedom based on that individual's perceived disability, handicap or age. Trying to reconcile a right to care and the right to refuse care is a current political and legal issue. There are always going to be circumstances that outstrip current legal and legislative developments. There are pressures to implement new therapies, to carry out clinical trials and research controversial treatments as well as the use of interventions that prolong life, perhaps at the cost of those ideals of choice, self-determination or quality of life.

Among the many areas that reflect these issues are:

- The right to die at a time and manner of choice.
- The right to all possible life-prolonging treatments.
- Who owns life? Tissue donation, sperm donation, surrogacy, abortion, cloning.
- What is death, when can machines be turned off?
- Denial of reproductive rights based on intellectual capacity or criminal history.

In Chapter 4 the issue of advance directives or living wills was discussed in relation to consent. The rights in law for an individual with legal capacity to make decisions for their future treatment in the event of their being unable at the time to give direction are entrenched, yet we know that the families and health providers often find it difficult or unethical to obey these directives or accept refusal of treatments.

Refusals of treatment - including life-support treatment or artificial hydration and nutrition - and provision of necessary treatment for the relief of pain or other symptoms of serious physical distress are not euthanasia, even if they do shorten life. In the latter case, the primary intention is to respect the right to inviolability - the right not to be touched without consent - or to relieve pain, not to inflict death (Sommerville, 2013).

Another area of anxiety is the pressure sometimes brought to bear on health professionals by a client who is unable or unwilling to end their life themselves but seeks help and support from another to do this for them. Recall the definition of homicide: any deliberate act to end another person's life is murder. Suicide is not a crime – there are no legal consequences from suicide – but the shock, loss and investigations to establish that it was suicide take a terrible toll on those left who are required to give an account and pick up the pieces.

Euthanasia

In legal terms euthanasia, that is, an active or passive enabling of a person to end their life, is quite simple. It is illegal. What keeps it in the news is the desire of some to remove the stigma and risks to health professionals or others who choose to provide this final care to their client or loved one. An example of such media coverage is 'Court may set right-to-die precedent', ABC Radio Broadcast AM, Thursday, 29 May 2003, Reporter: Rachel Carbonell, at <www.abc.net.au/am/content/2003/s867063.htm> (accessed 4 August 2014).

The controversy continues; another media report showing the conflict between a choice and how the state responds is <http://www.theaustralian.com.au/national-affairs/senate-euthanasia-candidate-max-bromson-takes-his-own-life/story-fn59niix-1227007026625> (accessed 4 August 2014).

There have been and there continue to be attempts, to pass legislation to make euthanasia legal. As recently as June 2014 a draft bill to legalise euthanasia was tabled in the Senate by Greens Senator and health spokesperson, Richard Di Natale (Medical Services (Dying with Dignity) Exposure Draft Bill 2014). This bill - A Bill for an Act relating to the provision of medical services to assist terminally ill people to die with dignity, and for related purposes - would make it legal for doctors to prescribe and administer an `end of life' substance. Two doctors and a psychiatrist would have to sign off on the prescription of the lethal drug to people dying of terminal diseases.

The debate is more than just one case or one state's dilemma. There have been extensive inquiries and law reform discussions over this issue. Below is an extract from an excellent but fairly large document produced by the Tasmanian government. Should you have the time and interest the author would suggest you spend some time reviewing the whole document, which looks at legal concepts and legislative issues and will provide an opportunity to bring together many of the ideas presented throughout this textbook. The language, arguments and content will give you a chance to see how legal concepts are addressed and an awareness of the enormous resources and time spent dealing with all of the issues raised in this chapter.

COMMUNITY DEVELOPMENT COMMITTEE
REPORT ON THE NEED FOR LEGISLATION ON VOLUNTARY EUTHANASIA
REPORT NO. 6
HOUSE OF ASSEMBLY
TASMANIA

SUMMARY

2.42 Having outlined the main arguments proposed by those on both sides of the debate it is clear that questions of moral social principles and individual autonomy dominate the debate.

2.43 The practical considerations of implementing safe legislation to allow active voluntary euthanasia are also matters of debate. Proponents suggest that the Northern Territory legislation demonstrated the feasibility of safe implementation. Opponents however argue that there is no foolproof way to guarantee free consent has been given, nor can the inherent corrupting effects of voluntary euthanasia be contained.

2.44 Furthermore opponents argue that it is ironic for advocates of voluntary euthanasia to campaign for its legalisation on the grounds that it is already a common practice and then suggest that it could be safely regulated to prevent abuse.

2.45 Overarching this debate is the necessity to balance the rights of the individual against those of society for the protection of the public good.

2.46 The Committee heard anecdotal evidence illustrating the desperate plight of many individual cases where prolonged suffering could not be alleviated with palliative care and patients were forced to endure painful lingering deaths. When confronted with such instances of human suffering we feel empathy and compassion for our fellow human beings, but the Committee had to consider whether public policy can be based on individual cases. It can be argued that if the general principle of prohibition against intentional killing is qualified by exceptions for individual cases there is a risk of compromising the safety of all individuals in society, especially those on the margins such as people with disabilities, the aged and vulnerable minorities.

2.47 Individuals presently enjoy equality as participants of society with equal protection under the law. If voluntary euthanasia were to be legalised an inequality would arise where one category of individual is deemed to be of less value than another and could therefore be killed.

(Report of the Community Development Committee, House of Assembly (Tasmania), <www.parliament.tas.gov.au/ctee/old_ctees/euth.htm> (accessed 4 August 2014)).

Another paper that should help you apply many of the ethical principles from Chapter 1 is worth a read. The author, Margaret Sommerville articulates historical and philosophical arguments particularly in relation to propositions put forward for physician assisted suicide. Somerville M. (2013) *What would we lose by legalising euthanasia?* ABC Religion and ethics 24 May. http://www.abc.net.au/religion/articles/2013/05/24/3766685.htm (accessed 4 August 2014)

Most students are aware of the fact that some countries have legislation protecting medical staff who assist clients to die with dignity and remain pain free at a time of their choosing when facing a terminal illness. There has been legislation in Australia in the Northern Territory which, under very strict conditions, legalised euthanasia but this was overturned by Commonwealth legislation in 1997.

Euthanasia is not a legal term; its current usage implies a compassionate but hastened death. Actively assisting someone to die is a crime, therefore it is not surprising that there is confusion when the term is used. In practice, palliative care staff deal with the problem every day and health care staff reconcile the need for medications to alleviate suffering with the fact that the medication will has a 'double effect', that is, it will hasten death. (This concept is also discussed in Chapter 4.)

Doctrine of double effect

The doctrine of double effect has not surprisingly been argued within the context of the arguments for euthanasia. Ethicists have grappled with the idea and there have been claims this is assisted death by another name. The doctrine of double effect holds that intentionally causing death is not acceptable but prescribing high doses of sedatives and opioids to relieve pain is, even if the resulting death is foreseen.

Another option in treating a terminally ill client is Terminal Sedation, this is sometimes called the "last resort therapy". Assessment identifies there is no relief gained by any other intervention so medications that induce sleep or unconsciousness until such time as death occurs as a result of the underlying illness or disease.

It gets more troublesome when the issue is to withhold food or fluids or remove life support technology. There are regular media reports of 'test cases', where the decision to stop feeding a client is based on the client's own directives, family decisions or medical advice. At this point the question is often whether the individual is totally dependent on that treatment to remain alive and if withdrawal of the treatment will cause death. This is a difficult area for the law, not to mention health professionals.

An extensive review of cases and legislation is available in:

Willmott, Lindy, White, Benjamin P., & Downie, Jocelyn (2013) Withholding and withdrawal of 'futile' life-sustaining treatment : unilateral medical decision-making in Australia and New Zealand. *Journal of Law and Medicine*, 20(4), pp. 907-924.

Common law and legislation support the principle that a doctor can on the grounds of "futility" make a decision to withhold life sustaining treatments.

A document that aims to give health staff clear guidelines is the Queensland Health policy; Implementation Guideline-Withholding and Withdrawing Life-Sustaining Measures Part 1 – Legal Framework and Clinical Considerations; (page 7) states:

Life-sustaining medical treatment can only be withheld or withdrawn where consent is obtained or where legislative authority is given to make the decision without consent.

Where the patient lacks capacity to make health care decisions, except in some acute emergency situations, consent is required before any life-sustaining treatment can be withheld or withdrawn.

Known objections by the patient to the provision or withholding of medical treatment can affect the consent provisions.

Consent must be obtained through the following, in order:

1. The patient's valid Advance Health Directive. If none, then:
2. Guardian/s appointed by the Tribunal or Order of the Tribunal.15 If none, then:
3. Attorney/s appointed under most recent enduring document. If none, then:
4. A statutory health attorney/s. If none, then;
5. The Adult Guardian.

Establishing death

Technology can overcome failure of tissue perfusion as the use of various chemicals and cardiac stimulants, artificial ventilation and parenteral feeding can maintain adequate circulation. Death was once defined as failure of tissue perfusion leading to 'cardiac death'. Today that definition is problematic as cessation of breathing or cardiac function can be compensated for.

Since the latter part of the twentieth century the concept of brain death has been used. Again with technological advances the risk of brain tissue death secondary to failure of tissue perfusion has lessened and the increased ability to monitor brain activity has led to constant debate of this criterion. Legislation in most Australian jurisdictions specifies in almost identical language that death is:

1. irreversible cessation of all function of the brain of the person; or
2. irreversible cessation of circulation of blood in the body of the person.

This all gets difficult when the brain functions sufficiently to maintain organ functions but is so damaged that consciousness, independence and awareness (often called a 'persistent vegetative state') are lost. The legislation does not address this situation where parts of the brain continue to function.

Most hospitals have very clear policies and in practice it is usually after consultation with neurologists who have carried out extensive testing that the decision is made to remove life-sustaining technology. Most hospitals have a policy that two doctors must make the diagnosis. In addition, two doctors are required in most states as a matter of law where there is any tissue harvesting for donation purposes (see below).

Optional reading

The ANZICS statement on death and organ donation Edition 3.2 2013. Australian and New Zealand Intensive Care Society (ANZICS).

Home page: <http://www.anzics.com.au/contact.htm>

On the menu on the right side of the page is DOD Death and Organ donation. Click on this to go to the Committee page and scroll down to find the link. (accessed 4 August 2014)

While most of this large report has little bearing on the activities of nurses or (truth be told) legal issues as such, the coverage of policies and protocols for establishing brain death is comprehensive and informative and is the procedure followed in the majority of hospitals. Pages 9–11 are recommended.

Tissue removal after death

All states have legislation to cover issues of tissue transplantation but not all legislation provides a precise definition of death. The main pieces of state and territory legislation relating to organ donation and transplantation are the:

- Transplantation and Anatomy Act 1978 (ACT)
- Human Tissue Act 1983 (NSW)
- Human Tissue Transplant Act 1979 (NT)
- Transplantation and Anatomy Act 1979 (QLD)

- Transplantation and Anatomy Act 1983 (SA) • Human Tissue Act 1985 (Tas)
- Human Tissue Act 1982 (Vic) and the
- Human Tissue and Transplant Act 1982 (WA).

Generally, in law, irreversible cessation of all brain function and irreversible cessation of circulation of blood throughout the body, defines death.
Post mortem removal of tissue for donation relies on establishing whether or not the deceased had given express or implied consent for this during their lifetime. Before taking tissue it is policy to determine that the deceased would have wanted this. Often it is the next of kin who is asked when there is no written or verbal evidence that the deceased had contemplated the matter. In situations where there is no next of kin to ask, legislation provides for the removal of tissue on the approval of a 'designated officer'. Some institutions have a nominated specialist, others a team aimed at providing a balance of medical and community representatives.

Here again society has moved faster than legislation. To raise public awareness, increase the availability of donor organs and lessen the burden on survivors obliged to make such decisions in 2005 the Commonwealth government established a national registry where a record of consent or refusal to donate would be kept. In 2008 there was legislation passed. *Australian Organ and Tissue Donation and Transplantation Authority Act 2008.*

Activity

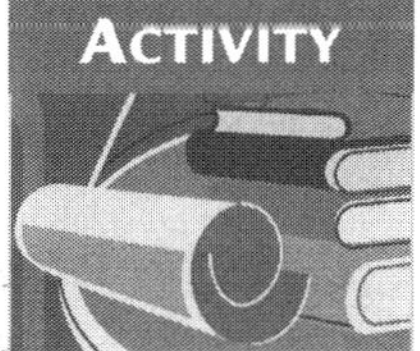

To read the current guidelines on tissue transplantation, go to <http://www.medicareaustralia.gov.au/public/services/aodr/index.jsp #N10057> (accessed 4 August 2014) Tissue transplantation was discussed above.
This area of complex legal issues raises the need to be able to define death and of course consent. Imagine you are asked by a family member of a dying patient for advice and guidance about tissue donation options.

- What is your understanding of death? Can you define it?
- Who at your local health facility is responsible for donor information and support?
- Who would you turn to for appropriate information or referral of this family?

Live organ donation and human tissue banking

Living donation is only possible if the person who donates (the donor) can still live healthily without that organ or tissue. To be a living donor, a person must be in good physical and mental health. They also need to be free from diseases that may affect the health of the person who receives the transplant. Living donors are usually aged between 18 and 60 years old. In some cases, children may donate regenerative tissue, such as bone marrow, to a close relative.

A number of new practices have developed overseas to help people without suitable living donors. Paired donation aims to help people go through with living donation even when the kidney donor and potential recipient are not matched. The unmatched pair is combined with another unmatched pair. The two pairs 'exchange' organs and both avoid the waiting list. Paired donation currently takes place in the US and the Netherlands. In Australia, this type of donation is only legal in WA.

List Exchange acts as an organ 'matching' service. A donor who does not have a match with his or her intended recipient offers to donate to a stranger on the waiting list. In return, the intended recipient is given priority for an organ from a deceased donor. This practice does not currently occur in Australia.

For living donors willing to donate non-regenerative organs there are extensive physical, mental and social assessments undertaken (Source: National Health and Medical Research, 2009).

Human tissue and umbilical cord blood have become valuable in the treatment of many diseases and it is readily evident that this trend will continue. Legally tissue donation assumes that the process of informed consent must involve the person from whom the tissue is being taken (in living donation), or their representative (in some types of posthumous donation). Such an assumption is problematic in cord blood banking because it is not clear whether the mother or the child is the donor.

There have been several areas of increased or new commercial activity involving human tissue products, including the manufacture of products from human tissue. Questions have been raised about the ownership of blood from standard newborn screening, (Guthrie test) heel prick cards which provide critical health information on newborns but these have been used by researchers without permission of the families.

The commercial value of human organs and increasingly tissue and blood products has the potential for abuse of process and fraudulent misuse of the byproducts of treatment.

Legal and ethical restrictions prohibit payments to donors of tissue and their families, but once the tissue has been subjected to some kind of manufacturing process, it is considered freely available for commercial applications as a human tissue product.

In Australia, organisations like blood, bone marrow and eye banks, and organ transplantation programs, are dependent on altruism and the willingness of individuals to contribute to their fellow man. Regulation of commercial applications may limit or restrict these programs. This is a current dilemma and reviews and debate as to the solution are ongoing. Ownership of tissue and blood may, if Australia follows the UK be controlled by property law, therapeutic uses of tissue products are controlled by the *Therapeutic Goods Act* (1989).

Abortion

Abortion in Australian jurisdictions was always covered by the criminal law rather than the civil law. As a consequence there are criminal penalties and attendant social stigma attached to a guilty finding in those states that have not decriminalised abortion. Western Australia is one state that has removed abortion from the criminal code; however, the *Acts Amendment (Abortion) Act 1998* does specify that the criteria described in cases discussed below must be fulfilled. Abortion is also discussed in Chapter 11.

Recall that criminal cases are usually brought in the name of the Crown so the monarch's title 'Regina' (R) is identified as in the case *R v. Jane Smith* or the name of the prosecuting public law official such as the Director of Public Prosecutions (DPP) or Attorney-General resulting in a case title such as *AG v. John Smith*.

Abortion is an area where the legal position (it is a crime) in various state and territory legislation has been subject to interpretation by courts to reflect the changing attitudes prevailing in society. An example of how courts have interpreted such law is found the English case of *R v. Bourne* (1939). Dr Bourne was a well-known and respected obstetrician, who acted openly (and without cost) to terminate the pregnancy of a 14-year-old girl who was a rape victim. The trial judge came to the view that not all abortions were automatically unlawful and the jury acquitted Dr Bourne. This case recognised a defence where 'the probable consequence of the continuance of the pregnancy will be to make the woman a physical or mental wreck'.

In Australia the Victorian Court followed this stance in *R v. Davidson* (1969). This case became the precedent for the proposition that the law allowed an abortion to be performed if it was 'necessary to preserve the woman from a serious danger to her life or physical or mental health'. In 1971 this view was extended in the New South Wales decision of *R v. Wald* (1971) when Levine J held that 'it would be for the jury to decide whether there existed in the case of each woman any economic, social or medical ground or reason which in their view would constitute reasonable grounds upon which an accused could honestly and reasonably believe there would result a serious danger to her health (physical or mental) if the pregnancy continued'. (© State of New South Wales through the Attorney General's Department of NSW.)

The law in Queensland and other common law jurisdictions was examined in 1986 in *R v. Bayliss and Cullen*. In his judgment Judge Maguire held that s. 282 of the Queensland Criminal Code could be read as a defence to those sections of the code that prohibited abortion. Section 282 cites 'the preservation of the mother's life . . . having regard to the patients' state at the time and to all the circumstances of the case' as a reason to excuse criminal responsibility.

These cases indicate that there are considerations that can be taken into account in the face of legislation making abortion a crime but there is still uncertainty and this restricts access to abortion on demand. There have been ongoing attempts to decriminalise abortion, removing it from a legal construct to being a matter of choice or ethics.

The sometimes very heated debate that surrounds abortion involves not only whether abortion should be a choice but at what point in a pregnancy an abortion is justified. The age of the foetus is certainly always going to be a serious ethical and medical consideration. In Western Australia, for example, after 20 weeks the *Acts Amendment (Abortion) 1998 Act* requires:

- That 2 medical practitioners must agree that there are significant risks to the mother or that the unborn child has such a severe medical condition that the procedure is warranted.
- Further, the abortion can only be carried out in a facility approved by the Minister. [This means a hospital rather than a clinic.]

There are social implications about the rationale for abortion where decisions are taken based on the presence or absence of some trait in the foetus. It may be that the law will move to tackle such matters in the future. Certainly in countries where there is a cultural/social pressure to abort females, the resulting imbalances in populations has led to active prevention and penalties.

The morning-after pill was a matter for the courts in 2002. The issue has been raised in the media on numerous occasions. The fact that this pill prevents pregnancy rather than causes abortion/miscarriage led the court to conclude it did not fall within the 'unlawful act' and its supply and use was not unlawful.

Counselling and consent

It is a requirement that a woman be given sufficient information to ensure that her decision to go forward and consent to an abortion is informed. She must know about the risks of the procedure and either be referred to a qualified counsellor or can access such a service to ensure informed consent. The fact that issues in reproductive health matters involve personal values and ethical and legal considerations make it particularly important that the health professional provides information in a manner that allows the client to make decisions without outside influence. Health professionals have a legal duty to be non-judgmental. Meeting clients' needs may require the health professional to recognise and accommodate sexual practices that they could feel are immoral and even unnatural. The professional's attitudes must not deny or deter clients from requesting the reproductive or sexual health care they need in their circumstances. The World Health Organization states:

> Legal doctrine on free decision-making concerns patients' freedom from any bias exercised, consciously or unconsciously, by those to whom they turn for reproductive health advice or care. Providers' recommendations are liable to be influential and perhaps decisive, but recommendations must be made on the basis only of patients' best interests, directed by patients' reproductive health status and their expression of their wishes, goals and preferences. Patients' informed choices may not appear to be in their medical interests, but since health relates to physical, mental and social well-being, providers must tolerate their patients to exercise informed choices according to patients' own ranking of their physical, psychological and social interests. Patients are not obliged to put their medical interests first (World Health Organization (2000) *Considerations for Formulating Reproductive Health Laws*).

Free decision making

In addition to providers ensuring that clients are adequately informed for decision making, providers must also be alert to how far patients are free to exercise independent choice. Many clients are never entirely free, because they are subject to factors in their social and family surroundings that are liable to influence their choices. Clients' hopes and fears, the well-being of those they care for and who depend on them and, for instance, their material resources and their dreams for the future will limit the options from which they may feel themselves free to choose.

Occasionally there are cases where a woman seeks to have an abortion but the father is opposed to the procedure. A case that explored this, where the husband had sought to prevent the wife proceeding, was *F v. F* (1989) in which the finding was that where there was a marriage break down the husband had no rights to prevent the abortion. Generally as long as the procedure satisfies the law on the basis of 'risk to the mother's health – emotionally or physically' the court will not support another party seeking to prevent abortion. It has been held that neither the father nor the foetus have rights in law in various cases in Australia.

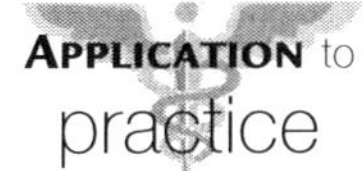

Application to practice

Like euthanasia the issue of abortion will be subject to legislative and judicial review during your career. While there are considerably fewer legal issues in early termination taken on the basis of health of the mother, physically and emotionally, there are medical and legal obligations that must be satisfied before a termination in late pregnancy is undertaken.

An individual or a facility with strong religious or ethical beliefs can choose not to work in the area or provide the service. However, that personal/professional choice cannot be made at the expense of a woman who is at risk. Referral of the client would be essential and, in an emergency, active measures including, if necessary, termination to save the mother's life must be carried out.

Whether or not the professional agrees with the woman's decisions, professional standards dictate that the care and treatments, communication and responsibilities to that client be satisfied.

Wrongful birth

The issue of wrongful birth and wrongful life is a new legal issue to the common law. Above you read that abortion is potentially a criminal offence yet there have been successful cases in civil jurisdictions claiming that allowing a pregnancy and not performing a termination was a negligent act. Below is an extract that defines and explains the term 'wrongful birth'.

1 **Wrongful birth defined**

Wrongful birth occurs where an act of medical negligence causes the birth of an unplanned child. The child may be 'healthy' (non-disabled) or disabled. The negligence may involve a doctor's failure to:

(a) warn of the risk that a competently performed sterilisation may naturally reverse or otherwise fail; so that the plaintiffs, unaware of that risk, cease using contraception;

(b) diagnose or advise of pregnancy, where diagnosis or advice would have led to lawful termination;

(c) diagnose a condition in either the parents or the foetus that will cause the child to be disabled, where diagnosis would have led to effective contraception or lawful termination;

(d) take reasonable care in performing an attempted sterilisation or abortion; or

(e) take reasonable care in giving advice on, or supplying, contraceptives.

Each of (a)–(e) creates a risk that an unplanned pregnancy will occur or continue. If the risk eventuates, and the pregnancy is carried to term – because pregnancy was discovered too late to terminate safely or legally, or because the plaintiffs feel morally or emotionally unable to terminate – then wrongful birth has occurred.

In a *wrongful birth action*, the parent or parents sue the doctor in negligence in respect of the damage resulting from the pregnancy and birth.

The terms 'wrongful birth', 'wrongful pregnancy' and 'wrongful conception' have been variously defined, sometimes interchangeably. Here, only 'wrongful birth' is used, and has the meaning given above. Strictly, what is 'wrongful' is the *negligence*, not the birth; but the label is a convenient shorthand (Stretton, 2005).

Cloning and reproductive technology

Reproductive technology involves many technologies including artificial insemination, in-vitro fertilisation (IVF), embryo and gamete transfer and, potentially, cloning technology. In Australia there is relevant legislation: Research Involving Human Embryos Act 2002 and the Prohibition of Human Cloning Act 2002 which prohibited research cloning, therapeutic as well as reproductive cloning. Embryo production containing DNA from more than two people as well as the development of embryos in laboratories in excess of 14 days after the fertilization was prohibited.

However the Commonwealth government repealed the research cloning prohibition in November 2006. This permitted research on stem cells to be carried out if the stem cells were derived from redundant embryos before 2002. In 2006 the Prohibition of Human Cloning for Reproduction and the Regulation of Human Embryo Research Amendment Act came into effect. In 2008 the law was revised and affirmed. Reproductive cloning remains prohibited in Australia. However, individual states can decide whether they approve cloning for research- and therapeutic ends. For example, research-cloning is permitted in the states of: Victoria, New South Wales, Queensland. NSW, Human Cloning for Reproduction and Other Prohibited Practices Act 2003 and Research Involving Human Embryos (New South Wales) Act 2003; Queensland, Research Involving Human Embryos and Prohibition of Human Cloning for Reproduction Act 2003. Legally it is a complex and daunting area. To give you an insight into some of the considerations an extract from very large report is provided below.

> The regulation of human cloning and the use of human embryos in research has evolved as part of the regulation of assisted reproductive technologies. The use of the human embryo in the course of assisted reproductive technologies has been premised on the consent of the genetic parents. There is no comprehensive and consistent approach in Australia to the regulation of human cloning and its related research. This variation between jurisdictions

creates frustration and confusion for researchers, practitioners and the general public.

New Commonwealth provision

8.21 The recently enacted Commonwealth *Gene Technology Act 2000* contains a prohibition on the cloning of whole human beings. It also prohibits placing human cells into animal eggs or placing a combination of animal and human cells into a human uterus. Section 192B of the Act provides:

Cloning of human beings is prohibited

(1) A person is guilty of an offence if:

(a) the person engages in conduct; and

(b) the person knows that, or is reckless as to whether, the conduct will result in the cloning of a whole human being.

(2) In this section:

cloning of a whole human being means the use of technology for the purpose of producing, from one original, a duplicate or descendant that is, or duplicates or descendants that are, genetically identical to the original.

(House of Representatives Standing Committee on Legal and Constitutional Affairs Human Cloning, 2001, *Scientific, Ethical and Regulatory Aspects of Human Cloning and Stem Cell Research*, pp. 1–28.)

You can expect changes to legislation and controversies will continue; research opens new avenues and therapeutic advances continue to pressure governments. In 2010 the Prime Minister Gillard commissioned a formal review into legislation affecting cloning and research on human embryos. That review recommended that there should continue to be a criminalisation of human cloning for reproduction, and of the other conduct specified in the Prohibition of Human Cloning for Reproduction Act 2002.

Research involving human embryos should only be permitted under license and with ongoing monitoring by the NHMRC Embryo Research Licensing Committee (the Licensing Committee).

Surrogacy

This is when a woman offers to carry a child to term for others. It may be that the surrogate carries the fertilised egg of both parents or is also the donor of an egg fertilised by the father. In these cases there have been problems of custody and legal parenthood, and the issues of 'selling a baby' and contracts between parties. Some states (e.g. Queensland) have enacted legislation making it illegal to induce, request or act as a surrogate parent.

At common law the case of *Re Evelyn* (1998) decided that a surrogacy agreement would not be enforced, that it was the welfare of the child that was the important issue. In that case, the child remained with the biological mother. This means that even if a fertilised egg was carried to term or only the father's sperm was provided, the woman who bore the child has sole rights.

The act of surrogacy introduces so many legislative considerations that it is a minefield. Adoption, custody, child welfare and family law legislation have all at some point a section that will be relevant to the parties. Most states have Acts that support altruistic surrogacy. Strict rules about who can seek a surrogate and on what grounds apply. Section 60HB of the Family Law Act 1975 recognises orders of state and territory courts that transfer the legal parentage of children who are born as a result of surrogacy arrangements for the purposes of legal proceedings under the Family Law Act. No state supports or encourages commercial surrogacy but where it is not a crime, should there be disputes between parties, historically no matter whether the infertile couple has paid for or contributed genetic material they will rarely have rights at law. New South Wales, Queensland and the Australian Capital Territory have made it an offence for residents to enter into international commercial surrogacy arrangements with potential penalties extending to imprisonment for up to two years.

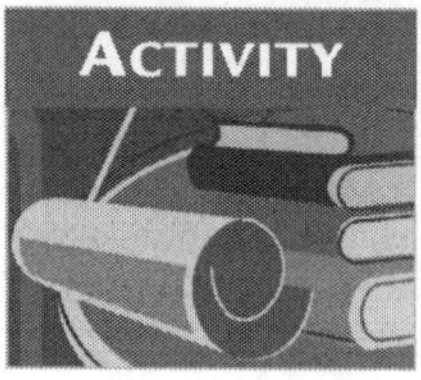

Activity

- Under what circumstances do the issues of surrogacy tend to come before the courts?
- What position should the health professional take if asked for advice by people contemplating entering into a contract for surrogacy?

Genetics and privacy issues

Genetic testing and the issues of privacy and discrimination are something society and thus governments are coming to grips with. The genetic basis of almost 2,000 different familial conditions has been determined (Forrest et al 2007). Genetic information resulting from assessment of an individual may be relevant not only to that person but also to genetic relatives, due to the shared genetic heritage within families. Conflict arises when information is deemed private and there is no consent by the person identified as a genetic carrier to allow dissemination of this fact. The Office of the Privacy Commissioner guidelines on health privacy 5 states that a "serious" threat "must reflect significant danger to the individual and could include a potentially life-threatening situation or one that might reasonably result in serious illness or injury." With changes to the Privacy Act incorporating National Privacy Principles (NPP) the current situation is:

- changes to the Privacy Act and to NPP 2 that provide for disclosure of genetic information to genetic relatives without the consent of the patient in certain circumstances.

The additional exception introduced through National Privacy Principle 2.1:

- allows use or disclosure of a patient's genetic information, without the patient's consent, in circumstances when there is reasonable belief that disclosure is necessary to lessen or prevent a serious threat to the life, health or safety of his or her genetic relatives
- applies to private sector organisations that have obtained genetic information in the course of providing health services to individuals

(these include private medical practices, pathology services, private hospitals) and their employees
- applies only to genetic information concerning a living person that was collected by an organisation on or after 21 December 2001
- does not apply to situations concerning genetic information that presents a serious threat to an unborn child (Source: National Health and Medical Research Council, 2009). (Privacy Act 1988 Cth section s95AA deals with disclosure of genetic information to relatives).

Release of genetic information may affect the individual by leading to discrimination. Refusal of insurance is one example.

The reading in the activity below should provide you with a chance to draw together some earlier learning about privacy issues as well as raise your awareness about this area.

Activity

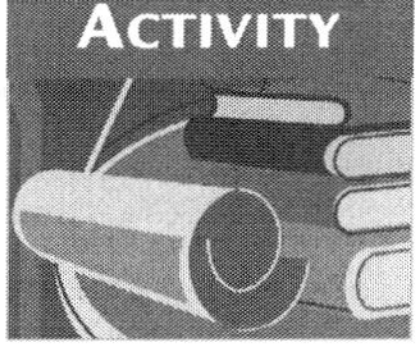

First, go to the homepage of the Australasian Legal Information Institute at <www.austlii.edu.au/> and search for genetic testing. Read 'Genetic testing: the potential for genetic discrimination in insurance' (found at number 18 on the menu) (1999) by Pamela Jensen (accessed 4 August 2014).

It should be noted that Australian life insurers are permitted to use an applicant's genetic information to assess applications for life insurance. This is based on an exemption under s 46 of the *Disability Discrimination Act 1992 (Cwlth)*, which prohibits disability discrimination; underwriting for life insurance involves assessing individual risk, and applicants have a duty to fully disclose all health information relevant to the insurer. However, to come within the scope of the legislative exemption, life insurance companies need to be able to provide actuarial or statistical data to justify their underwriting decisions (Keogh & Otlowski, 2013)

Second, the whole case transcript of the case below is recommended reading; the way a case is reported and the issues are considered and the legal reasoning and complexities involved will be apparent.

Case re consent for sperm: MAW v. Western Sydney Area Health Service (2000) NSWSC 358 (3 May 2000), New South Wales Supreme Court, Judgment date: 03/05/2000, judgement of: O'Keefe J, <www.austlii.edu.au/au/cases/nsw/supreme_ct/2000/358.html>.

New law or changes to precedents

There are many areas of the law and changes in society give rise to new and different public concerns hence new legislation or changes to precedents in case law occur all of the time. Many of these changes have an ethical as well as legal component.

The law is part of society and reflects that society. The inclusion of what once might have been 'welfare' issues into the broader legal structures is common today. Focus on the needs of victims, alternative dispute handling, alternatives to incarceration and inclusion of many controls and regulations in legislation is evidence of the dynamic nature of the law.

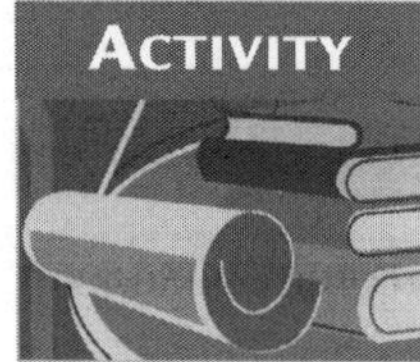

Activity

An excellent paper that attempts to explain the possible future intersections between health and law, the moral and economic conflicts that need to be addressed and the part genetics will have in future choices is worth a read.

"Will there be a broadening of medicine's focus beyond the individual patient, and a winding back of medical law's preoccupation with the individual, and its protection of his or her choices within the clinical sphere and health care market? If such a shift is likely, genetics might be one place where it will become apparent. Genes are often seen as irreducibly tied to a person's identity and future prospects" (Magnusson 2003 p.748).

The full article: Magnusson, R.S. (2003) A short history of the next thirty years: genetic testing, clinical care and personal choices. *UNSW Law Journal* Volume 26(3) available on-line http://www.unswlawjournal.unsw.edu.au/sites/default/files/49_magnusson_2003.pdf (accessed 4 August 2014).

While these chapters have focused on areas of law that are clearly relevant to health practice you can appreciate that the law is far broader and much more complex than the areas we have covered. Specialty areas of legal practice grow or decline with changes in society. Crimes of one era are no longer to be found on statute books. The rapid changes to law relating to refugees and asylum seekers that occurred after 11 September 2001 is an example of how legislation can alter almost overnight in keeping with new policies.

The growth in Family Law Courts is a good example of the way society has shaped the legal institutions. The recognition that neither the common law nor legislation could meet the needs of families and children has brought about the development of a completely new area of law. The growth in control and regulations through centralised government agencies has underpinned the growth in administrative law and tribunals to review and monitor decisions that affect our lives.

Summary

While reading these chapters no doubt you have recalled your own clinical activities and life experiences and you may have concluded that those clinical examples indicate that there are times when staff have had poor judgment about legal or professional risks. Some of your assessments may be entirely accurate but other judgments made about colleagues and situations might need to be considered in the light of other information, expertise or knowledge. Always make sure that you have all the facts before you judge a situation. You should see that in our work there are situations arising constantly where there is no obvious legal or professional governance rule.

This final chapter highlights just how ethical dilemmas have been taken up by the legislation and matters that were once private family issues are now increasingly brought before the courts. The various concepts covered in the chapter evidence that there are tensions between the rights of the individual and the law, between ethics and legal principles. Science and societies are always moving forward, the need to certainty and justice for individuals and nations in ordering their lives and protecting their rights is increasingly left to legal respresentatives working with governments. The law is always changing, in this chapter you have explored cases and concepts that have been examined as a result changing expectations and beliefs about rights, control and fairness.

Possible assignment question

Length 500 words

Refer to NMBA Code of ethics to identify issues in the scenario.

Twins Joseph and Paul are 9 years old. Joseph suffered severe burns and needs donor skin grafts.

Paul is the nominated donor. Paul is terrified and tells the nurse he does not want to do this. The nurse reassures him telling him it is a very good thing he is doing and he must help his brother.

The nurse spends considerable time with him and explains everything that will happen and why things will be done.

The nurse leaves him with a hug when he has stopped crying and after he says he has no further questions. When the boy's parents arrive the nurse tells them that Paul is now OK about proceeding to be the donor.

Sources

Australian Government, National Health & Research Council, (2014) *Genetic Discrimination. https://www.nhmrc.gov.au/your-health/genetics-and-human-health/ethical-legal-and-social-issues/genetic-discrimination*

Australian Government, NHMRC, (2009) Use and disclosure of genetic information to a patient's genetic relatives under Section 95AA of the *Privacy Act* 1988 (Cth). Guidelines for health practitioners in the private sector. Canberra.

Australian Government, National Health & Research Council, (2007) *Making a decision about living organ and tissue donation*. Canberra.

Commonwealth of Australia (2011) Report of the Independent Review of the *Prohibition of Human Cloning for Reproduction Act 2002* and *Research Involving Human Embryos Act 2002*. Canberra.

Cook, R. J. & Dickens, B. M., World Health Organization (2000) *Considerations for Formulating Reproductive Health Laws*, previously located at <www.who.int/reproductive-health/publications/rhr_00_1/index.html> (accessed 28 June 2006).

Everingham, S. (2014) Use of surrogacy by Australians: Implications for policy and law reform, Chapter 8 in *Families, policy and the law: Selected essays on contemporary issues for Australia*. Eds by Alan Hayes and Daryl Higgins. Australian Institute of Family Studies. Melbourne.

Forrest, L.E., Delatycki, M.B. & Skene, L. et al. (2007) Communicating genetic information in families -a review of guidelines and position papers. *Eur J Human Gen* 15: 612 -18.

Forrester, K. & Griffiths, D. (2005) *Essentials of Law*, 2nd edn, Harcourt, Sydney.

Guirguis, A. (2001) 'Retention of body parts following post mortem in New South Wales', *Health Law Update*, June.

Jensen, P. (1999) 'Genetic testing: the potential for genetic discrimination in insurance', <www.austlii.edu.au> (accessed 15 December 2005).

Kennedy, R. & Richards, J. (2004) *Integrating Human Service Law and Practice*, Oxford University Press, Melbourne.

Keogh, L.A. & Otlowski, M.F.A. (2013) Life insurance and genetic test results: a mutation carrier's fight to achieve full cover. *Med J Aust* 199 (5): 363-366

Lynch, V. A. (1995) 'Clinical forensic nursing: a new perspective in the management of crime victims from trauma to trial', *Critical Care Nursing Clinics of North America*, **7**(3): 489–507.

MacFarlane, P. (1995) *Health Law*, 2nd edn, The Federation Press, Sydney.

MacFarlane, P. J. & Reid, S. J. (2003) *Queensland Health Law Handbook*, Queensland Dept of Health, Brisbane.

Mainsbridge, A. (2002) 'Employers and genetic information: a new frontier for discrimination', *Macquarie Law Journal*, <www.austlii.edu.au> (accessed 27 June 2006).

Office of the State Coroner, Department of Justice and Attorney-General, previously located at <www.justice.qld.gov.au/courts/coroner/fs4care.htm> (accessed 10 June 2005).

Somerville, M. (2013) *What would we lose by legalising euthanasia?* ABC Religion and ethics 24 May. <http://www.abc.net.au/religion/articles/2013/05/24/3766685.htm> (accessed 4 August 2014)

Staunton, P. & Chiarella, M. (2003) *Nursing and the Law*, 5th edn, Elsevier, Sydney.

Staunton, P. & Whyburn, B. (1997) *Nursing and the Law*, 4th edn, Harcourt Australia Pty Ltd, Sydney.

Stuhmcke, A. (1995) 'For love or money: the legal regulation of surrogate motherhood', *Australian Journal of Family Law*, **2**(3) <www.murdoch. edu. au/elaw/issues/v2n3/stuhmcke23.html > (accessed 15 April 2011).

Stretton, D. (2005) 'The birth torts: damages for wrongful birth and wrongful life', *Deakin Law Review*, **10** (1).

World Health Organization (2000) 'Considerations for formulating reproductive health laws', 2nd edn, previously located at <www.who.int/reproductive-health/publications/rhr_00_1/index.html> (accessed 20 November 2006).

Cases

R v. Bourne (1939) 1KB 687.
R v. Davidson (1969) VR 667.
R v. Wald (1971) 3NSW DCR 25.
R v. Bayliss and Cullen (1986) 9 Qld Lawyer Reps 8.
MAW v. Western Sydney Area Health Service (2000) NSWSC 358.
Re Evelyn (1998) Fam CA 55.
F v. F (1989) FLC 92–031.

Index